Research Issues in Learning Disabilities

Sharon Vaughn   Candace Bos
Editors

Research Issues in Learning Disabilities

Theory, Methodology,
Assessment, and Ethics

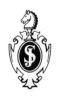

Springer-Verlag
New York Berlin Heidelberg London Paris
Tokyo Hong Kong Barcelona Budapest

Sharon Vaughn, Ph.D.
School of Education and
  Department of Psychology
University of Miami
Coral Gables, FL 33124, USA

Candace S. Bos, Ph.D.
Department of Special Education
  and Rehabilitation
University of Arizona
Tucson, AZ 85721, USA

With 6 Illustrations

Library of Congress Cataloging-in-Publication Data
Research issues in learning disabilities: theory, methodology,
  assessment, and ethics / [edited by] Sharon Vaughn, Candace Bos.—
  1st ed.
      p.   cm.
    Includes bibliographical references and index.
    ISBN 0-387-94079-0
    1. Learning disabilities—Research—United States.   2. Learning
  disabled children—Research—United States.   I. Vaughn, Sharon,
  1952–   .   II. Bos, Candace S., 1950–   .
  LC4705.R48   1993
  371.9—dc20   93-24815

Printed on acid-free paper.

© 1994 Springer-Verlag New York Inc.
Copyright is not claimed for works by U.S. Government employees.

Production coordinated by Chernow Editorial Services, Inc., and managed by
  Christin R. Ciresi; manufacturing supervised by Jacqui Ashri.
Typeset by Best-set Typesetter Ltd., Hong Kong.
Printed and bound by Edwards Brothers, Inc., Ann Arbor, MI.
Printed in the United States of America.

9 8 7 6 5 4 3 2 1

ISBN 0-387-94079-0 Springer-Verlag New York Berlin Heidelberg
ISBN 3-540-94079-0 Springer-Verlag Berlin Heidelberg New York

Contents

Contributors

Candace S. Bos, Ph.D., Department of Special Education and Rehabilitation, University of Arizona, Tucson, AZ 85721, USA

Donald D. Deshler, Ph.D., Center for Research on Learning, University of Kansas, Lawrence, KS 66045, USA

Carol Sue Englert, Ph.D., College of Education, Michigan State University, East Lansing, MI 48824, USA

Steven R. Forness, Ph.D., Neuropsychiatric Institute, University of California, Los Angeles, CA 90024, USA

Douglas Fuchs, Ph.D., George Peabody College, Vanderbilt University, Nashville, TN 37203, USA

Lynn S. Fuchs, Ph.D., George Peabody College, Vanderbilt University, Nashville, TN 37203, USA

Steve Graham, Ed.D., Department of Special Education, University of Maryland, College Park, MD 20742, USA

Diane Haager, Ph.D., School of Education, University of Miami, Coral Gables, FL 33124, USA

Karen R. Harris, Ph.D., Department of Special Education, University of Maryland, College Park, MD 20742, USA

Kenneth A. Kavale, Ph.D., Division of Special Education, University of Iowa, Iowa City, IA 52242, USA

B. Keith Lenz, Ph.D., Center for Research on Learning, University of Kansas, Lawrence, KS 66045, USA

John Wills Lloyd, Ph.D., Curry School of Education, University of Virginia, Charlottesville, VA 22903, USA

G. Reid Lyon, Ph.D., Johnson State College, Underhill Center, VT 05490, USA

Margo A. Mastropieri, Ph.D., Department of Educational Studies, Purdue University, West Lafayette, IN 47907, USA

James D. McKinney, Ph.D., School of Education, University of Miami, Coral Gables, FL 33124, USA

John E. Obrzut, Ph.D., Department of Educational Psychology, University of Arizona, Tucson, AZ 85721, USA

Marilyn Ransby, Doctoral Student, Ph.D. Candidate, Department of Educational Psychology and Special Education, University of British Columbia, Vancouver, British Columbia, V6T 1Z1, Canada

Ruth Perou, Ph.D., Centers for Disease Control and Prevention, Atlanta, GA 30341, USA

Virginia Richardson, Ph.D., Department of Teaching and Teacher Education, University of Arizona, Tucson, AZ 85721, USA

Marcia Strong Scott, Ph.D., Department of Psychology, University of Miami, Coral Gables, FL 33124, USA

Thomas E. Scruggs, Ph.D., Department of Educational Studies, Purdue University, West Lafayette, IN 47907, USA

Deborah L. Speece, Ph.D., Department of Special Education, University of Maryland, College Park, MD 20742, USA

H. Lee Swanson, Ph.D., School of Education, University of California, Riverside, CA 92521, USA

Elizabeth Talbott, M.A., Curry School of Education, University of Virginia, Charlottesville, VA 22903, USA

Melody Tankersley, Ph.D., Curry School of Education, University of Virginia, Charlottesville, VA 22903, USA

Joseph K. Torgesen, Ph.D., Department of Psychology, Florida State University, Tallahassee, FL 32306, USA

Anne Uecker, Ph.D., Department of Psychology, University of Arizona, Tucson, AZ 85721, USA

Sharon Vaughn, Ph.D., School of Education and Department of Psychology, University of Miami, Coral Gables, FL 33124, USA

Part I
Models and Theories

1
Learning Disabilities Theory: Issues and Advances

Joseph K. Torgesen

In 1984, a survey of many of the leaders in our field was commissioned by the *Journal of Learning Disabilities* to identify the most widespread beliefs and concerns about the learning disabilities field at that time (Adelman & Taylor, 1985). One of the most frequently cited concerns in the survey centered on the need to improve both theory and research on learning disabilities. In response to some of these concerns, I wrote a relatively optimistic paper titled "Learning Disabilities Theory: Its Current State and Future Prospects," which appeared in *JLD* in 1986 (Torgesen, 1986). The paper was optimistic because it identified some of the reasons for past difficulties in theory development and showed that at least some of these difficulties (those involving a lack of adequate scientific concepts and methodology to support the study of learning disabilities) were well on the way to being overcome. I remain optimistic about the future of theory development in our field, not only because the supporting scientific methodology has continued to advance, but also because we are moving toward greater clarity in our discussion of issues that have frequently produced theoretical confusion about learning disabilities.

In the first section of this chapter, I will briefly describe three issues that must be understood as context for the discussion of learning disabilities (LD) theory. Second, I will identify four elements that should be a part of any fully developed theory of learning disabilities, and I will also suggest certain a priori constraints to theory development within the cognitive domain. Finally, I will briefly outline what I consider to be the two most completely developed current theories of learning disabilities.

Issues in the Development and Validation of Learning Disabilities Theory

Definitional Constraints

One of the first things required for theory development in any field is a clear definition that delimits the phenomena to be described and explained by theory. Definitional confusion has been a chronic part of the

3

history of our field (Torgesen, 1991a), but we now have a definition that appears to enjoy a broad current consensus (Hammill, 1990). This is the definition proposed by the National Joint Committee on Learning Disabilities, and it states:

Learning disabilities is a general term that refers to a heterogeneous group of disorders manifested by significant difficulties in the acquisition and use of listening, speaking, reading, writing, reasoning, or mathematical abilities. These disorders are intrinsic to the individual, presumed to be due to central nervous system dysfunction, and may occur across the life span.

Problems in self-regulatory behaviors, social perception, and social interaction may exist with learning disabilities but do not by themselves constitute a learning disability.

Although learning disabilities may occur concomitantly with other handicapping conditions (for example, sensory impairment, mental retardation, serious emotional disturbance) or with extrinsic influences (such as cultural differences, insufficient or inappropriate instruction), they are not the result of those conditions or influences (NJCLD Memorandum, 1988).

If we take this definition seriously, it places a number of important boundaries on theory development in our field. For present purposes, the important elements of the definition are: (a) recognition that the term "learning disabilities" refers to more than a single type of learning disorder; (b) the assumptions that these learning disorders are intrinsic to the individual and the result of central nervous system (CNS) dysfunction; and, (c) the assertion that they are different from those caused by pervasive or general mental deficiency or lack of opportunities to learn. These elements direct our attention to learning disabilities that are specific, or limited, in their impact on cognitive development, and that are caused by brain-based differences in cognitive functioning that are intrinsic to the individual. While it is undoubtedly true that there are many types of learning problems *not* covered by this definition, if our intent is to develop theories of learning disabilities, then our efforts should focus on the kinds of problems identified in this definition.

The first element of the definition suggests that eventually, we may have many different and equally valid theories of learning disability. Efforts to identify a single, general theory of learning disability are inconsistent with the definition. Since the definition covers a heterogeneous group of disorders, we will clearly need more than a single theory to describe them.

The second element of the definition contains what have been previously referred to as the foundational assumptions of the field (Hallahan & Cruickshank, 1973; Wiederholt, 1974). Stated another way, this definitional element indicates that learning disabilities result from intrinsic cognitive differences that are, in turn, the result of variation in brain function resulting from genetic influences or damage from accident or disease. The assumptions about the intrinsic nature of the disabilities, as well as their origin in CNS differences, have been a part of the fabric of our field since its earliest beginnings, and they provide the core of the rationale for creating special programs for children with learning disabilities. As I shall show later, these assumptions also make it impossible to have a complete theory of learning disabilities derived from a single methodological or theoretical paradigm. That is, it is not possible to have a viable, complete theory of learning disabilities derived solely from the behavioral, cognitive, or neuropsychological point of view. Although one may develop a behavioral theory of learning problems that adequately describes some kinds of learning difficulties, these are not the kind of problems described in the LD definition. It is also possible to describe learning difficulties from the point of view of information processing (cognitive) psychology, but this theory can never be complete without explanatory constructs at the neurological level.

The third important element of the definition, that learning disabilities are not the same as those caused by pervasive mental deficiency or by lack of opportunities to learn, places constraints on the type of intrinsic cognitive limitations that can be proposed as the cause of learning disabilities. This point will be discussed more fully in the second section of this paper.

Learning Disabilities as Science and Social Movement

The definition of learning disabilities presented above contains both descriptive and theoretical elements. The foundational assumptions contained within the definition are clearly theoretical; they need to be validated by careful empirical work. A problem arises, however, from the fact that this definition is used in two significantly different ways. First, it identifies a particular kind of learning disorder for further scientific study. Used in this way, it has given rise to a research area that focuses on special kinds of individual differences in learning and performance. Second, and equally important, the definition has also stimulated development of the field of learning disabilities in special education, which is more similar to a political/social movement than a field of scientific study (Torgesen, 1991a).

In order to validate the theoretical elements in the definition of learning disabilities from a scientific perspective, all that is required is to show that children with neurologically based, intrinsic learning disabilities do, in fact, exist. Even one case of a child with this type of disorder can serve as an "existence proof" for the definition and concept.

However, validation of the definition from the perspective of learning disabilities as a field in special education is much more difficult. This type of validation requires nothing less than evidence that a significant portion of children currently being served in learning disabilities programs fit the essential elements of the definition. It is on this point that the theoretical assumptions of the definition are most frequently attacked. For example, Jim Ysseldyke and his colleagues have reported on a program of research showing that school-identified learning disabled children cannot be differentiated from other kinds of poor learners on the basis of their patterns of intellectual abilities (Ysseldyke, Algozzine, Shinn, & McGue, 1982). In his book *The Learning Mystique*, Gerald Coles (1987) has mounted an extensive attack on the idea that most school-identified LD children have neurological problems as the basis of their learning difficulties. In fact, he is right in showing that the evidence for this idea is exceedingly weak.

The central point here is that the concept of learning disabilities, from a scientific point of view, is not threatened by our current inability to show that a majority of school-identified LD children have intrinsic cognitive limitations resulting from neurological impairment. Historically, it is possible to argue that learning disabilities as a social/political movement has overgeneralized the concept of learning disabilities in order to create improved educational opportunities for the largest possible number of children (Senf, 1986; Torgesen, 1991a). Given that school-identified LD children are a group defined by shifting political realities, local expediencies, and questionable psychometrics (Ysseldyke, 1983), they are hardly a population about which we can hope to make coherent theoretical statements.

Primary verses Secondary Characteristics

Usually when we think of theories of learning disabilities, we think of causal theories that attempt to identify the intrinsic, preexisting (before schooling starts) factors that limit the ability to learn. However, we also know that early failure in school has, itself, profound effects on the child's continuing development (Stanovich, 1986a). That is, the early and consistent failure caused by a primary, or intrinsic learning disorder frequently results in the development of secondary characteristics that further interfere with the child's ability to perform successfully in school, on the job, or in social situations (Kistner & Torgesen, 1987; Schumaker, Deshler, & Ellis, 1986). Although such characteristics as a limited knowledge base, low self-esteem, or confused and inactive learning style might be secondary consequences of early reading failure, these characteristics could easily be primary causes of school dropout, delinquency, or even poor grades in middle school.

Our present knowledge of the development of secondary characteristics in learning disabilities is at least as primitive as our knowledge of the primary causes of learning difficulties. Preliminary work has begun on such topics as attributional styles (Licht, 1983), self-efficacy (Schunck, 1989), social behavior (McKinney, 1990), knowledge-base deficits (Ceci & Baker, 1990), and schooling changes (Brown, Palincsar, & Purcell,

1986) that can help to understand the development of secondary characteristics in children with learning disabilities. Substantial work has also been done on LD children's difficulties in selecting and utilizing effective cognitive strategies on a variety of intellectual and academic tasks (Ryan, Weed, & Short, 1986). However, there is still some confusion as to whether strategic inefficiencies in LD children should be considered primary (Swanson, 1988), or secondary (Torgesen & Licht, 1983) characteristics.

The study of secondary characteristics in LD children is an area ripe for the development of systematic theories to guide further study. Such theories promise to be equally important as those focusing on primary characteristics in helping us to understand the development of children with learning disabilities. However, theories about the development of secondary characteristics need to be clearly differentiated from those that seek to identify primary, intrinsic learning disabilities. Theories about primary learning disabilities must meet the particularly difficult challenge of showing that the "intrinsic" disabilities they identify are, in fact, causes rather than results of failure to learn in school. We turn now to a discussion of the essential elements in any fully developed theory of learning disabilities.

Important Elements of Learning Disabilities Theory

To be complete, any causal theory of learning disabilities needs to address at least four points. These points will be described in the order they should probably be addressed in theory development.

Identification of Specific Behavioral Outcome

The first requirement is a clear specification of the academic or behavioral outcome to be explained by the theory. Having a detailed and specific description at this level is essential to further theory development. Such descriptions as "reading difficulties," "learning problems," or "math disabilities" are not a good starting point for the development of useful theoretical explanations. A good example of the level of specificity required can be found in the area of reading. At the simplest level, reading skills can be divided into those involved in translating from visual to oral or semantic representations of words (word identification), and those involved in constructing the meaning of text (comprehension). Fundamental problems in acquiring word identification skills should require quite different theoretical explanations than difficulties in language comprehension. Even within the relatively narrow area of word identification, it is possible to identify different kinds of skills, such as those involved in alphabetic reading or whole-word identification (Frith, 1985).

The point here is that our starting point should be as specific as possible, and take full advantage of all we know about academic tasks, in order to specify a coherent family of skill deficits to be explained by our theory (Brown & Campione, 1986).

Formulation of an Information Processing Model

The next step in theory development should be formulation of an information processing model to identify the "intrinsic" processing limitations that underlie failure on the academic or developmental learning task. This model is essential to further theory development because it should help pinpoint the phenomena to be explained by deeper layers of theory involving brain-behavior relationships. That is, a specific academic difficulty might potentially be caused by several different factors. Having a well-validated conceptualization of the specific processing limitations responsible for the learning problems would provide substance and specificity to the behavior side of the brain-behavior link.

Recently, Butterfield and Ferretti (1987) have summarized research on individual differences in cognition by identifying five kinds of cognitive differences that are most frequently used to explain learning and performance variations on intellectual tasks. This framework provides a useful context within which to consider the kinds of "intrinsic" cognitive limitations that might cause learning disabilities. According to information processing analyses of performance, important areas of cognitive difference among children and adults occur in:

1. The operational efficiency of basic, or elemental, processing operations as measured by speed, capacity, or perceptual accuracy.
2. The size and organization of the knowledge base.
3. The range, complexity, and activity of strategies selected and utilized.
4. The degree of metacognitive understanding of their own cognitive systems and their relationship to the environment.
5. Completeness and flexibility of executive processes in controlling thinking.

The first category of differences involves *elemental information processing operations* that are closely tied to the biological substrate, have a strong hereditary component, and are relatively impervious to change through educational programming. Although these operations are very difficult to measure in isolation (Brown, Bransford, Ferrara, & Campione, 1982), it is reasonable to assume that they do play a role in creating individual differences in cognitive performance among children (Torgesen, Kistner, & Morgan, 1987).

Base knowledge is all of the information contained in long-term memory about facts, concepts, and relationships among concepts. It is sometimes referred to as "content" knowledge, and it is usually considered to be organized into domains. For example, we have domains of knowledge concerned with chemistry, elementary math operations, soccer, and family life. Psychologists have recently begun to appreciate more fully the enormous influence that previously acquired knowledge has on an individual's ability to learn new information within a domain, or to engage in efficient problem-solving activities (Flavell, Miller, & Miller, 1993).

Strategies are sequences of processing operations that are used to manipulate base knowledge in accomplishing specific tasks. Strategies may be domain-specific, such as a strategy used to help solve two-digit addition problems, but they are usually considered to apply across several domains (Torgesen, 1982). For example, a reading comprehension strategy could contribute to understanding of both social studies and biology texts, and could also be used to prepare for a class as well as to increase general enjoyment in reading. One of the characteristics of good instruction with children with learning disabilities has long been to teach them specific strategies to use in compensating for their cognitive weaknesses. Some of these strategies might be applicable to only a single task, while others would have application across several domains (Ellis, Lenz, & Sabornie, 1987).

The next two terms are more difficult to define than the previous two terms. *Metacognitive knowledge* is information about how, when, and why to use various strategies on specific tasks. Our awareness of the actual strategies we have in our cognitive repertoire is also part of metacognitive knowledge. It also involves awareness of the extent of one's own base knowledge, such as, for example, the fact that I know a great deal more about psychology than I do about chemistry. Also a part of my metacognitive knowledge is the fact that I would usually have to apply different reading strategies, and allow more study time, to understand an article on chemistry than one on psychology. *Executive procedures* provide overall control of strategic processing. These are general strategies for information processing that include planning, selecting, and self-monitoring functions. They have broad utility across all problem domains.

Our current definition of learning disabilities constrains our choice of cognitive explanations of learning disabilities in two ways. First, and most obviously, any theory of learning disabilities must explain in what specific ways the processing limitation or limitations it focuses on can lead to problems in acquiring the academic or developmental skills identified in the first stage of theory development. Second, and equally important, the theory must also show how these particular processing limitations exercise only a limited, or specific effect on cognitive performance. Since, by definition, learning disabilities are not the result of pervasive, or general learning problems, any processing limitation identified as a core disability must be shown to have a strictly limited impact on intellectual functioning. This brings us back to the framework outlined above.

We cannot for example, propose differences in background or base knowledge to be a primary cause of learning disabilities, because this, by itself, could not be an "intrinsic" disability. Ceci and Baker (1990) have shown how knowledge-base deficiencies might easily limit the performance of LD children on many types of tasks. However, these deficiencies should be considered a secondary, rather than primary characteristic of LD children. There is also clear evidence from many sources (Ellis, Lenz, & Sabornie, 1987; Ryan, Weed, & Short, 1986) that LD children, as a group, are less metacognitively and strategically sophisticated than their normal learning peers. However, I prefer to view these strategic inefficiencies as being either a cognitive-affective consequence of early and chronic academic failure (Kistner & Torgesen, 1987; Torgesen & Licht, 1983), or as resulting from improper educational programs assigned to children with reading difficulties (Brown, Palincsar, & Purcell, 1986). Anyone who views strategic inefficiencies as resulting from intrinsic cognitive limitations accepts the difficult theoretical task of showing why these limitations in executive functioning affect only a very narrow range of tasks. Of course, as Stanovich (1986b) has pointed out, many children classified as LD do show mild and pervasive cognitive problems. However, accepting such a characterization of LD children in general will fundamentally alter the nature of our field.

As the reader may have already guessed, I prefer to search for the "intrinsic" cognitive limitations of LD children within the first category of individual differences in the framework. Our conceptualization of this kind of difference suggests that it will be difficult to remediate directly, which is consistent with the results of long-term follow-up studies (Gottfredson, Finucci, & Childs, 1982; Horn, O'Donnell, & Vitulano, 1983). If the particular elemental operation involved affected processing of only one kind of information, or limited the general processing of information in only one way, then it would also have some reasonable hope of being specific in its impact on learning and development.

Identification of Locus of Central Nervous System Dysfunction

The third part of any complete causal theory of learning disabilities should involve identification of the locus or pattern of brain abnormality that is responsible for the intrinsic cognitive limitations described earlier. Much of the current excitement in the field of learning disabilities derives from the development of new technologies that will allow collection of better data relevant to theory development at this level. In fact, the National Institute of Child Health and Human Development (NICHHD) has recently funded several large program projects whose specific aim is to employ recently developed brain imaging technology to examine brain-behavior links in learning disabilities.

Development of Etiological Hypotheses

The last element in a fully adequate theory of learning disabilities should address the etiology of the CNS dysfunction that is part of the theory. Here, it is important to show that the dysfunction itself could not be caused by the learning failure it is used to explain. For example, in explaining specific kinds of reading disability by reference to CNS dysfunction, we must be sure that the failure to learn to read was not itself the cause of the apparent CNS abnormality (Coles, 1987).

Current Theories of Learning Disabilities

I will now birefly outline the two most completely developed and best supported current causal theories of learning disabilities. The first to be discussed is the theory of nonverbal learning disabilities (NLD) developed by Byron Rourke (1989), and the second is the theory of reading disabilities involving difficulties in phonological processing. I will discuss the completeness of each theory in terms of the four points I have just outlined.

The Theory of Nonverbal Learning Disabilities

NLD children were originally identified by their particularly poor performance on mechanical arithmetic tasks (Rourke & Finlayson, 1978; Rourke, Young, & Flewelling, 1971). Over the past 19 years, Rourke and his colleagues have expanded their description of these children's developmental and academic difficulties to include problems with graphomotor skills, difficulties in reading comprehension, mathematical reasoning, and tasks in science that involve complex concept formation. They have also identified specific areas of strength in these children to include word identification skills in reading, spelling, and verbatim memory for both oral and written material. Children with nonverbal learning disabilities have also been shown to have quite severe social/behavioral problems.

Rourke's theory does not identify intrinsic cognitive deficits within an information processing moded of mechanical arithmetic. However, he does describe NLD children's intrinsic limitations from a neuropsychological perspective. The theory indicates how a core of primary processing difficulties involving tactile perception, visual-spatial-organizational skills, and complex psychomotor functions lead to a variety of higher-level cognitive deficits. Rourke specifically links these higher-level cognitive deficits to many of the academic deficits shown by NLD children that involve complex reasoning and problem solving. Rourke is also careful to indicate how NLD children's cognitive limitations cause their social/behavioral problems (Rourke, Young, & Leenaars, 1989).

Rourke's theoretical description of NLD children also includes explicit discussion of areas of normal cognitive development. Early in development, these areas of strength include auditory perception, simple motor behaviors, and rote memory ability. Later, these intact areas of functioning produce normal levels of skill in phonological processing, receptive language, verbal knowledge and associations, and verbal output.

The major locus of neurological impairment in NLD children, according to Rourke's theory, is in the right cerebral hemisphere. Specifically, he states that the necessary condition for the production of the NLD syndrome is the destruction or dysfunction of white matter that is required for intermodal integration. (For example, a significant reduction of callosal fibers or any other neuropathological state that interferes substantially with "access" to right hemispheral systems [and thus, to those systems that are necessary for intermodal integration] would be expected to eventuate in the NLD syndrome.) (Rourke, 1988, p. 312). According to the theory, each individual will manifest specific aspects of the NLD syndrome depending upon both the total amount of white matter that is affected and upon the location and stage of development at which the white matter was damaged.

In terms of etiology, Rourke views the NLD syndrome to be the "final common pathway" for a number of different conditions that produce white matter disease or dysfunction (Rourke, 1987). Examples of such conditions include head injury involving shearing of white matter, hydrocephaly, treatment of acute lymphocytic leukemia with large doses of X-irradiation for a long period of time, congenital absence of the corpus callosum, or significant tissue removal from the right cerebral hemisphere. Other etiologies that might produce the kind of white matter destruction or dysfunction associated with the NLD syndrome include teratogenic effects between conception and birth, and extremely low birth-weight itself. At present, there is no evidence that NLD is transmitted genetically, except as specific diseases that produce white matter damage may be transmitted genetically (Rourke, 1990).

In terms of the theoretical framework outlined earlier in this paper, the theory of nonverbal learning disabilities has a number of significant strengths. It was developed within a comprehensive model of brain-behavior relationships that not only has a strong developmental emphasis, but also provides a clear rationale for both cognitive strengths and weaknesses. The goals of the theory are very ambitious. In Rourke's words, ". . . the clear aim was to develop and refine a comprehensive theoretical model of brain-behavior relationships that would be capable of encompassing the life-span developmental/adaptive dimensions of learning abilities and disabilities in all of their complex manifestations" (Rourke, 1988, p. 327).

The theory also makes an important contribution by its focus on both the cognitive and social development of children with NLD. Rourke is very careful to show how the primary cognitive limitations of the syndrome alter the normal developmental sequence. Although NLD theory is a causal theory of learning disabilities, it is also sensitive to the ways that secondary characteristics can develop from primary disabilities. In particular, the model pays careful attention to the ways in which primary cognitive limitations can lead to serious social/behavioral problems in NLD children.

In terms of the theory itself, a major weakness at present is the failure to clearly specify how the cognitive limitations of NLD children actually produce the primary academic symptom, difficulties with mechanical arithmetic. A useful addition to the theory would be the development of a more complete information processing model of their problems acquiring arithmetic skills. This model would add to the theory in two ways. First, it would help to refine our understanding of NLD children's specific difficulties in acquiring arithmetic skills in a way that might suggest remedial interventions. Second, it might also help to clarify or validate theoretical statements about the underlying cognitive limitations of NLD children. Such a model is important if tight theoretical links are to be established between the defining academic performance problem and the intrinsic cognitive disabilities of NLD children.

Theory of Phonological Reading Disabilities

Both the initial formulation and major development work on this theory have come from the research of Isabelle Liberman and her colleagues at Haskins laboratories (Mann, 1986; Shankweiler & Liberman, 1989). However, in contrast to Rourke's theory, many other investigators have also made, and continue to make, important contributions to the theory (cf. Bradley & Bryant, 1985; Lundberg, Frost, & Peterson, 1988; Morais, Alegria, & Content, 1987; Perfetti, 1985; Stanovich, 1988; Vellutino & Scanlon, 1987; Wagner & Torgesen, 1987).

The most important academic disability of children with phonological reading disabilities (PRD) involves difficulties acquiring fluent word identification skills. In particular, these children have great difficulty learning to use the phonological structure of words to translate between visual and oral language. They are often unable to attain fully alphabetic (Frith, 1985) reading skills. Through careful instruction and practice, they can frequently learn to recognize a useful vocabulary of words as wholes, and may even attain fairly high levels of comprehension of text (Snowling & Hulme, 1989), but their ultimate progress in reading is usually severely curtailed by their difficulties in attaining flexible word identification skills. Areas of cognitive strength for children with PRD frequently include average to high levels of general intelligence along with at least average skills in mathematics and nonverbal tasks.

In their attempts to explain the kind of reading problems outlined above, Liberman and her associates began by asking the question, "What is required of the child in reading a language but not in speaking or listening to it?" (Liberman, Shankweiler, & Liberman, 1989, p. 4). They suggest that the child must master the alphabetic principle: This entails an awareness of the internal phonological structure of words of the language, and awareness that must be more explicit than is ever demanded in the ordinary course of listening and responding to speech. If this is so, it should follow that beginning learners with a weakness in phonological awareness would be at risk (p. 5).

Research testing this hypothesis has generally found that delays in the development of phonological awareness, even before school begins, are strongly predictive of difficulties acquiring alphabetic reading skills (Liberman, Shankweiler, & Liberman, 1989; Stanovich, Cunningham, & Cramer, 1984; Wagner, Torgesen, & Rashotte, in press). Further research has also found that children with PRD have subtle difficulties in speech perception, speech production, and naming. These children also frequently show difficulties on short-term memory tasks involving verbal materials (Torgesen, 1991b). Although there are still unanswered questions about whether these processing difficulties actually derive from a common source (Wagner & Torgesen, 1987), they are usually regarded as reflecting a specific disability in processing the phonological aspects of language.

The theoretical links between phonological processing disabilities and early difficulties acquiring alphabetic reading skills are very tight (Liberman et al., 1989). Furthermore, in suggesting that the processing difficulties of children with PRD are limited to the phonological structures of language, the theory also allows for generally normal cognitive development in many other areas. For example, the ability of these children to process the semantic aspects of language is relatively unaffected.

Studies of normal brain function locate phonological processing operations in the left temporal region of the brain (Damasio & Geschwind, 1984). Thus, this is a likely locus of brain dysfunction in children with PRD. In fact, three converging strands of research provide strong evidence that children with PRD do frequently show anomalies of development in this region of the brain. First, Al Galaburda's micro-examinations of the brains of diseased individuals with PRD consistently found disturbances of brain development in this region (Galaburda, 1988). Furthermore, the particular anomalies identified in his work arise very early in development, and thus could not be the result, rather than the cause, of reading problems. Furthermore, studies involving measurement of regional cerebral blood flow during reading have also verified that this same temporal region of the brain is differentially affected in dyslexics than in normal readers (Flowers, Wood, & Naylor, in press). Finally, a recently reported study using magnetic resonance imaging technology to examine a carefully selected sample of children with PRD provides quite strong evidence of differences in brain structure along the temporal plane between reading disabled and normal children (Hynd, Semrud-Clikeman, Lorys, Novey, & Eliopulos, 1990). These three sources of information, taken together, provide convincing evidence of disturbances in development of the left temporal region of the brain in children with PRD.

The primary etiological factor for the kinds of brain anomalies associated with PRD is thought to be genetic transmission. The Colorado Twin study of reading disabilities has provided very convincing evidence that phonological processing ability is highly heritable (Olsen, Wise, Conners, Rack, & Fulker, 1989).

A major strength of the theory of phonological reading disabilities is its conceptualization of the intrinsic cognitive limitations of these children and the way these limitations affect acquisition of early reading skills. Already, this information processing analysis has suggested intervention procedures that are effective in both a preventive (Bradley & Bryant, 1985; Lundberg, Frost, & Peterson, 1988) and remedial (Alexander, Anderson, Voeller, & Torgesen, 1991) role. Studies have shown that explicit training in phonological awareness can help to reduce the number of children who show reading difficulties in the early grades, and it can also help older children with severe reading problems learn to read words more effectively.

An important weakness of the theory is that its conceptualization of developmental changes in the PRD syndrome is relatively undeveloped. Very little is actually known about the course of development of phonological processing difficulties. For example, it is possible that this type of difficulty is much more widespread among young children than older children (Torgesen, 1991b). Further, possible changes in symptoms with development is also in need of further study and theoretical elaboration. For example, the most reliable symptom of PRD in young children is delay in development of phonological awareness (Felton & Wood, 1990). However, as children grow older, other kinds of phonological processing disabilities, such as naming or short-term memory problems, may be more characteristic of the syndrome (Torgesen, Wagner, Simmons, & Laughon, 1990).

A Comparison of the Theories

An important strength of both of these theories is that they address all the points of concern for complete causal theories of learning disabilities. They identify specific academic difficulties, and they contain explanations for these difficulties in terms of intrinsic cognitive limitations. They also propose specific areas or processes of CNS dysfunction that cause the cognitive deficits, and they both address a range of possible etiologies for these neural pathologies. Of course, anyone who has studied the history of the field of learning disabilities will recognize that the same things could be said about other theories that are no longer accepted as plausible.

However, these theories are an advance over previous theories for a variety of reasons. First, they are both based on a much more extensive data base than previous theories. The empirical research on which they are based has employed more sophisticated methodologies than were available to pioneering theorists in the field. Finally, they are both derived from more fully developed scientific paradigms than have been available until recently (Torgesen, 1986). Undoubtedly, both PRD and NLD theory will undergo alterations based on future research. However, both theories provide a solid framework that can help future research to be more systematic. The evidence to date helps me to be optimistic that they may be the first in a series of theories that ultimately prove useful in the prevention and treatment of learning disabilities.

The individual strengths of each theory reflect the dominant scientific paradigm within which it was developed. Because most of the supporting research for NLD theory was conducted within the neuropsychological paradigm, it is relatively strong and complex in its conceptualization of the brain-behavior relationships involved in the disorder. The theory itself is embedded within a more complete neuropsychological framework than is the theory about phonologically based reading disabilities.

In contrast, the dominate research paradigms used to develop PRD theory have come from information processing psychology. Thus it is relatively complete in its analysis of the academic tasks on which failure occurs, and the links between intrinsic cognitive deficits and academic failure are much better developed than in NLD theory.

The greatly enlarged scope of information processing research on reading that has taken place over the past 20 years has been very helpful in the development of PRD theory.

It is frequently difficult for researchers operating within different scientific paradigms to communicate with one another because of the differing assumptions, methodologies, and concepts that are used in their research. However, LD theory is clearly a place where such communication is vital to the enterprise. NLD theory can clearly profit from more attention to information processing analysis of academic and cognitive tasks, while PRD theory can benefit from more complete utilization of developmental neuropsychological concepts in its formulation.

Although both NLD and PRD theory help to validate the definition of learning disabilities from a scientific point of view, they do not provide much comfort for the learning disabilities movement in special education. The point at issue is prevalence. At present, the safest assumption about the problems described in each theory is that they are continuously distributed in a multidimensional space (Stanovich, 1988). This makes answers to questions about prevalence entirely dependent upon the degree of severity, or specificity, we are concerned with. However, as a reasonable starting point, it seems likely that children who are clearly described by each theory are relatively rare within populations of school-identified children with learning disabilities. For example, research we have conducted (Torgesen, 1988) indicates that, among children in the middle elementary grades, only about 15% of school-identified LD children continue to show severe problems with the representation of phonological information in short-term memory. Two other empirical classification studies showed that about 15% of samples of LD children had specific problems with phonological representation, while another 15% had similar problems in the context of broader intellectual impairment (Lyon & Watson, 1981; Speece, 1987).

In a personal communication, Byron Rourke (Rourke, 1990) indicated that for every 20 childen with a phonological reading disability referred to his clinic, they see one child with nonverbal learning disabilities. Although this makes these problems very rare, Rourke also indicated that this incidence rate has doubled in the last 20 years due to the increased survivability of children who have problems associated with white matter disease or injury.

Although both of these prevalence estimates must be considered extremely tentative, they suggest that learning disabilities of the type described in the NJCLD definition may be much rarer than is commonly estimated. Of course, school-identified populations may contain many children with other types of learning disabilities that will eventually be described by additional viable theories, but there is not currently available a coherent body of research findings to identify or describe these children. At present, it seems clear that both scientific integrity and advancement of theory will be best served by careful discipline in our claims about the extent of these problems in samples of school aged children.

References

Adelman, H.S. & Taylor, L. (1985). The future of the LD field: A survey of fundamental concerns. *Journal of Learning Disabilities*, *18*(7), 423–427.

Alexander, A., Anderson, H., Voeller, K.S., & Torgesen, J.K. (1991). Phonological awareness training and remediation of analytic decoding deficits in a group of severe dyslexics. *Annals of Dyslexia, 41*, 193–206.

Bradley, L. & Bryant, P. (1985). *Rhyme and reason in reading and spelling*. Ann Arbor: University of Michigan Press.

Brown, A.L., Bransford, J.D., Ferrara, R.A., & Campione, J.C. (1982). Learning, remembering, and understanding. In J.H. Flavell & E.M. Markman (Eds.), *Handbook of child psychology* (4th ed.): *Cognitive development* (Vol. 3) (pp. 315–345). New York: Wiley.

Brown, A.L. & Campione, J.C. (1986). Psychological theory and the study of learning disabilities. *American Psychologist, 14*, 1059–1068.

Brown, A.L., Palincsar, A.S., & Purcell, L. (1986). Poor readers: Teach, don't label. In U. Neisser (Ed.), *The school achievement of minority children: New perspectives* (pp. 105–143). Hillsdale, NJ: Erlbaum.

Butterfield, E.D. & Ferretti, R.P. (1987). Toward a theoretical integration of cognitive hypotheses about intellectual differences among children. In L. Borkowski & L.D. Day (Eds.), *Cognition in special children: Comparative approaches to retardation, learning disabilities, and giftedness* (pp. 195–234). New York: Ablex.

Ceci, S.J. & Baker, J.G. (1990). On learning . . . more or less: A knowledge × process × context view of learning disabilities. In J.K. Torgesen (Ed.), *Cognitive and behavioral characteristics of children with learning disabilities* (pp. 159–178). Austin, TX: PRO-ED.

Coles, G.S. (1987). *The learning mystique: A critical look at "learning disabilities".* New York: Pantheon.

Damasio, A.R. & Geschwind, N. (1984). The neural basis of language. *Annual Review of Neurosciences, 7,* 127–147.

Ellis, E.S., Lenz, B.K., & Sabornie, E.J. (1987). Generalization and adaptation of learning strategies to natural environments: Part 2: Research into practice. *Remedial and Special Education, 8,* 6–23.

Felton, R.H. & Wood, F.B. (1990). Cognitive deficits in reading disability and attention deficit disorder. In J.K. Torgesen (Ed.), *Cognitive and behavioral characteristics of children with learning disabilities* (pp. 89–114). Austin, TX: PRO-ED.

Flavell, J.H., Miller, P.H., & Miller, S.A. (1993). *Cognitive development* (3rd ed.). Englewood Cliffs, NJ: Prentice-Hall.

Flowers, L., Wood, F.B., & Naylor, C.E. (in press). Regional cerebral blood flow in adults diagnosed as reading disabled in childhood. *Archives of Neurology.*

Frith, U. (1985). Beneath the surface of developmental dyslexia. In K. Patterson, J. Marshall, & M. Coltheart (Eds.), *Surface dyslexia* (pp. 301–330). London: Erlbaum.

Galaburda, A.M. (1988). The pathogenesis of childhood dyslexia. In F. Plum (Ed.), *Language, communication, and the brain* (pp. 127–137). New York: Raven Press.

Gottfredson, L.S., Finucci, J.M., & Child, B. (1982). *The adult occupational success of dyslexic boys: A large-scale, long-term follow-up* (Report No. 334). Baltimore: Johns Hopkins University, Center for Social Organization in the Schools.

Hallahan, D.P. & Cruickshank, W.M. (1973). *Psycho-educational foundations of learning disabilities.* Englewood Cliffs, NJ: Prentice Hall.

Hammill, D.D. (1990). On defining learning disabilities: An emerging consensus. *Journal of Learning Disabilities, 23,* 74–84.

Horn, W.F., O'Donnell, J.P., & Vitulano, L.A. (1983). Long-term follow-up studies of learning disabled persons. *Journal of Learning Disabilities, 16,* 542–555.

Hynd, G.W., Semrud-Clikeman, M., Lorys, A.R., Novey, E.S., & Eliopulos, D. (1990). Brain morphology in developmental dyslexia and attention deficit disorder/hyperactivity. *Archives of Neurology, 47,* 919–926.

Kistner, J. & Torgesen, J.K. (1987). Motivational and cognitive aspects of learning disabilities. In A.E. Kasdin & B.B. Lahey (Eds.), *Advances in clinical child psychology*. New York: Plenum Press.

Liberman. I.Y., Shankweiler, D., & Liberman, A.M. (1989). The alphabetic principle and learning to read. In D. Shankweiler & I.Y. Liberman (Eds.), *Phonology and reading disability: Solving the reading puzzle* (pp. 1–34). Ann Arbor: University of Michigan Press.

Licht, B.G. (1983). Cognitive-motivational factors that contribute to the achievement of learning disabled children. *Journal of Learning Disabilities*, *16*, 483–493.

Lundberg, I., Frost, J., & Peterson, O. (1988). Effects of an extensive program for stimulating phonological awareness in pre-school children. *Reading Research Quarterly*, *23*, 263–284.

Lyon, R. & Watson, B. (1981). Empirically derived subgroups of learning disabled readers: Diagnostic characteristics. *Journal of Learning Disabilities*, *14*, 256–261.

Mann, V.A. (1986). Why some children encounter reading problems: The contribution of difficulties with language processing and phonological sophistication to early reading disability. In J.K. Torgesen & B.Y.L. Wong (Eds.), *Psychological and educational perspectives on learning disabilities* (pp. 133–160). New York: Academic Press.

McKinney, J.D. (1990). Longitudinal research on the behavioral characteristics of children with learning disabilities. In J.K. Torgesen (Ed.), *Cognitive and behavioral characteristics of children with learning disabilities* (pp. 115–138). Austin, TX: PRO-ED.

Morais, J., Alegria, J., & Content, A. (1987). The relationships between segmental analysis and alphabetic literacy: An interactive view. *Cahiers de Psychologie Cognitive*, *7*, 415–438.

National Joint Committee on Learning Disabilities. (1988). Letter to NJCLD member organizations.

Olsen, R., Wise, B., Conners, F., Rack, J., & Fulker, D. (1989). Specific deficits in component reading and language skills: Genetic and environmental influences. *Journal of Learning Disabilities*, *22*, 339–348.

Perfetti, C.A. (1985). *Reading ability*. New York: Oxford University Press.

Rourke, B.P. (1987). Syndrome of nonverbal learning disabilities: The final common pathway of white-matter disease/dysfunction? *The Clinical Neuropsychologist*, *1*, 209–234.

Rourke, B.P. (1988). The syndrome of nonverbal learning disabilities: developmental manifestations in neurological disease, disorder, and dysfunction. *The Clinical Neuropsychologist*, *2*, 293–330.

Rourke, B.P. (1989). *Nonverbal learning disabilities: The syndrome and the model*. New York: Guilford.

Rourke, B.P. (1990). Personal communication. Sept. 19, 1990.

Rourke, B.P. & Finlayson, M.A.J. (1978). Neuropsychological significance of variations in patterns of academic performance: Verbal and visual-spatial abilities. *Journal of Abnormal Child Psychology*, *6*, 121–133.

Rourke, B.P., Young, G.C., & Flewelling, R.W. (1971). The relationships between WISC Verbal-Performance discrepancies and selected verbal, auditory-perceptual, and problem-solving abilities in children with learning disabilities. *Journal of Clinical Psychology*, 27, 475–479.

Rourke, B.P., Young, G.C., & Leenaars, A.A. (1989). A childhood learning disability that predisposes those afflicted to adolescent and adult depression and suicide risk. *Journal of Learning Disabilities*, 22, 169–175.

Ryan, E.B., Weed, K.A., & Short, E.J. (1986). Cognitive behavior modification: Promoting active, self-regulatory learning styles. In J.K. Torgesen & B.Y.L. Wong (Eds.), *Psychological and educational perspectives on learning disabilities* (pp. 367–397). New York: Academic Press.

Schumaker, J.B., Deshler, D.D., & Ellis, E.S. (1986). Intervention issues related to the education of learning disabled adolescents. In J.K. Torgesen & B.Y.L. Wong (Eds.), *Psychological and educational perspectives on learning Disabilities* (pp. 329–365). New York: Academic Press.

Schunk, D.H. (1989). Self-efficacy and cognitive achievement: Implications for students with learning problems. *Journal of Learning Disabilities*, 22, 14–22.

Senf, G.M. (1986). LD research in sociological and scientific perspective. In J.K. Torgesen & B.Y.L. Wong (Eds.), *Psychological and educational perspectives on learning disabilities* (pp. 27–53). New York: Academic Press.

Shankweiler, D. & Liberman, I.Y. (1989). *Phonology and reading disability*. Ann Arbor: University of Michigan Press.

Snowling, M. & Hulme, C. (1989). A longitudinal case study of developmental phonological dyslexia. *Cognitive Neuropsychology*, 6, 379–401.

Speece, D.L. (1987). Information processing subtypes of learning disabled readers. *Learning Disabilities Research*, 2, 91–102.

Stanovich, K.E. (1986a). Matthew effects in reading: Some consequences of individual differences in the acquisition of literacy. *Reading Research Quarterly*, 21, 360–406.

Stanovich, K.E. (1986b). Cognitive processes and the reading problems of learning-disabled children: Evaluating the assumption of specificity. In J.K. Torgesen & B.Y.L. Wong (Eds.), *Psychological and educational perspectives on learning disabilities* (pp. 87–131). New York: Academic Press.

Stanovich, K.E. (1988). Explaining the differences between the dyslexic and the garden-variety poor reader: The phonological-core variable-difference model. *Journal of Learning Disabilities*, 21, 590–604.

Stanovich, K.E., Cunningham, A.E., & Cramer, B.B. (1984). Assessing phonological awareness in kindergarten children: Issues of task comparability. *Journal of Experimental Child Psychology*, 38, 175–190.

Swanson, H.L. (1988). Toward a metatheory of learning disabilities. *Journal of Learning Disabilities*, 21, 196–209.

Torgesen, J.K. (1982). The learning disabled child as an inactive learner: Educational implications. *Topics in Learning and Learning Disabilities*, 2, 45–52.

Torgesen, J.K. (1986). Learning disabilities theory: Its current state and future prospects. *Journal of Learning Disabilities*, 19, 399–407.

Torgesen, J.K. (1988). Studies of children with learning disabilities who perform poorly on memory span tasks. *Journal of Learning Disabilities*, 21, 605–612.

Torgesen, J.K. (1991a). Learning disabilities: Historical and conceptual issues. In B.Y.L. Wong (Ed.), *Learning about learning disabilities* (pp. 3–37). San Diego: Academic Press.

Torgesen, J.K. (1991b). Subtypes as prototypes: Extended studies of rationally defined extreme groups. In L.V. Feagans, E.J. Short, & L.J. Meltzer (Eds.), *Subtypes of learning disabilities: Theoretical perspectives and research* (pp. 229–246). Hillsdale, NJ: Erlbaum.

Torgesen, J.K., Kistner, J.A., & Morgan, S. (1987). Component processes in working memory. In J. Borkowski & J.D. Day (Eds.), *Memory and cognition in special children: Perspectives on retardation, learning disabilities, and giftedness* (pp. 49–86). Norwood, NJ: Ablex.

Torgesen, J.K. & Licht, B. (1983). The learning disabled child as an inactive learner: Retrospect and prospects. In J.D. McKinney & L. Feagans (Eds.), *Topics in Learning Disabilities, Vol. 1* (pp. 3–32). Rockville, MD: Aspen Press.

Torgesen, J.K., Wagner, R.K., Simmons, K., & Laughon, P. (1990). Identifying phonological coding problems in disabled readers: Naming, counting, or span measures? *Learning Disabilities Quarterly*, *13*, 236–243.

Vellutino, F. & Scanlon, D.M. (1987). Phonological coding, phonological awareness, and reading ability: Evidence from longitudinal and experimental study. *Merrill-Palmer Quarterly*, *33*, 321–364.

Wagner, R.K. & Torgesen, J.K. (1987). The nature of phonological processing and its causal role in the acquisition of reading skills. *Psychological Bulletin*, *101*, 192–212.

Wagner, R.K., Torgesen, J.K., & Rashotte, C.A. (in press). The development of reading-related phonological processing abilities: New evidence of bi-directional causality from a latent variable longitudinal study. *Developmental Psychology*.

Wiederholt, J.L. (1974). Historical perspectives on the education of the learning disabled. In L. Mann & D.A. Sabatino (Eds.), *The second review of special education* (pp. 103–152). Austin, TX: PRO-ED.

Ysseldyke, J.E. (1983). Current practices in making psycho-educational decisions about learning disabled students. *Journal of Learning Disabilities*, *16*, 209–219.

Ysseldyke, J.E., Algozzine, B., Shinn, M., & McGue, M. (1982). Similarities and differences between underachievers and students labeled learning disabled. *Journal of Special Education*, *16*, 73–85.

Theory to Practice

2
Neuropsychological Theories Associated with Learning Disorders

JOHN E. OBRZUT AND ANNE UECKER

Introduction

Although the term "learning disabilities" has been in existence for little over 25 years (Duane, 1991; Morrison & Siegel, 1991), the condition itself has aroused considerable interest for well over a century. Originally identified as congenital word blindness, learning disabilities and developmental dyslexia have long been suspected to be a result of a neural substrate located in the posterior left cerebral hemisphere (Satz, 1991). Observations such as anomalous hand preference, male predominance, and underachievement in subjects such as spelling have been consistently made since the turn of the century (Duane, 1991). A particularly persisting line of research has concerned the topic of language lateralization. Recent technological advances allow new approaches to an old problem.

Recent investigations continue to provide insight concerning the neurological and neuropsychological underpinnings of specific disabilities (see Obrzut & Hynd, 1991 for a review). These studies have indicated differences in brain structure and functioning between normal and dyslexic readers, as well as providing information into specific neuropsychological profiles associated with learning difficulties. A number of different theories provide speculation regarding the etiology of specific learning disabilities; many of these theories rest upon unavailable empirical support. Researchers agree that the population with learning disabilities (LD) is both complex in nature and heterogenous in composition. The purpose of this chapter is to discuss the assumptions and concepts underlying neuropsychological theories associated with learning disorders. In particular, anatomical, physiological, and behavioral evidence supporting the view that group differences in hemispheric organization tend to characterize the population with LD will be presented. In so doing, applications of neuropsychological theories to interpreting and conducting research in learning disabilities may become more evident.

Theories of Hemisphere Specialization and Cognitive Performance

One of the central issues of neuropsychology is the asymmetrical organization of functions in the brain. Ever since physical differences in the two hemispheres were noted, researchers have been attributing function to structure. Most studies have shown lateralization, or the presence of hemispheric specialization of task. Tasks that require processing of verbal stimuli are lateralized to the left hemisphere, and those performances that require processing of nonverbal stimuli are lateralized to the right hemisphere (see Hynd & Cohen, 1983 for review, p. 41). There are many ideas or models about laterality and asymmetry of function. Several of these neuropsychological models are outlined below.

Zaidel (1986) recognized three major models that explain functional hemispheric asymmetry. He stated that the first two are anatomically motivated and the third model is more psychologically motivated.

Zaidel's first model is called "direct access." This model reflects the belief that the hemisphere that receives the sensory input first, processes it. Laterality differences are attributed to differences in the perceptual cognitive competencies of the two hemispheres.

The second model is called "callosal relay." Kimura (1967) called it the "verbal-nonverbal model." This theory assumes the specialization of each hemisphere to perform specific functions. Verbal stimuli, whether presented to the right or left side of the body, will be processed by the left hemisphere. Thus verbal stimuli presented to the right side of the body will be directly processed by the left hemisphere, but verbal stimuli presented to the left side of the body will be presented to the right hemisphere and transferred across the corpus callosum to the left hemisphere to be processed. Direct routes would appear more efficient; therefore, it would explain the right-ear, right visual field and right-hand advantage for verbal stimuli. The right hemisphere is considered specialized for nonverbal information directly.

The third model is called "dynamic shift." Kinsbourne (1974) called it the "attention model." Kinsbourne agrees with Kimura that hemispheres are functionally specialized, but according to Kinsbourne, hemispheric specialization does not explain lateral advantages. Kinsbourne believes that an aroused hemisphere "primes" the attention centers to focus on perceptions in that particular perceptual field of the body. Overloading of hemispheric activation can lead to eventual shift of control to the other hemisphere (Hellige, 1983). This mode, dynamic shift, accommodates both direct access of bilateral competencies and the callosal relay of lateral specialization. Split-brain and lesion studies support the direct access model, but hemispheric lesion studies also support the callosal relay.

Individual differences in structural function, according to the direct access model, would be attributed to individual hemispheric specialization, or inherent variability. Individual differences in structural function, according to the callosal relay model could be attributed to the individual differences in callosal connectivity.

Several other models that seek to explain lateralization in relation to behavior have also been presented by other researchers. Another behavioral model, "novel information," presented by Goldberg and Costa (1981) suggests that the verbal-nonverbal theory is too simplistic. They believe that the right hemisphere is functionally specialized to process new information and the left hemisphere is specialized to process familiar information. Bakker (1979) supports this theory in finding that beginning readers process written stimuli primarily with the right hemisphere.

Lenneberg (1967) believes that the left hemisphere gradually gains control over language and that lateralization is established around puberty. Krashen (1973) altered this "developmental" model by changing the age of left hemisphere establishment to 5 years of age.

Although some research has provided support for each of the theoretical positions, there has been little concensus regarding a theoretical explanation for the condition known as learning disabilities. The following section outlines the progress that has been made to this point in the neuropsychological study of learning disabilities and suggests contemporary theories and research directions in the neuropsychology of learning disabilities.

Laterality, Cognitive Deficits, and Learning Disabilities

One way to study functional asymmetries is to look at a population that has deviant cognitive abilities. Looking at the deviation, where normal lateralization or hemispheric specialization may have failed to occur, is one way to draw conclusions about normal lateralization of function. It is hypothesized that the population with LD has an anomalous pattern of cerebral language lateralization as compared to the majority of right-handed individuals. Orton (1937) originally asserted the idea that disordered language processes in individuals with LD were due to faulty development within the left hemisphere. The original theory was premised on the observation that since a very small area of destruction in the controlling or dominant hemisphere resulted in an extensive loss of speech or reading skills, and that since an equally small area of destruction in exactly the same part of the opposite or nondominant hemisphere was followed by no language disorder at all, language disorders in children must be preceded by some sort of maldevelopment or lack of development in the dominant hemisphere. It was on the basis of this logic that Orton (1937) proclaimed that language disorders of children might be better understood. A primary assertion was that the many delays and defects evident in the development of language and related functions arose during the process of establishing unilateral brain superiority in individual areas of the brain.

The suggestion that dyslexia resulted from incomplete or mixed cerebral dominance (Orton, 1925) was contrary to the previous theory of a deficiency in the center for visual images. Theories that can be considered to have developed from Orton's original proposals include the deficit and delay models. The deficit model proposes that cerebral dysfunction underlies the inability to acquire appropriate reading skills. Cerebral dysfunction, or deficit, may take the form of faulty hemispheric organization, of abnormal development of neural cells, or of patterns of abnormal cellular connections. On the other hand, the maturational lag or delay model is a developmental theory proposing that dyslexia is due to difficulties in the establishment of cerebral dominance. Although the delay model continues to enjoy a moderate level of acceptance, current research has shown the beginnings of hemispheric specialization to be present at or near birth (Spreen, Tupper, Risser, Tuokko, & Edgell, 1984).

Orton's original theory (1925, 1937) has generated a considerable amount of subsequent research and controversy. Much of the controversy has remained unresolved due to a lack of precise measuring techniques. Answers regarding individual and group differences in hemispheric organization remain elusive. Even with today's more sophisticated technology, neither agreement nor disagreement has been convincingly demonstrated. With the recent development and availability of neuroimaging techniques (i.e., computerized topography [CT] and positron emission tomography [PET]) both Orton's and subsequent theories are able and need to be put to more convincing tests. Thus, technological advances have lessened the constraints to conducting this type of research.

Anatomical and Behavioral Differences

Due to the lack of hard evidence, early theories of cerebral dominance centered upon the study of functional asymmetry. It is only recently that technology has allowed for the parallel finding of anatomical asymmetry, enabling more tangible speculations regarding the neuroanatomical basis for language. Data from Geschwind and Levitsky (1968) offer proof that the language areas in the left hemisphere are significantly larger than the corresponding areas in the right hemisphere. Specifically, the planum temporale, the area of the brain containing the auditory association cortex, was larger in the left hemisphere. The planum temporale comprises a portion of Wernicke's area. Since the study of Geschwind and Levitsky (1968), it has been demonstrated that lesions involving the planum temporale on the left side are likely to produce Wernicke's aphasia. This finding makes more robust the suggestion that the left planum temporale contains functional areas necessary for language (Galaburda, 1983).

Subsequent studies have confirmed the finding of an anatomical asymmetry in the left hemisphere. For example, Witelson and Pallie (1973), in measurements of adult and neonatal postmortem brains, again found the left planum to be significantly larger than the right. In addition to offering an anatomical basis for functional asymmetry, it is suggested that the language area in the human infant is larger either at birth or shortly thereafter. Wada, Clark, and Hamm (1975) also offered subsequent confirmation of left hemisphere anatomical dominance in both infant and adult postmortem brains. These authors found the left hemisphere to be larger than the right hemisphere in approximately 90% of both samples. The finding of Wada and associates correlated well with the presumed incidence of cerebral language lateralization in the general population.

The previous studies provide evidence showing that the majority of brains, when free of neurological disease, show asymmetry of the planum temporale in favor of the left side. This side is larger in roughly two-thirds of brains; reverse asymmetry is present in about 10%, and brains with asymmetrical plana make up about 25% of the total (Geschwind & Levitsky, 1968; Wada et al., 1975; Witelson & Pallie, 1973). These findings render the fact of hemispheric asymmetry of the temporal speech region in the area of the planum temporale well established (Falzi, Perrone, & Vignolo, 1982). Additional evidence for hemispheric asymmetry is found in research demonstrating the left frontal operculum to have a greater total surface area than the right side (Falzi et al., 1982). Lesions in this area have been known to cause Broca's aphasia (Kertesz, Lesk, & McCabe, 1977).

Wada and colleagues (1975) provide evidence for individual differences in hemispheric organization. Variations in morphological asymmetry in early gestational stages were observed; the degree of hemispheric development differed across individuals at different ages. That morphological maturation takes place at variable speeds is suggested. It is likely that functional maturation mimics anatomical maturation. In other words, both language and its responsible structures are likely to show variability at different stages in development.

Analyses of individuals with dyslexia and LD often suggest abnormalities in brain structures. Drake (1968), for example, performed a postmortem study on a 12-year-old dyslexic boy. He discovered an abnormal corpus callosum and an abnormal convolutional pattern in both parietal lobes. Galaburda and Kemper (1979) examined a 19-year-old dyslexic boy and discovered abnormalities in the left planum temporal. Reportedly the patient had a well-documented history of developmental dyslexia; severe problems in reading, moderate difficulties with arithmetic, and mild disturbance in right-left discrimination. Prior testing revealed a

Stanford-Binet intelligence score of 105. Reading problems were seen in other male members of the immediate family.

Upon examining the brain, it was found that this patient lacked the asymmetry found in the majority of people. Most people have a large left temporal (planum temporale) region different than that of the right region. The planum temporale regions in the patient with dyslexia were discovered to be symmetrical in the two hemispheres. The abnormality was defined to the left region only (Galaburda & Kemper, 1979; Hynd & Hynd, 1984).

These abnormalities were not due to brain damage but attributable to a number of speculative causes: congenital factors, autoimmune disease, or perhaps to cytomegalovirus (CMV). Hynd and Hynd (1984) state that this abnormal pattern appears primarily in the region involved in reading.

In examination of four other brains of men with developmental dyslexia, Galaburda, (1986) and Galaburda, Sherman, Rosen, Aboitiz, & Geschwind (1985) located similar hemispheric anomalies. All four showed deviation from the standard asymmetry found in the majority of the general non-dyslexic population.

It is pointed out that roughly 25% of the population have symmetrical plana, the pattern of dyslexia. However, as mentioned earlier, the pre-valency rate for dyslexia is reportedly half that number. An explanation offered is that symmetrical plana is causally related to full-blown dyslexia but that a proportion of persons with similar brain structure are able to compensate. Still, "the probability of finding four consecutive brains (for this study) with symmetrical plana is close to ¼ to the fourth power (i.e., less than 0.004), so it is not likely to (have been) a chance occurrence" (Galaburda et al., 1985, p. 228).

Hynd, Semrud-Clikeman, Lorys, Novey, & Eliopulos (1990) used a magnetic resonance imaging (MRI) procedure to test 10 dyslexic, 10 attention deficit/hyperactive (ADD/H), and 10 normal age- and sex-matched control children. The dyslexic group was distinguished from the normal subjects in that a significantly smaller left planum temporale was found. The study of Hynd and colleagues represents an attempt to resolve problems from earlier research. For example, in a critical review of past neuroimagings studies, Hynd et al., (1990) note that poorly documented dyslexic populations are employed. Also questionable are the control populations. Hynd and colleagues assert that it may be necessary to include populations with other clinical syndromes in order to document the uniqueness of deviations in the patterns of brain asymmetry in dyslexics. An additional fault in brain morphology studies is a failure to examine whether or not a relationship is evident between left-handedness and autoimmune disease. The study of Hynd and colleagues (1990) at-tempts to improve on these methodologic weaknesses by the inclusion of a clinical population of ADD/H children without significant learning problems.

In Hynd's study, both the normal and ADD/H children were found to have a more typical pattern of cerebral lateralization. Seventy percent of these populations showed left-greater-than-right asymmetry, and 30% showed a pattern of plana symmetry or reversed asymmetry with the right side being greater than the left. In contrast, 90% of the dyslexic children had either symmetrical or reversed asymmetry of plana length. Assuming that the 30% left-is-less-than-or-equal-to-right plana length morphology is normal, the 90% incidence of this pattern in the dyslexic children represents a very significant departure from normal patterns of differential brain maturation. The results of symmetrical or asymmetrical hemispheres in the study of Hynd and colleagues (1990) occurred primarily due to the significantly smaller left planum temporale. A definite pattern of deviant hemispheric specialization emerged in the dyslexic population.

Further support for neuroanatomical abnormality in developmental disorders was recently obtained by Plante, Swisher, Vance, and Rapcsak (1991). These researchers found atypical perisylvian asymmetries in male subjects who were diagnosed as specific language impaired (SLI). Atypical perisylvian asymmetries also were documented in a majority of the parents of SLI subjects, and were frequently associated with a history of communication difficulty (Plante, 1991).

The preceding studies provide support for the conclusions of Galaburda et al. (1985) regarding the notion that the mechanisms of corticogenesis and possibly the processes associated with the elimination of unwanted cells is implicated in dyslexia. The deviation in corticogenesis seems to affect the left planum temporale during development. These neuroanatomical findings also suggest that a prenatal alteration of brain development underlies specific language impairment and may even reflect a transmittable, biological factor that places some families at risk for language impairment (Plante, 1991).

Anatomical and Physiological Asymmetries Examined through Neuroimaging

Using CT scans Hier, LeMay, Rosenberger, and Perlo (1978) proposed a "mismatch between hemispheric specialization for language and structural asymmetry of the hemispheres" (p. 92). Heir et al. viewed this pattern of reversed asymmetry as a potential contributor to the possibility of dyslexia. These authors based their theory on 24 developmental dyslexics, 10 of which had a wider right parietal occipital area. Heir et al. found that the verbal intelligence of the atypical asymmetric group was significantly less than the normal group, while performance did not vary significantly. Also, the atypical group reported more delay in the acquisition of speech than the asymmetrical group. This could be interpreted to mean that a particular group of developmental dyslexics have a deviant pattern of neurological organization.

CT scan irregularities are not universally seen in children with LD (Denckla, LeMay, & Chapman, 1985). Denckla and colleagues utilized a CT procedure with a group of 32 individuals with LD. Of these children, ages 7 to 15, most were found to have normal scans. Independent radiologists read 25 of the scans; only 5 of these (20%) were read as "slightly abnormal" by both radiologists. At this time, no CT abnormalities are considered to be diagnostic of learning disability; however, cases exist in which a structural basis appears to be present. Common findings in individuals with LD include cerebral asymmetries or more specific pathology in the posterior association cortical areas (Bigler, 1989). For example, Haslam, Dalby, Johns, and Rademaker (1981) found no reversed asymmetry, but only symmetry in the brains of dyslexics. Parkins, Roberts, Reinarz, and Varney (1987) found no difference in reversed asymmetry or symmetry in the right-handed dyslexics, but in left-handed dyslexics normal asymmetry was not as prevalent.

One might hypothesize that left-handed dyslexics present abnormal patterns of asymmetry more often than right-handed dyslexics. Hynd and Semrud-Clikeman (1989) agree that dyslexic learners are not a homogeneous group, and that asymmetry may vary with handedness as well as with the severity and type of the problem. For example, Rosenthal (1982) used event-related potentials (ERPs) with dyslexics and found left hemispheric abnormality with language deficit subtypes and right hemispheric abnormality with visual-spatial deficit subtypes. Though CT studies discriminate the density of tissue, cellular irregularities need further examination.

Duffy, Denckla, Bartels, and Sandini (1980), using the brain electrical activity mapping (BEAM) technique, found differences in dyslexic subjects and normal subjects in every state dependent task, in the supplementary motor area, Broca's area, the left temporal region, and parietal and visual association areas. Between group differences in the dyslexics were found in the medial frontal lobe, a supplementary motor area, sometimes associated with speech deficits.

Using magnetic resonance imaging (MRI) Hynd et al. (1990) reported finding frontal regions of dyslexic subjects to be symmetrical. These authors suggested that normal growth patterns of development may be interrupted causing certain areas of the dyslexics' brains to be smaller than normal children's brains, or symmetrical in shape.

The argument could be made that dyslexics have difficulty with reading and that their EEG readings are indicating the lack of skills in processing the written language. If this were so, then the dyslexic's EEG readings should be similar to the younger normal reader. This is not the case, however. Dyslexics have been found to exhibit longer waveform and peak-to-peak latencies (Pirozzolo & Hansch, 1982). Also, regional cerebral blood flow (rCBF) (Hynd, Hynd, Sullivan, & Kingsbury, 1987) techniques showed bihemispheric activation when normal and dyslexic subjects engaged in reading narrative passages, but the dyslexics showed less activation in the right hemisphere or both hemispheres.

Behavioral Asymmetries: Visual Half Field and Dichotic Listening Evidence

Historically, learning disability has been attributed to neurological impairments (Geschwind & Behan, 1982; Orton, 1937), or more specifically, the lack of left language lateralization in the brain. Within this approach the visual right field advantage should be lacking and this has been indicated in some studies (Olson, 1973; Zurif & Carson, 1970), but other studies have shown that this is not the case (Bouma & Legein, 1977; Caplan & Kinsbourne, 1982; Marcel & Rajan, 1975; McKeever & Van Deventer, 1975).

Many explanations have been offered to confirm the studies. Satz, Rardin, and Ross (1971) theorized that the brain exhibits increases in lateralization with age, and that dyslexic readers do so at a slower rate. To demonstrate this effect of maturation these authors used dichotic listening with two different-aged groups of dyslexic boys. The groups of dyslexic boys were individually matched for age, sex, race, and intelligence level, with two normal-reader control groups. There was a significant right-ear advantage (REA) in all groups; however, left hemisphere lateralization for speech was pronounced. The REA was greater in the older normal group as compared to the older dyslexic group while no significant differences were found between the younger normal group and the younger dyslexic group. Satz, Orsini, Saslow, and Henry (1985) theorized skills that develop earlier (visual-motor and auditory-visual integration) would be delayed in older dyslexic children. Satz's model is founded on the ontogenetic development of lateralization of function.

Obrzut, Hynd, Obrzut, and Pirozzolo (1981) found dyslexic children better able to switch attention from one ear to the other in a study of 7- to 13-year-olds. This left-ear advantage (LEA) could mean that dyslexics lack efficient bilateral communication, which is the responsibility of the corpus callosum. Obrzut, Hynd, and Zellner (1983) supported this theory in the perceptual field of visual laterality, also.

When subtypes of LD are used to discriminate laterality, again, the answers are unclear (Dalby & Gibson, 1981; Obrzut, 1979). For example, Alyward (1984) used three subtypes of dyslexic children: dysphonetic, dyseidetic, and nonspecific. She found no laterality differences among the subtypes, but when the three subtypes were combined she found a REA in dichotic listening.

Perhaps the most work linking dichotic listening performance in populations with LD has been conducted by Obrzut and his associates (see Obrzut, 1991). Through systematic study with listening asymmetries, the relationship between cognitive deficits in children with LD and cerebral organization is becoming clearer. Based on a review of studies that have used the dichotic selective-attention paradigm, it can be inferred that children with LD, in comparison to age-matched, normal control children, are deficient in their ability to process auditory receptive language unilaterally in the left hemisphere. Clearly, the systematic control of subject and task parameters has allowed for more direct tests of specific learning disability models of abnormal lateralization. These particular studies have indicated it is likely that right hemisphere attentional activation interferes with left hemisphere verbal processing in children with LD. In addition, children with LD experience a greater imbalance in activation between hemispheres suggestive of an attentional-control dysfunction. Thus, hemispheric processes involved in selective-attention strategies as employed in the dichotic task may share common neuronal mechanisms with cognitive processes that are important for successful completion of academic tasks.

Contemporary Theories Associated with Learning Disorders

No work would be complete without some discussion of Geschwind's autoimmune theory of learning disorders as well as providing some mention of the relationship between reading disability and genetics.

Autoimmune Theory of Learning Disorders

Geschwind (1984) has stated that there is very strong evidence of a link between left-handedness and learning disorders, such as dyslexia. Gerschwind and colleagues also have found learning disorders to be linked as well to migraine and autoimmune diseases.

Autoimmunity occurs when the immune system begins attacking the body's own tissue, which is associated with childhood allergy problems and is the cause of such disorders as ulcerative colitis, atopic diseases such as asthma, myasthenia gravis, celiac disease, and inflammation of the thyroid and the colon (Geschwind, 1984; Geschwind & Behan, 1982; Geschwind & Galaburda, 1985; Marx, 1982). It is proposed that a common origin may account for the anomaly in the immune system as is already understood in the case of learning disorders. As impairment of the left hemisphere is noted in disturbance of language function and in a significant number of left-handers, so it is hypothesized that autoimmunity's roots may be traced to left hemisphere malformation (Geschwind & Behan, 1982; Marx, 1982).

Further, testosterone slows the growth of the convexity of the left hemisphere *in utero* (italics in original), accounting for a greater number of left-handers in males. When the testosterone effects are more marked, abnormalities in the formation of the left hemisphere will result. This would account for the greater frequency of learning disorders in males. During development, *in utero*, the immune system is also developing. Testosterone has suppressive effects on the thymus gland. The thymus gland is where the T-cell lymphocytes mature. One of the functions of these particular lymphocytes is the distinction of self from nonself, or foreign invading bodies, which may result in the maladaptive attack of the immune system on the body (Geschwind & Behan, 1982; Marx, 1982).

In two related studies by Geschwind and Behan (1982), they found the frequency of immune disease among left-handed subjects to be 2.7 times that in the control group of right-handers. The frequency of bowel and thyroid disorders was said to be notable. Also found was a significant number of left-handers reporting learning disorders. In the second study, conducted under stricter guidelines, a higher percent of severe migraine was found among the left-hand group. The possibility that stress, as a result of the learning disorder, is the cause of the immune disorders is difficult to accept, however, in view of the fact that increased frequency of immune disorder is found among relatives without learning disorders (Geschwind & Behan, 1982).

Reading Disability and Genetics

As reported by Decker and Bender (1988), Tarnopol and Tarnopol (1981) estimated the prevalence rates for reading disability in a survey of 26 countries to be from 1% in Japan and China to as much as 33% in Venezuela. The overall median was found to be 7%.

A number of common characteristics have been recognized among those with the disability, which have suggested a biological and possibly a genetic link: Critchley (1970) demonstrates a male-to-female ratio of three or four males to each affected female; Spreen (1982) points out that reading and spelling deficits persist well into adulthood despite remedial methods; Decker and Vandenberg (1985) report greater risk for the disorder among monozygotic twins as compared with dizygotics; and Finucci (1978) has verified the presence of nonrandom familial aggregations of reading problems within certain families.

The evidence seems to point to the conclusion that "reading disability appears to be a heterogenous language disorder with multiple subtypes, some of which may have a genetic etiology and some of which do not" (Decker & Bender, 1988, p. 198). Some support of this statement is provided by Smith, Kimberling, Pennington, and Lubs (1983) in research on specific reading disability, who report on the identification of an inherited form through "linkage analysis."

Smith et al. (1983) stated that if a trait, such as reading disability, can be demonstrated to be linked to a known genetic marker locus, then it is assumed that a major gene for that trait is located on the same chromosome as the marker. Smith et al. (1983) proposed to look for this marker among selected families identified to have positive generational histories of reading disability, in an "autosomal dominant fashion" (p. 1346).

Each family member was administered various standardized achievement tests to ensure that the disability was confined to reading and spelling. The tests used were the Gray Oral Reading Test, the spelling subtest of the Wide Range Achievement Tests (WRAT), and the Peabody Individual Achievement Tests (PIAT). Subsequent chromosomal analyses were performed and the linkage analysis revealed a connection between specific reading disability and chromosome 15. Obviously there is a need to confirm these findings through validation studies before a linkage is considered proven. This is reasonable considering the fact other specific disorders, such as cleft lip and palate, are more easily defined and diagnosed than reading disorder and have been found to have various causes. It is likely the identification of a specific gene as cause for specific reading disability may not be found. Thus, evidence of a specific gene located on chromosome 15 speculated to be related to reading disorder by Smith et al. (1983) is considered tentative. If confirmed, however, it will likely be found to account for a minute sample of subjects with reading disability (Decker & Bender, 1988).

There are many diverse explanations and theories to explain learning disorders (i.e., dyslexia), as presented in this chapter. At the present, although there is little agreement over diagnostic definitions, methods and measurements of research, and experimental designs (Obrzut, 1989), a neuropsychological and neurobiological approach to this cognitive disability is needed to fully understand its nature and etiology.

The Promise of the Future

Several predictions regarding the course human neuropsychology will take in the 1990's are offered. More sophistication is expected not only of the neuroimaging techniques, but also of neuropsychological assessment in general. Specifically, Rourke (1991) suggests that theory-driven techniques such as Q-type factor analysis, confirmatory factor analysis, and structural equations modeling can be expected to generate new models of conditions such as learning disabilities. Of great importance is the longitudinal study: How does the condition develop, how can its course be altered, and who really is at risk? In addition, as the close of the century approaches, it would not be surprising to see the focus turn from neurological-behavioral relationships to neurochemical-behavioral relationships.

A major problem needing to be beset is an understanding of how the normal brain develops. Though much has been learned from the study of brain-damaged adults, the models enjoy only modest success when applied to children (Rourke, 1991). Whereas, research has traditionally focused upon exclusive parameters of development (i.e., language), the advantage of an interactive approach is to provide focus on everything from genetics to environment as determiners of function.

Neuropsychological theory, when viewed with all its respective ramifications, offers an important avenue for understanding the brain-behavior interface. Through continued study, subtleties of broad disorders such as "learning disability" can be harnessed and better defined, specific interventions can be more appropriately targeted, and procedures providing accurate identification of individuals at risk can be developed.

References

Aylward, E.H. (1984). Lateral asymmetry in subgroups of dyslexic children. *Brain and Language*, *22*, 221–231.

Bakker, D.J. (1979). Hemispheric differences and reading strategies: Two dyslexias? *Bulletin of the Orton Society*, *29*, 84–100.

Bigler, E.D. (1989). Radiologic techniques in neuropsychological assessment. In C.R. Reynolds & E. Fletcher-Janzen (Eds.), *Handbook of clinical child neuropsychology* (pp. 247–264). New York: Plenum Press.

Bouma, H. & Legein, C.P. (1977). Foveal and parafoveal recognition of letters by dyslexics and average readers. *Neuropsychologia*, *15*, 69–80.

Caplan, B. & Kinsbourne, M. (1982). Cognitive style and dichotic asymmetries of disabled readers. *Cortex*, *18*, 353–366.

Critchley, M. (1970). *The dyslexic child*. Springfield, IL: Charles C. Thomas.

Dalby, J.T. & Gibson, D. (1981). Functional cerebral lateralization in subtypes of disabled readers. *Brain and Language*, *14*, 34–48.

Decker, S. & Bender, B. (1988). Converging evidence for multiple genetic forms of reading disability. *Brain and Language*, *33*, 197–215.

Decker, S.N. & Vandenberg, S.G. (1985). Colorado twin study of reading disability. In D. Gray & J. Kavanaugh (Eds.), *Biobehavioral measures of dyslexia* (pp. 123–135). Baltimore: York Press.

Denckla, M.B. LeMay, M., & Chapman, C.A. (1985). Few CT scan abnormalities found even in neurologically impaired learning disabled children. ·*Annals of Dyslexia*, *18*, 132–135.

Drake, W.E. (1968). Clinical and pathological findings in a child with developmental learning disability. *Journal of Learning Disabilities*, *1*, 486–502.

Duane, D.D. (1991). Biological foundations of learning disabilities. In J.E. Obrzut & G.W. Hynd (Eds.), *Neuropsychological foundations of learning disabilities: A handbook of issues, methods, and practice* (pp. 7–27). San Diego: Academic Press.

Duffy, F.H., Denckla, M.B., Bartels, P.H., & Sandini, G. (1980). Regional differences in brain and electrical activity by topographic mapping. *Annals of Neurology*, *7*, 412–420.

Falzi, G., Perrone, P., & Vignolo, L.A. (1982). Right-left asymmetry in anterior speech region. *Archives of Neurology*, *39*, 239–240.

Finucci, J.M. (1978). Genetic considerations in dyslexia. In H.R. Myklebust (Ed.), *Progress in learning disabilities* (pp. 41–63). New York: Grune & Stratton.

Galaburda, A.M. (1983). Developmental dyslexia: Current anatomical research. *Annals of Dyslexia, 33*, 41–53.

Galaburda, A.M. (1986, November). *Human studies on the anatomy of dyslexia.* Paper presented at the annual conference of the Orton Dyslexia Society, Philadelphia.

Galaburda, A.M. & Kemper, T.L. (1979). Cytoarchitectonic abnormalities in developmental dyslexia: A case study. *Annals of Neurology, 6*, 94–100.

Galaburda, A.M., Sherman, G.F., Rosen, G.D., Aboitiz, F., & Geschwind, N. (1985). Developmental dyslexia: Four consecutive patients with cortical anomalies. *Annals of Neurology, 18*, 222–233.

Geschwind, N. (1984). Cerebral dominance in biological perspective. *Neuropsychologia, 22*(6), 675–683.

Geschwind, N. & Behan, P. (1982). Left-handedness: Association with immune disease, migraine, and developmental learning disorder. *Proceedings of the National Academy of Science, 79*, 5097–5100.

Geschwind, N. & Galaburda, A. (1985). Cerebral lateralization. *Archives of Neurology, 42*, 428–459.

Geschwind, N. & Levitsky, W. (1968). Human brain: Left-right asymmetries in temporal speech region. *Science, 161*, 186–187.

Goldberg, E. & Costa, L. (1981). Hemisphere differences in the acquisition and use of descriptive systems. *Brain and Language, 14*, 144–173.

Haslam, R.H.A., Dalby, J.T., Johns, R.D., & Rademaker, A.W. (1981). Cerebral asymmetry in developmental dyslexia. *Archives of Neurology, 38*, 679–682.

Hellige, J.B. (1983). *Cerebral hemisphere asymmetry, method, theory, and application.* New York: Praeger.

Hier, D.B., LeMay, J., Rosenberger, P.B., & Perlo, V.P. (1978). Developmental dyslexia: Evidence for a subgroup with a reversal of cerebral asymmetry. *Archives for Neurology, 35*, 90–93.

Hynd, G.W. & Cohen, M. (1983). *Dyslexia: Neuropsychological theory, research, and clinical differentiation.* New York: Grune & Stratton.

Hynd, G.W. & Hynd, C. (1984). Dyslexia: Neuroanatomical/neurolinguistic perspectives. *Reading Research Quarterly, 19*(4), 482–498.

Hynd, G.W., Hynd, C.R., Sullivan, H.G., & Kingsbury, T.B. (1987). Regional cerebral blood flow (rCBF) in developmental dyslexia: Activation during reading in a surface and deep dyslexic. *Journal of Learning Disabilities, 20*(5), 294–300.

Hynd, G.W. & Semrud-Clikeman, M. (1989). Dyslexia and brain morphology. *Psychological Bulletin, 106*, 447–482.

Hynd, G.W., Semrud-Clikeman, M., Lorys, A., Novey, E.S., & Eliopulos, D. (1990). Brain morphology in developmental dyslexia and attention deficit disorder/hyperactivity. *Archives of Neurology, 47*, 919–926.

Kertesz, A., Lesk, D., & McCabe, P. (1977). Isotope location of infarcts in aphasia. *Archives of Neurology, 34*, 590–601.

Kimura, D. (1967). Functional asymmetry of the brain in dichotic listening. *Cortex, 3*, 163–178.

Kinsbourne, M. (1974). Mechanisms of hemispheric interaction in man. In M. Kinsbourne & W.L. Smith (Eds.), *Hemispheric disconnection and cerebral function.* Springfield, IL: Charles C. Thomas.

Krashen, S. (1973). Lateralization, language, learning, and the critical period: Some new evidence. *Language and Learning, 23*, 63–74.

Lenneberg, E.H. (1967). *Biological foundations of language*. New York: Wiley.

Marcel, T. & Rajan, P. (1975). Lateral specialization for recognition of words and faces in good and poor readers. *Neuropsychologia, 13*, 489–497.

Marx, J. (1982). Autoimmunity in left-handers. *Science, 217*(9), 141–144.

McKeever, W.F. & Van Deventer, A.D. (1975). Dyslexic adolescents: Evidence of impaired visual and auditory language processing associated with normal lateralization and visual responsivity. *Cortex, 11*, 361–378.

Morrison, S.R. & Siegel, L.S. (1991). Learning disabilities: A critical review of definitional and assessment issues. In J.E. Obrzut & G.W. Hynd (Eds.), *Neuropsychological foundations of learning disabilities: A handbook of issues, methods, and practice* (pp. 79–97). San Diego: Academic Press.

Obrzut, J.E. (1979). Dichotic listening and bisensory memory skills in qualitatively diverse dyslexic readers. *Journal of Learning Disabilities, 12*, 304–314.

Obrzut, J.E. (1989). Dyslexia and neurodevelopmental pathology: Is the neuro-diagnostic technology ahead of the psychoeducational technology? *Journal of Learning Disabilities, 22*, 317–318.

Obrzut, J.E. (1991). Hemispheric activation and arousal asymmetry in learning disabled children. In J.E. Obrzut & G.W. Hynd (Eds.), *Neuropsychological foundations of learning disabilities: A handbook of issues, methods, and practice* (pp. 179–198). San Diego: Academic Press.

Obrzut, J.E. & Hynd, G.W. (Eds.). (1991). *Neuropsychological foundations of learning disabilities: A handbook of issues, methods, and practice*. San Diego: Academic Press.

Obrzut, J.E., Hynd, G.W., Obrzut, A., & Pirozzolo, F.J. (1981). Effect of directed attention on cerebral asymmetries in normal and learning-disabled children: Evidence from visual half-field asymmetries. *Developmental Psychology, 17*, 118–125.

Obrzut, J.E., Hynd, G.W., & Zellner, R.D. (1983). Attentional deficit in learning-disabled children: Evidence from visual half-field asymmetries. *Brain and Cognition, 2*, 89–101.

Olson, M.E. (1973). Laterality differences in tachistoscopic word recognition in normal and delayed readers in elementary school. *Neuropsychologia, 11*, 343–350.

Orton, S.T. (1925). Word-blindness in school children. *Archives of Neurology and Psychiatry, 14*, 581–615.

Orton, S.T. (1937). *Reading, writing, and speech problems in children*. London: Chapman and Hall.

Parkins, R.A., Roberts, R.J., Reinarz, S.J., & Varney, N.R. (1987). *CT asymmetries in adult developmental dyslexics*. Paper presented at the annual meeting of the International Neuropsychological Society, Washington, DC.

Pirozzolo, F.J. & Hansch, E.C. (1982). The neurobiology of developmental reading disorders In R.N. Malatesha & P.G. Aaron (Eds.), *Neuropsychological and neurolinguistic aspects of reading disorders* (pp. 224–256). New York: Academic Press.

Plante, E. (1991). MRI findings in the parents and siblings of specifically language-impaired boys. *Brain and Language, 41*, 67–80.

Plante, E., Swisher, L., Vance, R., & Rapcsak, S. (1991). MRI findings in boys with specific language impairment. *Brain and Language, 41*, 52–66.

Rosenthal, J.H. (1982). EEG-event related potentials in dyslexia and its subtypes. In D.A.B. Lindenberg, M.F. Collen, & E.E. Van Brunt (Eds.), *AMIA Congress*, 82. New York: Masson.

Rourke, B.P. (1991). Human neuropsychology in the 1990s. *Archives of Clinical Neuropsychology*, *6*, 1–14.

Satz, P. (1991). The Dejerine hypothesis: Implications for an etiological reformulation of developmental dyslexia. In J.E. Obrzut & G.W. Hynd (Eds.), *Neuropsychological foundations of learning disabilities: A handbook of issues, methods, and practice* (pp. 99–112). San Diego: Academic Press.

Satz, P., Orsini, D.L., Saslow, E., & Henry, R. (1985). The pathological left-handedness syndrome. *Brain and Cognition*, *4*, 27–46.

Satz, P., Rardin, D., & Ross, J. (1971). An evaluation of a theory of specific developmental dyslexia. *Child Development*, *42*, 2009–2021.

Smith, S.D., Kimberling, W.J., Pennington, B.F., & Lubs, H.A. (1983). Specific reading disability: Identification of an inherited form through linkage analyses. *Science*, *219*, 1345–1347.

Spreen, O. (1982). Adult outcome of reading disorders. In R.N. Maletsha & P.G. Aaron (Eds.), *Reading disorders: Varieties and treatments* (pp. 473–492). New York: Academic Press.

Spreen, O., Tupper, D., Risser, A., Tuokko, H., & Edgell, D. (1984). *Human developmental neuropsychology*. New York: Oxford University Press.

Tarnopol, L. & Tarnopol, M. (1981). *Comparative reading and learning difficulties*. Lexington, MA: Lexington Books.

Wada, J.A., Clarke, R., & Hamm, A. (1975). Cerebral hemispheric asymmetry in humans: Coretical speech zones in 100 adult and 100 infant brains. *Archives of Neurology*, *32*, 239–246.

Witelson, S.F. & Pallie, W. (1973). Left hemisphere specialization for language in the newborn. *Brain*, *96*, 641–646.

Zaidel, E. (1986). Callosal dynamics and right hemisphere language. In F. Lepore, M. Ptito, & H.H. Jasper (Eds.), *Two hemispheres-one brain: Functions of the corpus callosum*. Neurology and Neurobiology (Vol. 17). New York: Alan R. Liss.

Zurif, E.B. & Carson, G. (1970). Dyslexia in relation to cerebral dominance and temporal analysis. *Neuropsychologia*, *8*, 351–361.

3
Models and Theories:
Their Influence on Research in
Learning Disabilities

KENNETH A. KAVALE AND STEVEN R. FORNESS

The field of learning disabilities (LD) seems to be marked by a constant state of crisis characterized by disagreement, confusion, and ambiguity. This turmoil, however, has not abated the growth of LD research (Summers, 1986). Yet, research findings have not successfully resolved long-standing disputes. It would seem that an expanding data base would permit greater problem resolution but instead it only seems to aggravate the situation. A number of problems in the research process appear to contribute to the lack of resolution and the purpose of this chapter is to explore these problems.

Paradigm Wars in Learning Disabilities

Setting aside the research process for a moment, it seems that the LD field has recently been engaged in its own "paradigm wars." Gage (1989) discussed paradigm wars related to research on teaching and demonstrated how criticisms leveled by antinaturalists, interpretivists, and critical theorists resulted in the demise of objective and quantitative research in teaching. Gage (1989) then discussed possible resolutions for the paradigmatic conflicts that affect rapprochement among paradigms and that take seriously the moral obligations of educational research.

Heshusius (1982, 1989) criticized the Newtonian mechanistic paradigm predominate in special education and called for its replacement by a holistic paradigm. Similarly, Iano (1986) called for the replacement of the "natural science–technical model" with a human science model. Rosenberg and Jackson (1988) discussed a number of "world views" and demonstrated how they influence research activities. Similarly, Warner and Bull (1986) discussed the necessity of grounding LD in systems of educational thought. They advocated a cognitive-field approach because of its non-reductionist nature. Poplin (1988) has advocated strongly for the elimination of the reductionist foundation of the LD field and the many fallacies it has produced. These papers initiated sometimes heated discussion (e.g., Forness & Kavale, 1987; Kimball & Heron, 1988; Licht & Torgesen, 1989; Ullman & Rosenberg, 1986).

It is not clear, however, whether discussions about paradigms have had significant impact on the LD field. It would seem that regardless of the passion these discussions generate, the LD field finds comfort in the status quo. This observation in no way minimizes the importance of theoretical discussion. In fact, we have argued that theoretical development is of paramount importance if the LD field is to ever resolve its most fundamental concerns (Forness & Kavale, 1987; Kavale, 1987). Another point of view holds that theory is relatively unimportant for an applied field such as LD. Because of its limited value, theory becomes secondary to research and the LD field should emphasize research.

Research Wars in Learning Disabilities

While theoretical development may be shunted to the sidelines in favor of research, the nature of that research has also been the subject of debate. For example, the issue of basic versus applied research has been discussed (see Wong in the *Journal of Learning Disabilities*, 1988). In the lead paper, Swanson (1988) argued for basic research that can contribute to metatheoretical development. Responses were about equally divided between those supporting Swanson's position (e.g., Kavale, 1988) and those in disagreement (Carnine & Woodward, 1988). The disagreement centered around the role of applied research. For enhanced instruction and learning, applied research, because it takes place in context, is viewed as the best model. Such debate is not unique to LD but rather reflects a basic tension in behavioral science between understanding and helping.

The nature of research is also seen in debate about the role of quantitative and qualitative research. Stainback and Stainback (1984) discussed limitations of quantitative research methodology and called for the use of qualitative methodology to broaden the perspective of research in special education. Simpson and Eaves (1985) suggested that a shift towards more qualitative research is fraught with danger and that the real need is not more quantitative or qualitative research but rather better research.

The Interface of Paradigm and Research Wars

The discussion of paradigms and research methodology are not mutually exclusive. In fact, one's position in the paradigm wars has a direct bearing on one's perspective about the research wars. For example, those supporting a holistic paradigm (e.g., Poplin, 1988) also support qualitative methodology (e.g., Poplin, 1987). Qualitative methods are assumed to provide an insider's perspective, a dynamic reality, a discovery orientation, subjective data, naturalistic conditions, and valid results (Stainback & Stainback, 1984). Simpson and Eaves (1985) questioned qualitative methodology on the grounds of not being as well defined, not as well systematized, and not as open to independent verification as quantitative methods.

Resolution of such issues is difficult because debate is waged on an emotional rather than scholarly level. This is primarily because such debate is cast in terms of basic philosophical notions (Smith & Heshusius, 1986). Howe (1985) suggested that discussion about the relative merits of quantitative and qualitative research is difficult to resolve because the issues are discussed (sometimes unwittingly) within a positivistic epistemological framework. In a later paper, Howe (1988) discussed qualitative and quantitative differences in terms of three levels of research practice: data, design and analyses, and interpretation. Pragmatically, it was then argued that no incompatibility exists between methodologies and debate typically ignores the underlying positivistic and interpretivistic paradigms undergirding quantitative and qualitative methods, respectively.

What do these paradigm and research wars say about the research process in LD? They should say much but, in actuality, they say little because of the way the research process has come to be viewed. The different models describing paradigms and methodologies are important, but research activity in LD has taken on a quite independent existence. Research in LD shares many commonalities that are assumed required if it is to be deemed "good" research. For educational research in general, there is considerable attention directed at journal quality (e.g., Luce & Johnson, 1978) and LD is no exception (Swanson & Alford, 1987). Although the quality issue for journals is complex, at a fundamental level it is related to the quality of the research articles received (Yoels, 1974), and in this regard there appears to be only one model that is consistently viewed as the standard. This model is termed the *scientific method* and the typical form is outlined in Table 3.1.

TABLE 3.1. The scientific method (hypothetico-deductive paradigm).

Step 1: A *theory* about the phenomenon exists.

Step 2: The research detects a *research problem* within the theory and selects from it a research question to investigate.

Step 3: A *research hypothesis* is deduced from the propositions in the theory. The research hypothesis is a statement about the relationship between constructs.

Step 4: The researcher determines the *operations* (specific procedures or methods) by which the constructs will be defined and states a hypothesis that can be tested statistically. This hypothesis is called a *null hypothesis*. A *research design* is developed as a plan for implementing the operations and testing the null hypothesis. These operations, the null hypothesis, and the design make up the guidelines for the study.

Step 5: The researcher conducts the study according to the guidelines.

Step 6: The null hypothesis is tested based on the data from the study.

Step 7: The original theory is revised or supported based on the results of the hypothesis testing.

The scientific method is thus an empirical and experimental system that attempts to place data in a logico-mathematical system. It is a deductive system that attempts to specify cause and effect within a theoretical structure.

The Scientific Method

Even a cursory review of LD journals would show that most LD research approximates the scientific method. Although all facets of the scientific method are not explicitly stipulated, there is, at least, an implicit recognition that the scientific method has provided the structure for the research process and the dissemination of findings. Although the LD field produces much research (Summers, 1986), the quantity of research has little bearing on the resolution of basic problems (Forness & Kavale, in press; Kavale, 1987). The reason is found in the roots of the scientific method, which can be traced to the rise of logical positivism or logical empiricism developed during the 1920s by members of the Vienna Circle (Hanfling, 1981). The guiding theme was the idea that all knowledge could be accounted for from a perspective emphasizing empirical and logical components without resort to metaphysics (Achinstein & Barker, 1969). In line with this hostility towards metaphysics was the adoption of the verifiability principle which stated that something was meaningful if and only if it was validated empirically (i.e., directly) or is a tautology of mathematics or logic. What counts as evidence is usually deemed "rock-bottom" sense experience (i.e., positive knowledge). Theories, in the logical positivist context, because of difficulties in verification were neither true or false but rather served as conceptual tools for predicting and arranging facts.

The philosophy of logical positivism maintained that all the behavioral sciences needed to be like the natural sciences was simply to emulate the natural sciences—especially through the use of its empirical methodologies, the scientific method (Ayer, 1959). This was the early promise, but there has been relatively little progress in uncovering laws of human behavior as contrasted with the rapid and major advances in the natural sciences (Koch, 1981).

Yet, the hypothetico-deductive model of logical positivism carries the weight of authority. It is assumed that those who follow the prescribed sequence will produce credible findings. It is important to note that the sequence outlined in Table 1 represents *the* scientific method and any deviation is viewed as weakening the outcomes. The credibility of LD research is thus judged by the strength of its adherence to the scientific method. Especially for a field viewed as "soft," strict adherence to the scientific method is viewed as absolutely necessary if any useful knowledge is to be attained.

Critique of the Scientific Method

In the positivist sense, LD research must be empirical, objective, and value-free if it is to be useful. The scientific method is the avenue to that useful research. The positivist tradition, however, has come under close scrutiny and the "received view" of logical positivism is that it is no longer a predominant view (see Eisner, 1983; Phillips, 1983). In its place is a call for more open-mindedness about research traditions (Soltis, 1984), enhanced understanding about philosophical positions and empirical research (Macmillan & Garrison, 1984), and the development of principles to guide postpositivistic educational research (Garrison, 1986).

Although logical positivism as a philosophy might be considered dead, its influence remains and is seen most clearly in the research process. The scientific method promulgated by logical positivism is viewed as *the* research model for LD. Such "disciplined inquiry" (Cronbach & Suppes, 1969) is distinguished from other types of opinion and belief. Although disciplined inquiry does not imply a sterile, ritualized, and narrowly conceived form of investigation, it appears that LD research requires strict adherence to the scientific method to be viewed as disciplined inquiry (Swanson & Alford, 1987). In fact, research takes on a numbing sameness and scientific contributions are viewed, not by their content, but rather by the extent to which they parallel the scientific method (Smart & Elton, 1981).

At first glance, the scientific method appears sound and seems to possess a rigor that will insure successful research efforts. Barber (1976), however, discussed 10 pitfalls in human research that undermine objectivity and suggest that the scientific method is not as rigorous as it might appear. In fact, McGrath, Martin, and Kulka (1982) discussed the "judgment calls" necessary in research. The analogy is to baseball where, during a game, many decisions need to be made without the benefit of a fixed and objective rule that can be applied. These judgment calls are important because in baseball, such judgment calls accumulate in their effects; and indeed, they quite literally determine the outcome of most games. Similarly, in research, there are many crucial decisions that must be made without benefit of a hard and fast, "objective" rule, or even a good algorithm or general rule of thumb. And, as in baseball, the cumulative results of such judgment calls often determine the outcome of research (McGrath et al., 1982, p. 13).

The reasons for the lack of rigor and the necessity for making judgment calls are found in what Kaplan (1964) termed "logic-in-use" versus "reconstructed logic." A logic-in-use refers to the reasonable ways the research process proceeds and success of such inquiry is proof of its desirability. A reconstructed logic is the explicit formulation of a logic-in-use and may take many forms. For LD, the primary reconstructed logic is found in the "hypothetico-deductive paradigm" (i.e., the scientific method). Any reconstructed logic, however, is merely a hypothesis and, over time, it may become more awkward to "fit" the hypothesis to the facts (i.e., the research process). A reconstructed logic is an idealized view of scientific practice and LD should not slavishly initiate a particular reconstruction that claims to be science (especially physics). But, as Kaplan (1964) suggested, "where the reconstruction is mathematically elegant, precise, and powerful—as is true of the 'hypothetico-deductive' logic—its attractions are nearly irresistible" (p. 11). The primary question is not the value of the reconstructed logic itself but rather its usefulness in illuminating the logics-in-use. To illustrate, Kaplan (1964) relates the story of the drunkard's search. There is a story of a drunkard searching under a street lamp for his house key, which he had dropped some distance away. Asked why he didn't look where he had dropped it, he replied, "It's lighter here!" Much efforts, not only in the logic of behavioral science, but also in behavioral science itself, is initiated, in my opinion, by the principle of the drunkard's search (p. 11).

The consequences of a single reconstructed logic for LD research is a rigid and narrow system. Most influenced by logical positivism was research in educational psychology and, for some time, any educational research was defined as good or poor based on its proximity to educational psychology. In effect, research practice is focused on a single, sacrosanct, officially approved set of methods. The single, legitimate form of research is found in, for example, Campbell and Stanley (1967), which describes *the* way to do LD research. But, where research is defined in only one way and competence defined in terms of that research, competent research is the only type that will find its way to the journal page. However, such research has a too-predictable form as suggested by Eisner (1983): Consider our proclivity to write research reports in the third person; one does not use "I" in educational research articles. Because we seek objectivity, we camouflage our subjectivity with phrases such as "the researcher" or "we." We mask our voice. We do not refer to children as children, we refer to them as "subjects" or "Ss." The less human the better. We try to approximate the conditions of a laboratory by imitating the fields of chemistry and physics where laboratory conditions are possible and by conducting experiments in which the control of confounding variables is thought to be possible. The result is experimental treatments that are so brief that the achievement of educationally significant results is highly unlikely (p. 14).

Elements of the Scientific Method

Theory

The elements of the scientific method (see Table 1), on the surface, appear unobjectionable but each presents certain complexities that are not easily unraveled. For example, the foundation of the scientific method is theory. But the LD field does not possess a well-grounded theoretical base, suggesting that theory per se is not often tested (Kavale, 1987). Most often LD research tests hypotheses (from the Greek hypo—weak and thesis—something put forth), which are not as fully developed as theories. Hypotheses testing involves subjecting hypotheses to a number of comparisons against empirical evidence (Cook & Campbell, 1979). Theories differ from hypotheses in a scientific sense because they have survived a greater number and variety of attempts to disconfirm them. The theory referred to in the scientific method is thus far more circumscribed. For a field such as LD, "theories" tend to be more unparsimonious and noncumulative, suggesting that research investigates, at best, hypotheses that make for a more limited scope.

Research Questions

The limited theoretical development in LD also imparts limitations in the research questions asked. The scientific method stresses testing hypotheses over generating hypotheses (McGuire, 1973). Research activity should have the goal of investigating significant problems and findings should answer questions worth asking but this is too often not the case (Gergen, 1978). For the LD field, the lack of attention to hypotheses generation suggests that its research has done no more than to evaluate questions developed elsewhere. Design elegance is not a substitute for developing sound ideas and it would behoove the LD field to pay more attention to the "conceptual" level of inquiry by asking "good" questions (Brinberg & McGrath, 1985). Mitroff and Kilman (1978) showed that among scientists there are "experimenters" and "conceptualizers," who have different characteristics. Expecting LD researchers to fulfill both roles may inhibit progress in the field since the differentiated talents of members of our discipline are not exploited.

Campbell, Daft, and Hulin (1982) demonstrated that theory most often does not guide the generation of research questions and found only a limited number of questions that were stimulated by others' research or by previously asked questions. Too often, it was the case that questions were generated *after* the choice of method, which attempted to capture particular publication policies, and the questions either could not be answered or the answer was already known, or were faddish (i.e., "current"). Without an anchor in theory or even previous research, any and all questions may be deemed appropriate. The process of knowledge accumulation under these circumstances was considered akin to a large number of researchers throwing mud at a wall. Campbell et al. (1982) then suggested that the mud that sticks to the wall is knowledge and should be retained. That which falls off is indeed mud and should be discarded. This theory of knowledge accumulation suggests that the more individuals there are throwing different kinds of mud, the more likely it is that some of them will throw something that sticks (p. 19).

Research questions also need to be interesting. Davis (1971) argued that if research is to have significant impact it must be "interesting." Truth or empirical proof have little to do with impact or significance; rather, the critical variable is interest. If research findings deny certain widely held assumptions, then it qualifies as interesting. The findings must plow a middle ground because if all assumptions are denied then the research is not believable while, on the other hand, if no assumptions are denied, then the research is viewed as obvious. Therefore, research findings must differ moderately from expectations because then they will surprise and intrigue as in, for example, research where an assumed independent variable on a causal relationship is shown to be a dependent variable, or where assumed covariation on a positive direction between variables is shown to be in a negative direction. The emphasis here is not in "newness" but rather on being perceived as interesting in the sense developed.

Research versus Null Hypotheses

A research question does not, however, translate automatically into a research hypothesis. Instead, a null hypothesis is most often tested and it is not equivalent to a research hypothesis. A null hypothesis does not test a substantive question but rather represents a calculated description of uncertainty based on what has been observed (Grant, 1962). The problem lies in the fact that the null hypothesis, taken literally, is almost always false (see Morrison & Henkel, 1970). This state of affairs comes about because any dependent variable in LD will always be a function of a number of contributing influences. But, in any comparison (e.g., LD vs. non-LD), for two groups to be equal of a dependent variable, it must be the case that they are exactly equal or precisely counterbalanced on all contributing influences. Because the null hypothesis is almost always false in a field such as LD, the probability of refuting it is almost exclusively a function of sample size.

Fisher (1967) developed procedures for statistical significance testing in agronomy that is radically different from LD. In agronomy, there exists a much closer association between research and statistical (i.e., null) hypotheses. For example, if research is directed at knowing whether using fertilizer will increase soybean yields, then, because soybeans receive their nutrients from the soil, refutation of the null hypothesis means that the alternative (i.e., research) hypothesis is proved. Because the alternative hypothesis is an almost perfect approximation of the research hypotheses, direct interpretation is appropriate and it is possible to conclude, for example, that fertilizer has a positive effect on soybean yield.

The situation in LD is not at all equivalent and a variety of competing explanations are possible to explain non-null statistical differences (Bolles, 1962). The alternative hypothesis, in this case, is simply the obverse of the null hypothesis and, consequently, indicates little about the validity of the research hypothesis.

Research Methodology

The actual research methodology used in the scientific method presents many difficulties. Methodology refers to the study of methods, and not the methods themselves. The aim of methodology is to describe and to analyze particular techniques with the goal being to elucidate their assets and liabilities as well as their potential for contributing to knowledge (Kaplan, 1964). Thus, a field such as LD has developed its own methodology and this methodology takes on a normative character for the field. The methodological preferences are usually stipulated through, for example, journal editorial policies. Thus, adherence to "the methodology" is a necessary requirement to ensure that a researcher's findings are disseminated.

The LD field focuses much of its research efforts on comparative studies that examine LD performance in relation to the performance of an average (i.e., non-LD) performing group. The emphasis is on cataloging differences, but the problem of heterogeneity tends to obscure group comparisons (LD vs. non-LD) because of the possibility for sizable group overlap even when differences are found statistically significant (Weener, 1981). The scientific method attempts to overcome the overlap problem by comparing extreme groups (e.g., the 10% of the populations with the highest and lowest scores on the variable of interest). This procedure is presumed to increase power by attenuating heterogeneity based on the assumption that the 10% of LD students with the lowest scores are more similar to each other.

Besides sampling procedures, the scientific method also attempts to increase power by controlling confounding variables. For example, intelligence (IQ) is an influence on a number of variables and may be the source of variation on performance measures. Group differences may therefore reflect intellectual differences rather than performance differences. Besides IQ, in a similar fashion, socioeconomic status, family factors, school environment, and instruction, for example, may also influence performance and makes it difficult to determine the source of variation. The usual tactic is to control these factors through either design procedures (e.g., matching) or statistical procedures (e.g., ANCOVA). Although the effects of these variables are held constant and the variable of interest isolated, the price paid is a study that can explain only a very small proportion of the variation in LD performance. This situation is illustrated in Figure 3.1. Even if the group differences are significant, the

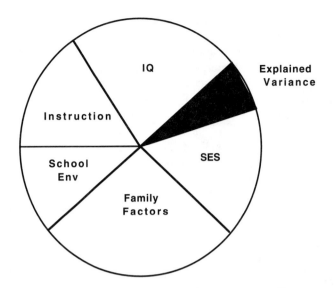

FIGURE 3.1. Proportion of explained variance in the typical study of learning disabilities investigating specific variables.

differences can explain only the variation not explained by the other contributing influences to the total variance. By focusing on specific variables, it is therefore difficult to determine their relative importance and makes for findings with limited application.

The LD research literature is replete with an extensive catalog of differences between LD and non-LD groups. But because of their narrow scope, not much should be invested in such studies, otherwise interpretation would become much like the story of the blind men who stumble upon different parts of an elephant and then describe the nature of the elephant. For example, research has demonstrated that some LD groups differ on perceptual discrimination tasks while other LD groups differ on verbal mediation tasks but not vice versa. This occurs because the scientific method permits different studies to glimpse only that aspect of LD that lies within its focus. But, as the focus of research narrows, it is probably the case that the number of "significant differences" between LD and non-LD groups will increase. Under these circumstances, it is also likely that the number of blind men touching different parts of an elephant will also increase significantly and, consequently, so too will the number of descriptions of LD.

Reductionism

The narrow focus of many LD research studies is necessary because of the logico-mathematical reductionism associated with the scientific method. Empirical analyses is contingent upon variables that can be made numerical and typically narrows the range of variables that can be studied because of difficulties in quantifying many contextual variables. Koch (1981) criticized this "single-principle imperialism" and described the pathology of knowledge produced when problems are reduced to a level of mathematical interpretation. The most usual mathematical interpretation of LD variables is found in tests where scores for LD and non-LD groups are compared. Tests, however, in and of themselves, are not mathematical interpretations. Tests need to be based on sound measurement, defined as the linking of empirical indicators with abstract concepts (see Blalock, 1982). Inherent in this definition is the theoretical function of linking concepts, not solely empirically, but also rationally and logically. Kavale and Mundschenk (1990) suggested that the LD field has not paid sufficient attention to the theoretical foundation of measurement. This means that LD concepts and indicators are connected only empirically making for a less than perfect isomorphism in the sense of a structural similarity between theoretical and observational levels. Thus, LD concepts remain essentially independent and are not meshed into a larger conceptual whole (Hempel, 1952).

Without a well-developed theoretical foundation, it is difficult for a test to be an appropriate and legitimate proxy for a trait (Messick, 1981). This is related to the notion of construct validity (Cronbach & Meehl, 1955) and a majority of tests in LD have been shown to lack adequate construct validity (e.g., Bennett, 1983; Berk, 1984) The generally poor construct validity for LD tests confounds the meaning of group differences because no inferences about ability based on observed performance are possible. Tryon (1979, p. 402) termed this the "test-trait fallacy" and said it begins with the assumption that test scores are trait measures. The second assumption is that trait measures are basic properties of the person. It easily follows that test scores reflect basic properties of the person. This sequence essentially converts a dependent variable into an independent variable; hence a measurement is reified into a causal force.

Operationism

The scientific method attempts to bypass the theoretical component of measurement through the use of an operational approach. Bridgman (1927) was among the first to declare that a theoretical concept is meaningful only if there is a repeatable operation through which it can be established. For any concept, there is a set of operations that defines its scientific status and to know these operations is to understand the concept fully. Besides providing meaning, operational approaches also indicate what meaning a particular concept possesses: One need only specify the operations that determine its application.

A primary difficulty with operational approaches is the creation of tautologies. The question, "How do we know that our attention measures, in fact, measure attention?" is without substance since one operational approach claims that attention is no more than its operations. Consequently, the test measures attention because "attention is what it measures." This is a low level of relationship with limited scope (Lundberg, 1942). Another problem surrounds the fact that the only meaning being conveyed is a particular set of operations to test for the presence of the thing to which the operations refer. But such meaning can be conveyed through any number of operations and there are no a priori rules to distinguish relevant from irrelevant operations (Bergmann, 1961). Consequently, the same concept can be specified with quite different operations. For example, research has demonstrated that LD students possess memory problems but the studies included a number of different memory measures. Operationally, it would be necessary to say that a number of different "memories" are being evaluated but such operational differences would obscure the significance of the conclusion. The obvious answer is that they all measure the same thing but an operational approach must deny this possibility.

Thus, operational approaches may involve a certain a priori plausibility, but the lack of a sound theoretical foundation soon undermines that plausibility upon analysis and results in meaningless or insignificant operations. The criteria for appropriate operations usually include items such as efficiency or ease in quantification but they are inappropriate and result in no more than "psychometric engineering" (Deese, 1972). It is little wonder then that operational approaches usually lack theoretical interest and technological power (Loevinger, 1957).

Data Analysis

Once data are collected, the analyses of that data is also a problematic component of the scientific method. The difficulty appears to surround the overreliance on statistical probabilities in deciding to accept or to reject hypotheses (Carver, 1978). Statistical inference is useful for eliminating chance findings but not so helpful in deciding subject matter issues (Berkson, 1942). Statistical decisions can enhance outcomes by making them more efficient and reliable, but this is not the same as reaching conclusions. The techniques of statistical analysis were designed for making practical decisions in applied work which should not be confused with conclusions. As Fisher (1956) stated: The Natural Sciences can only be successfully conducted by responsible and independent thinkers applying their minds and their imaginations to the detailed interpretations of verifiable observations. The idea that this responsibility can be delegated to a giant computer programmed with Decision Functions belongs to the phantasy of circles rather remote from scientific research (p. 100).

The LD field makes too much use of statistical decision techniques for qualitative decisions about hypotheses. Regardless of the sophistication of the analysis, the associated significant probabilities (e.g., $p < .05$) neither confirm nor refute a research hypothesis but only the null hypothesis (e.g., Lykken, 1968; Rozeboom, 1960). The findings may be "significant" but that significance should not be confused with importance. They should be taken to mean that the findings "signify" a basis for rejecting the null hypothesis. What is signified is simply the elimination of random findings, but no inference about the particular associations between variables is possible from a test of the null hypothesis itself. As Walberg (1984) pointed out, "Arbitrating results purely on statistical inference is like the false security of letting children play football on a busy street because they have had their polio shots" (p. 377).

The difficulty stems from the fact that caution about subject matter conclusions is rapidly abandoned when probabilities are less than .05. The reverse, however, is not as true because studies with probabilities greater than .05 are not often published and, consequently, the findings are not given serious consideration (Skipper, Guenther, & Nass, 1967). The choice of analytic technique is, however, a subjective matter and there are few rules to guide that choice (Strauss, 1987). While design considerations are evaluated in terms of internal validity (see Campbell & Stanley, 1969) and external validity (see Bracht & Glass, 1968), there has been a relative neglect of evaluating the validity of the chosen analytic method. Walberg (1984) outlined a number of threats to analytic validity and, in discussing each, demonstrated the complexity inherent in choosing analytic methods. It is not a ritualized, mechanical process and the LD field would be well served by paying greater attention to techniques of data analysis.

The consequences are not inconsequential. For example, consider the case where a new LD intervention is compared with a conventional treatment. Suppose the mean performance is higher for the new treatment but the probability of the null hypothesis (i.e., no difference between groups) is .06. The new treatment is probably considered a failure and, in all likelihood, the findings do not find themselves in print. In this case, the LD field has lost potentially valuable information because a piece of evidence that could aid a decision about whether or not to adopt the treatment is not available. It also eliminates the possibility of replication which, even if several investigations find probability levels above .05, might still contain useful information if individual findings were combined. Now imagine that one study (even if flawed) finds the conventional treatment more effective with a probability of .001 and is published. Even though it might be a chance finding, its publication makes it the standard and also makes it difficult to eliminate. In the meantime, the new treatment is placed in the background and considered "experimental" without the benefit of a fair and objective test.

An Evaluation of the Scientific Method

Interpretation of Findings

The goal of eliminating metaphysical contamination has been achieved through the scientific method. The difficulty, however, has been in putting the data collected into a coherent and unified whole. The emphasis on data collection and analysis has placed data interpretation in the background. Consequently, the scientific method tends to produce studies that remain isolated and independent. This "empiricism" places a premium on better observation (e.g., tests) and better analyses (i.e., more sophisticated) but pays far less attention to connecting findings logically and rationally (Toulmin & Leary, 1985). A problem is encountered, however, when it is realized that rigor in data collection provides no guarantee of producing "usable knowledge" (Lindblom & Cohen, 1979). For example, alchemy, astrology, and phrenology placed a premium on controlled observation, measurement, and prediction but all are recognized as exercises in futility and charlatanism (see Andreski, 1972).

The problem with interpretation in the scientific method is the need to be "scientific." Any interpretation beyond the data are deemed too subjective and by going outside the data, there exists the risk of becoming caught in a "web of interpretation" (Taylor, 1977). Moral and ethical judgments, however, can be judged true or false through "intuitionism," which suggests that humans have a faculty to intuit correctly the rightness or wrongness of actions. This moral theory, however, faces the difficulty of how to resolve the fact that given the same action, different human beings have incompatible intuitions. Resolution is problematic without an "objective," nonintuitionistic foundation. This was provided by John Stuart Mill ("On the Logic of Moral Sciences") where it was recommended that the empirical methods of the natural sciences be applied to the moral sciences. The outcome would be invariable laws of human behavior because human insight would play no role in testing hypotheses ("logic of confirmation") since confirmation would be based on data unencumbered by human interpretation.

The empiricist view would guarantee a strict correspondence between the way the world "really is" and our observation of it. It is easy to see that Mill's vision has not materialized. Perhaps the classic case in education is the decline and fall of a science of pedagogy based on the application of "general laws of learning" from psychology (see McKeachie, 1974). The difficulties encountered are many and varied. Kuhn (1970), for example, argued about the impossibility of drawing a distinction between theory and observation. All observations are theory-infected suggesting that there are no "basic" data (i.e., free of interpretation) with which to guarantee the objectivity of observational claims.

The difficulties are compounded by the values of researchers (Argyris, 1977; Laudan, 1984). The research process is not value-free and introduces the potential for bias in the outcomes (Rudner, 1953). Bias, in this sense, means having a prejudice (i.e., prejudgment), a conclusion arrived at prior to the evidence and justified independently of the evidence. The bias thus transcends the conclusion for a particular study and is rather the tendency to adhere to a certain belief no matter what evidence is brought to bear on the question (Ziman, 1968). The question of bias is therefore a deep-seated problem and not easily dismissed by only describing "what objectively happened." Kaplan (1964) argued that "keeping the facts" is not enough to eliminate bias and, in fact, may even induce more bias than attempts at "pure thought."

Alternative Interpretative Methods

The recognition of values playing a role in the scientific method has led to an attempt to reconstitute an empiricist view with a different conceptual foundation (Howard, 1985). Rosenberg (1980) argued for a sociobiological foundation because, when dealing with human behavior, the concepts of intention, belief, desire, and motive do apply. This is not to suggest a strict biological determinism or a belief in neurophysiological reductionism but rather the need for recognition of a biological basis for human action making for differences in human meanings. The human meaning can thus be approached only through an interpretive, nonempiricist science of interpretation (Ericson & Ellet, 1982). Plausibility should be a primary interpretative criteria and the goal should be understanding rather than a search for "hard" knowledge, prediction, and control. Much of the scientific method is acceptable (particularly with respect to data collection and analysis) but it is a mistake to believe that the data are a foundation for discovering invariable laws of human behavior. A science of interpretation demands the application of common sense and, as Ericson and Ellet (1982) suggested, "Good judgment will not yield certainty, but it can yield interpretations and analyses far more acute and powerful than even the most skilled application of the empiricist 'scientific method'" (p. 511).

Mook (1983) argued that too much attention to things like external validity can be a serious barrier to thought. External validity asks the question of generalizability of research findings but is not some absolute property without which results should be dismissed. Campbell and Stanley (1969) probably placed too much emphasis on external validity when it should serve merely to ask questions about the possibilities of generalizations. Mook (1983) suggested that, "It would then be easier to remember that we are not dealing with a criterion . . . but with a question like 'How can we get this sofa down the stairs?' One asks that question if, and only if, moving the sofa is what one wants to do" (p. 379). In place of external validity, Mook (1983) suggests "thinking through" where, on a case by case basis, decisions can be made about what conclusion we want to draw and whether the specifics of one sample or setting will prevent us from drawing it.

The idea of a different sort of interpretative base has been formalized in descriptions of hermeneutic or interpretive research (Hookway & Pettit, 1978). The application of hermeneutic approaches to human science was initiated by Heidegger (1962), who described it as an attempt to study meaningful human phenomena in a careful and detailed manner, as free as possible from prior theoretical assumptions, based instead on practical understandings. The object of study is what individuals actually do when engaged in practical tasks rather than in the artificial confines of an experimental task (Bleicher, 1980). Practical activity has two primary characteristics. The first is that it is "perspectival," meaning that an action has one meaning from one perspective; from a different perspective it has another. The second is its holistic character, meaning that understanding is not possible without reference to the context within which it occurs. Packer (1985) compared hermeneutics to the two other major modes of inquiry: rationalism (cognitive and structural) and empiricism (experimental and behavioral). They were compared with respect to the origins of knowledge, the proper object of study and the resulting types of explanation. A hermeneutic approach was considered useful for studying human behavior since it considers action in the context of complexity that is an integral part of human conduct. As Packer (1985) concluded: The end product of a hermeneutic inquiry—an interpretive account—is more modest in its aims than is a formal set of rules or a causal law, but at the same time it is, I believe, subtle and complex, intellectually satisfying, and more appropriate to human action, embracing the historical openness, the ambiguity and opacity, the deceptions, dangers, and delights that action manifests (p. 1092).

For the LD field, this means that a revitalization of phenomenology would not be inappropriate. Allender (1986) discussed research as a personal and social process whose goal is a construction of reality. To achieve that aim, a variety of "new paradigm" research methods have been proposed (see Morgan, 1983; Reason & Rowan, 1981). With a growing awareness about the subjectivity of science (Bronowski, 1965), there is greater recognition of methods that can interweave objectivity and subjectivity (see Sarason, 1981, 1984). Since subjectivity is an integral part of reality, knowledge is a product of a particular sociocultural system and its validity is probably limited to the particular system that created it (Scarr, 1985). To keep pace with ever-changing sociocultural patterns, it would behoove the LD field to choose methods that aid its advancement.

Any proposed change in the scientific method is immediately confronted with the problem of relativism. Does this imply that any sort of research strategy goes? One view holds that only an affirmative answer to such a question will not inhibit research progress (Feyerabend, 1975). Since there are no hard and fast rules for research and no set criteria for judging quality, it may be the case that the LD field will need to accept the fact that multiple research models may be equally appropriate (Labouvie, 1975). Moving beyond "what the data says" (since in and of itself it says little) and placing greater emphasis on interpretation, relativism, or the belief that judgments cannot be made, need not be a problem (Phillips, 1983). Soltis (1984) argued persuasively for tolerating a variety of research models but emphasized that open-mindedness should not be viewed as being synonymous with empty-mindedness. Donmoyer (1985) cautioned against resurrecting aspects of logical positivism to deal with the question of relativism and discussed Toulmin's (1972) notion that scientific rationality does exist. By emphasizing scientific purposes other than prediction, it is possible to rationally assess the relative worth of conflicting research findings.

The Consequences of the Scientific Method

The application of the scientific method presents problems with outcomes. What kind of confidence can be placed on study findings? Long ago, Tyler (1931) warned about confusing statistical significance with importance but the LD field seems to have focused on the word "significant" and confused it with an index of how strong and dependable the findings. The scientific method seems to emphasize alpha levels with the goal being the reduction of Type I error. But equally important is beta level and Type II error which surrounds the question of "statistical power" (Cohen, 1977). It appears, however, that power is given far less attention and, consequently, surveys of the power of research findings is usually found to be low (e.g., Brewer, 1972; Cohen, 1962).

The emphasis on elevating alpha levels leads to a variety of difficulties. With the scientific method being very good at collecting data, there exists the possibility of collecting a large amount of data without any preplanning about the way those data are to be analyzed. The difficulty here is that decisions about data analysis are made *after* the data has been "eyeballed" (Lipset, Trow, & Coleman, 1970). Data analyses in this situation become similar to a projective technique because individual expectancies and biases impinge on the analysis process and almost any "finding" can be extracted. The rigor in the scientific method may evaporate when "eyeballing" reveals that the data does not support the original hypothesis. This is easily remedied by deriving a new hypothesis and using the study to "verify" this new hypothesis.

What about a situation where a large number of comparisons are made but only a few are significant? Is the hypotheses supported? The question is difficult but is exacerbated when only significant findings are selected for reporting (McNemar, 1960). It also must be understood that multiple tests of significance can lead to erroneous conclusions. Feild and

Armenakis (1974) demonstrated this phenomenon and gave an example: Suppose an investigator set his significance level at .05 and conducted 10 independent tests. The investigator may think that the probability of Type I error (rejecting a null hypothesis when it is true) is .05. However, the actual probability of Type I error in one or more of the 10 decisions is .40 (p. 428).

This practice has been termed "probability pyramiding" (Neher, 1967) but seems to have little bearing on the number of comparisons made since, as Friedlander (1964) suggested, data analysis seems to accept the adage, "If you don't succeed at first, try and try again" (p. 199).

What about negative results that fail to confirm the original hypothesis? In all probability, nonsignificant findings do not find their way into print (e.g., Bozarth & Roberts, 1972; Greenwald, 1975; Sterling, 1959). If not supportive of a hypothesis, then data are assumed to be "bad" and are usually ignored (McNemar, 1960). A problem arises, however, when later investigations obtain positive findings and the earlier negative results are not mentioned since it is likely to be concluded wrongly that the positive results are more stable and more valid than is actually the case.

The motivation for positive results and the potential for data analysis efforts contributing to significant findings provides an answer to the question, "How come so many hypotheses in educational research are supported?" (Cohen & Hyman, 1979). This state of affairs has led to the observation that the results of educational research are obvious, that is, could have been predicted without doing the research (see Gage, 1990). Phillips (1985) termed this a "truism" and defined it as a statement whose truth is self-evident and does not require research to uncover it. With "truisms" the primary outcome of research, it is not surprising that LD research does little to enhance understanding. Cronbach and Suppes (1969) suggested that research should be "conclusion-oriented," meaning that its value should be judged in relation to what it does to the "prevailing view." The prevailing view in LD, however, seems to be firmly entrenched and research findings do not seem to be a primary means of replacing the conventional wisdom. The constricted nature of the scientific method makes findings ineffectual in changing the prevailing view. Jackson (1990) pointed out that research is viewed in many ways by saying that, "it [is seen] as important, frivolous, eye-opening, mind-boggling, serious, dull, elegant, sloppy, refreshing, interesting, boring, scientific, pseudo-scientific, pretentious, modest, ambitious, exciting, frustrating, puzzling, and more" (p. 8). Although research findings can be viewed in many ways, these views appear restricted to an initial reaction and soon dissipate because of the failure of most research to change substantially the prevailing view. Consequently, most research produced within the context of the scientific method are not "interesting" (see Davis, 1971) because the obviousness of findings makes for "truisms" (see Phillips, 1985) that do little to deny certain assumptions about the phenomenon.

Progress and the Scientific Method

When research findings produce few interesting results, progress is limited (Laudan, 1978). Mosenthal (1985) discussed progress in relation to the problem of partial specification. Literal interpretations of progress (see Soltis, 1984) assume a correspondence between the phenomenon in theory and in reality. The better the fit, the greater the progress and this represents "normal science" (Kuhn, 1970) whose goal is to refine existing theories. A problem is encountered, however, when theories and concepts are not "fully specified" but only "partially specified" (Mosenthal, 1985). Partial specification of educational phenomena refers to the fact that they are defined with only a select sample of distinguishing features and criteria. Research activity is the vehicle for providing full specification but it appears that the limitations of the scientific method have impeded the goal of full specification. The insistence on adherence to the scientific method seems to have produced a pattern of research activity that has limited progress in the LD field.

Meehl (1978) criticized the slow, noncumulative progress of psychology and suggested that this slow progress is the result of faulty scientific methodology and especially the reliance on null hypothesis testing. Full specification is difficult to achieve with a reliance on statistical significance testing and, as Lakatos (1970) suggested, one wonders whether the function of statistical techniques in the social sciences is not primarily to provide a machinery for producing phoney corroborations and thereby a semblance of "scientific progress" where, in fact, there is nothing but an increase in pseudo-intellectual garbage (p. 173).

Lakatos (1978) described the notion of a "research program" and discussed criteria for labeling the program as either "progressive" or "degenerating." A research program may be perceived as a succession of theories and the primary reason for replacing a theory is an experimental failure (Lakatos, 1970). A new theory must both accommodate the successes of its predecessor and explain the data that brought the earlier theory into question. The new theory should also do more: It should lead to new predictions that are verified experimentally. When these goals are met, the research program is said to be "progressive." An integral part of the process is "empirical progress" in the sense that some new predictions receive empirical support.

When a program is not progressive, it is termed "degenerating." This means that the research program has ceased to yield empirical successes. Initially, empirical anomalies can be met with ad hoc maneuvers but soon this process exhausts the "heuristic," the ability to develop more complex and adequate explanations and tests. A new research program may then be needed. It appears that the scientific method used by the LD field is not "empirically progressive," which means that it is not "theoretically progressive," and should be viewed as "degenerating." The lack of theoretical development (see Kavale, in press) in LD would suggest that very few areas of LD are progressive. The uniformity imposed by the scientific method is a major contributor to the degenerative nature of LD research.

Popper (1970) discussed the problem of distinguishing science from pseudoscience. One way to approach this "demarcation problem" is to classify a discipline as scientific if it conforms to the developmental structure of an acceptable model of pure science. This does not mean, however, that all sciences must conform to a single methodological pattern (i.e., the scientific method). In fact, LD does not have to conform to research practices in the physical sciences. The real question is whether or not the actual methodologies applied to research problems permit the field to be "progressive." Progress is not achieved, however, when there is the assumption that LD *must* conform to the pattern established by the physical sciences. In discussing this question, it is also important to avoid "disciplinary solipsism" (Toulmin, 1972) which is the view that LD is a science because of the reasons that make LD a science (e.g., showing features of LD that are shared by other sciences). The scientific method is certainly not enough to show LD to be a science and has probably done more harm than good by restricting the research process to questions and methods that have caused the degenerative nature of LD research. The method (i.e., scientific) may be perfectly appropriate but not for LD because at its most fundamental level its nature is much different from the physical sciences.

The Scientific Method and Learning Disabilities: Summary and Conclusions

Critiques of research in LD are not new (see Cohen, 1976 and responses following) and have been a continuing theme in the field (e.g., Keogh, 1986). The purpose of this chapter has been to show why that is the case. Legitimate problems can be shown to exist in, for example, sample selection (e.g., Smith et al., 1984) as well as other specific areas but the argument here has surrounded the very nature of the research process itself. The culprit seems to be that legacy of logical positivism termed the scientific method. It is the model for most LD research and adherence to its strictures is considered mandatory for publication in scholarly journals. But the scientific method is fraught with difficulties and, upon analysis, is not as "scientific" as it appears on the surface. The mechanistic mentality associated with the scientific method removes an important component from the research process: thought. Research is just as much a conceptual process as it is an empirical process but the scientific method has empha- sized the empirical over the conceptual. Wachtel (1980) has described the situation as encouraging activity at the expense of thought.

The problem is a lack of truly significant findings, not in any statistical sense but rather in the sense of propelling the LD field forward. It is said (perhaps apocryphally) that physicists rarely read their journals because anything published is obsolete by the time it appears in a journal. New findings have moved the field to another point by then. The point is that breakthroughs are common in a field such as physics. Although this view of physics (or the "hard" sciences) may be spurious, it would not be difficult to argue that LD studies tend to be far more enduring. It would not be difficult to conceive of a situation where an LD study from 1970, for example, could be easily published today (with some disguise) and be considered a noteworthy piece of research. The rate of obsolescence in LD is simply too low.

The obvious price paid is in the area of progress. Although some areas of LD show progress, as a whole the field reveals no real progress and the state of our field seems to leave considerable room for discontent. The discontent appears, unfortunately, to be manageable and not at a level where there is a willingness to do something about it. We seem convinced that the scientific method will resolve our problems but, in reality, without some modifications the sought-after progress will be elusive. The lack of thought in the search process leads to the tendency to think recurring ideas (see Crovitz, 1970). These "conceptual ruts" are a limiting factor and make for research being a process that simply reaffirms the same conclusions. Wicker (1985) outlined a number of strategies for expanding conceptual frameworks, including playing with ideas, considering contexts, probing and tinkering with assumptions, and clarifying and systematizing the conceptual frame. The benefits would be substantial because a single new insight can go a long way, particularly in specialties in which theoretical and methodological traditions are strong and in which most published contributions are variations in familiar themes. Properly developed, a fresh idea can have a lasting impact (Wicker, 1985, pp. 1101–1102).

None of this is to suggest that the scientific method be abandoned. Bernstein (1983) suggested instead that researchers need to overcome the "tyranny of method." At no point were alternative methodologies proposed as superior options because they probably are not and can engender considerable debate about their particular merits. The scientific method does, however, hold an advantage because of its pervasive influence on the research process. This influence is positive because the scientific method does impart standards of objectivity and rationality to empirical research. These standards, however, must be understood in a non-positivist way (see Howe & Eisenhart, 1990). In its positivist form, the scientific method does possess limitations that impede the research process. These limitations are only exacerbated through the mechanistic application of the scientific method. They may be avoided, however, if the element of thought is injected throughout the process. Research requires many decisions which introduces a cognitive component that, on the surface, the scientific method attempts to avoid but is really integral and critical to the success or failure of any particular investigation. Our goal should be to reach a point where our journals also represent "history" in the same way as physics journals. To do so, however, we must retain the best features of our present approach while, at the same time, entertaining greater diversity in method through the application of new modes of thought.

References

Achinstein, P. & Barker, F. (1969). *The legacy of logical positivism*. Baltimore: Johns Hopkins University Press.

Allender, J.S. (1986). Educational research: A personal and social process. *Review of Educational Research, 56*, 173–193.

Andreski, S. (1972). *Social sciences as sorcery*. London: Andre Deutsch.

Argyris, C. (1977). *Inner contradictions of rigorous research*. New York: Academic Press.

Ayer, A.J. (1959). *Logical positivism*. Glencoe, IL: Free Press.

Barber, T.X. (1976). *Pitfalls in human research: Ten pivotal points*. New York: Pergamon Press.

Bennett, R.E. (1983). Research and evaluation priorities for special education assessment. *Exceptional Children, 50*, 110–117.

Bergmann, G. (1957). *Philosophy of science*. Madison, WI: University of Wisconsin Press.

Berk, R.A. (1984). *Screening and diagnosis of children with learning disabilities*. Springfield, IL: Charles C. Thomas.

Berkson, J. (1942). Tests of significance considered as evidence. *Journal of the American Statistical Association, 37*, 325–335.

Bernstein, R. (1983). *Beyond objectivism and relativism*. Philadelphia: University of Pennsylvania Press.

Blalock, H.M. (1982). *Conceptualization and measurement in the social sciences*. Beverly Hills, CA: Sage.

Bleicher, J. (1980). *Contemporary hermeneutics: Hermeneutics as methods, philosophy and critique*. London: Routledge & Kegan Paul.

Bolles, R.C. (1962). The difference between statistical hypotheses and scientific hypotheses. *Psychological Reports, 11*, 639–645.

Bozarth, J.D. & Roberts, R.R. (1972). Signifying significant significance. *American Psychologist, 27*, 774–775.

Bracht, G.H. & Glass, G.V. (1968). The external validity of experiments. *American Educational Research Journal, 5*, 437–474.

Brewer, J.K. (1972). On the power of statistical tests in the *American Educational Research Journal*. *American Educational Research Journal, 9*, 391–401.

Bridgman, P.W. (1927). *The logic of modern physics*. New York: Macmillan.

Brinberg, D. & McGrath, J.E. (1985). *Validity and the research process*. Beverly Hills, CA: Sage.

Bronowski, J. (1965). *Science and human values* (rev. ed.). New York: Harper & Row.

Campbell, D.T. & Stanley, J.C. (1969). *Experimental and quasi-experimental designs for research.* Chicago: Rand McNally.

Campbell, J.P., Daft, R.L. & Hulin, C.L. (1982). *What to study: Generating and developing research questions.* Beverly Hills, CA: Sage.

Carnine, D. & Woodward, J. (1988). Paradigms lost: Learning disabilities and the new ghost in the old machine. *Journal of Learning Disabilities, 21,* 233–236.

Carver, R.P. (1978). The case against statistical significance testing. *Harvard Educational Review, 48,* 378–399.

Cohen, J. (1962). The statistical power of abnormal-social psychological research: A review. *Journal of Abnormal and Social Psychology, 65,* 145–153.

Cohen, J. (1977). *Statistical power analysis for the behavioral sciences* (rev. ed.). New York: Academic Press.

Cohen, S.A. (1976). The fuzziness and the flab: Some solutions to research problems in learning disabilities. *Journal of Special Education, 10,* 129–136.

Cohen, S.A. & Hyman, J.S. (1979). How come so many hypotheses in educational research are supported? (A modest proposal). *Educational Research, 9,* 12–16.

Cook, T.D. & Campbell, D.T. (1979). *Quasi-experimentation: Design and analysis issues for field settings.* Boston: Houghton-Mifflin.

Cronbach, L.J. & Meehl, P.E. (1955). Construct validity in psychological tests. *Psychological Bulletin, 52,* 281–301.

Cronbach, L.J. & Suppes, P. (1969). *Research for tomorrow's schools: Disciplined inquiry for education.* New York: Macmillan.

Crovitz, H.F. (1970). *Galton's walk.* New York: Harper & Row.

Davis, M. (1971). "That's interesting!" Towards a phenomenology of sociology and a sociology of phenomenology. *Philosophy of the Social Sciences, 4,* 309–344.

Deese, J. (1972). *Psychology as science and art.* New York: Harcourt Brace Jovanovich.

Donmoyer, R. (1985). The rescue from relativism: Two failed attempts and an alternative strategy. *Educational Researcher, 14,* 13–20.

Eisner, E.W. (1983). Anastasia might still be alive, but the monarchy is dead. *Educational Researcher, 12,* 13–24.

Ericson, D.P. & Ellet, F.S. (1982). Interpretation, understanding, and educational research. *Teachers College Record, 83,* 497–513.

Feild, H.S. & Armenakis, A.A. (1974). On the use of multiple tests of significance in psychological research. *Psychological Reports, 354,* 427–431.

Feyerabend, P. (1975). *Against method: Outline of an anarchistic theory of knowledge.* London: NLB.

Fisher, R.A. (1956). *Statistical methods and scientific inference.* New York: Hafner.

Fisher, R.A. (1967). *Statistical methods for research workers* (13th ed.). Edinburgh: Oliver & Boyd.

Forness, S.R. & Kavale, K.A. (1987). Holistic inquiry and the scientific challenge in special education: A reply to Iano. *Remedial and Special Education, 8,* 47–51.

Forness, S.R. & Kavale, K.A. (in press). Meta-analysis in intervention research: Methods and implications. In J. Rothman & E. Thomas (Eds.), *Intervention research: Effective methods for professional practice.* Chicago: Haworden Press.

Friedlander, F. (1964). Type I and Type II bias. *American Psychologist, 19,* 198–199.

Gage, N.L. (1989). The paradigm wars and their aftermath: A "historical" sketch of research on teaching since 1989. *Educational Researcher, 18,* 4–10.

Gage, N.L. (1990). The obviousness of social and educational research results. *Educational Researcher, 19,* 10–16.

Garrison, J.W. (1986). Some principles of post positivistic philosophy of science. *Educational Researcher, 15,* 12–18.

Gergen, K.J. (1978). Toward generative theory. *Journal of Personality and Social Psychology, 36,* 1344–1360.

Grant, D.A. (1962). Testing the null hypothesis and the strategy and tactics of investigating theoretical models. *Psychological Review, 69,* 54–61.

Greenwald, A.G. (1975). Consequences of prejudice against the hull hypothesis. *Psychological Bulletin, 82,* 1–20.

Hanfling, O. (1981). *Logical positivism.* New York: Columbia University Press.

Heidegger, M. (1962). *Being and time* (J. Marquarrie & E. Robinson, Trans.). New York: Harper & Row. (Original work published 1927)

Hempel, C.G. (1952). *Fundamentals of concept formation in empirical science.* Chicago: University of Chicago Press.

Heshusius, L. (1982). At the heart of the advocacy dilemma: A mechanistic world view. *Exceptional Children, 52,* 6–13.

Heshusius, L. (1989). The Newtonian mechanistic paradigm, special education, and contours of alternatives: An overview. *Journal of Learning Disabilities, 22,* 403–415.

Hookway, C. & Pettit, P. (Eds.). (1978). *Action and interpretation: Studies in the philosophy of the social sciences.* Cambridge, England: Cambridge University Press.

Howard, G.S. (1985). The role of values in the science of psychology. *American Psychologist, 40,* 255–265.

Howe, K.R. (1985). Two dogmas of educational research. *Educational Researcher, 14,* 10–18.

Howe, K.R. (1988). Against the quantitative-qualitative incompatibility thesis (or, dogmas die hard). *Educational Researcher, 17,* 10–16.

Howe, K. & Eisenhart, M. (1990). Standards for qualitative (and quantitative) research: A prolegomenon. *Educational Researcher, 19,* 2–9.

Iano, R.P. (1986). The study and development of teaching: With implications for the advancement of special education. *Remedial and Special Education, 7,* 50–61.

Jackson, P.W. (1990). The functions of educational research. *Educational Researcher, 19,* 3–9.

Kaplan, A. (1964). *The conduct of inquiry: Methodology for behavioral science.* San Francisco: Chandler.

Kavale, K.A. (1987). Theoretical quandaries in learning disabilities. In S. Vaughn & C.S. Bos (Eds.), *Research in learning disabilities: Issues and future directions* (pp. 19–29). Boston: Little, Brown/College-Hill.

Kavale, K.A. (1988). Epistemological relativity in learning disabilities. *Journal of Learning Disabilities, 21,* 215–218.

Kavale, K.A. & Mundschenk, N.A. (1990). A critique of assessment methodology. In H.L. Swanson (Ed.), *Handbook on the assessment of learning disabilities* (pp. 407–432). Austin, TX: PRO-ED.

Keogh, B.K. (1986). Future of the LD field: Research and practice. *Journal of Learning Disabilities, 19*, 455–460.
Kimball, W.H. & Heron, T.E. (1988). A behavioral commentary on Poplin's discussion of reductionistic fallacy and holistic/constructivistic principles. *Journal of Learning Disabilities, 21*, 425–428.
Koch, S. (1981). The nature and limits of psychological knowledge: Lessons of a century qua "science." *American Psychologist, 36*, 257–269.
Kuhn, T.S. (1970). *The structure of scientific revolutions* (2nd ed.). Chicago: University of Chicago Press.
Labouvie, E.W. (1975). The dialectical nature of measurement activities in the behavioral sciences. *Human Development, 18*, 205–222.
Lakatos, I. (1970). Falsification and the methodology of scientific research programs. In I. Lakatos & A. Musgrave (Eds.), *Criticism and the growth of knowledge* (pp. 91–196). Cambridge, England: Cambridge University Press.
Lakatos, I. (1978). *The methodology of scientific research programs.* Cambridge, England: Cambridge University Press.
Laudan, L. (1984). *Science and values: An essay on the aims of science and their role in scientific debate.* Berkeley, CA: University of California Press.
Licht, B.G. & Torgesen, J.K. (1989). Natural science approaches to questions of subjectivity. *Journal of Learning Disabilities, 22*, 418–419.
Lindblom, C.E. & Cohen, D.K. (1979). *Usable knowledge: Social science and social problem solving.* New Haven, CT: Yale University Press.
Lipset, S.M., Trow, M.A., & Coleman, J.S. (1970). Statistical problems. In D.E. Morrison & R.E. Henkel (Eds.), *The significance test controversy—A reader* (pp. 81–86). Chicago: Aldine.
Loevinger, J. (1957). Objective tests as instruments of psychological theory. *Psychological Reports, 9*, 635–694.
Luce, T.S. & Johnson, D.M. (1978). Rating of educational and psychological journals. *Educational Researcher, 7*, 8–10.
Lundberg, G.A. (1942). The operational definition in the social sciences. *American Journal of Sociology, 47*, 727–745.
Lykken, D. (1968). Statistical significance in psychological research. *Psychological Bulletin, 70*, 151–159.
Macmillan, C.J.B. & Garrison, J.W. (1984). Using the "new philosophy of science" in criticizing current research traditions in education. *Educational Researcher, 13*, 15–21.
McGrath, J.E., Martin, J., & Kulka, R.A. (1982). *Judgment calls in research.* Beverly Hills, CA: Sage.
McGuire, W.J. (1973). The yin and yang of progress in social psychology: Seven koan. *Journal of Personality and Social Psychology, 26*, 446–451.
McKeachie, W.J. (1974). The decline and fall of the laws of learning. *Educational Researcher, 3*, 7–11.
McNemar, Q. (1960). At random: Sense and non-sense. *American Psychologist, 15*, 295–300.
Meehl, P.E. (1978). Theoretical risks and tabular asterisks: Sir Karl, Sir Ronald, and the slow progress in soft psychology. *Journal of Consulting and Clinical Psychology, 46*, 806–834.
Messick, S. (1981). Constructs and their vicissitudes in educational and psychological measurement. *Psychological Bulletin, 89*, 575–588.

Mitroff, I.I. & Kilman, R.H. (1978). *Methodological approaches to social science.* San Francisco: Jossey-Bass.

Mook, D.G. (1983). In defense of external invalidity. *American Psychology, 38,* 379–387.

Morgan, G. (Ed.). (1983). *Beyond method: Strategies for social research.* Beverly Hills, CA: Sage.

Morrison, D.E. & Henkel, R.E. (Eds.). (1970). *The significance test controversy: A reader.* Chicago: Aldine.

Mosenthal, P.B. (1985). Defining progress in educational research. *Educational Researcher, 14,* 3–9.

Neher, A. (1967). Probability pyramiding, research error and the need for independent replication. *Psychological Record, 17,* 257–262.

Packer, M.J. (1985). Hermeneutic inquiry in the study of human conduct. *American Psychologist, 40,* 1081–1093.

Phillips, D. (1983). After the wake: Postpositivistic educational thought. *Educational Researcher, 12,* 4–12.

Phillips, D.C. (1985). The uses and abuses of truisms. In C.W. Fisher & D.C. Berliner (Eds.), *Perspectives on instructional time* (pp. 309–315). New York: Longman.

Poplin, M.S. (1987). Scientific method in education. A critique. *Remedial and Special Education, 8,* 31–37.

Poplin, M.S. (1988). The reductionistic fallacy in learning disabilities: Replicating the past by reducing the present. *Journal of Learning Disabilities, 21,* 389–400.

Popper, K.R. (1970). Normal science and its dangers. In I. Lakatos & A. Musgrave (Eds.), *Criticism and the growth of knowledge* (pp. 51–58). Cambridge, England: Cambridge University Press.

Reason, P. & Rowan, J. (Eds.). (1981). *Human inquiry: A sourcebook of new paradigm research.* New York: Wiley.

Rosenberg, A. (1980). *Sociobiology and the preemption of social science.* Baltimore: Johns Hopkins University Press.

Rosenberg, M.S. & Jackson, L. (1988). Theoretical models and special education: The impact of varying world views on service delivery and research. *Remedial and Special Education, 9,* 26–34.

Rozeboom, W.W. (1960). The fallacy of the null hypothesis significance test. *Psychological Bulletin, 57,* 416–428.

Rudner, R. (1953). The scientist qua scientist makes value-judgments. *Philosophy of Science, 20,* 1–6.

Sarason, S.B. (1981). *Psychology misdirected.* New York: Free Press.

Sarason, S.B. (1984). If it can be studied or developed, should it be? *American Psychologist, 39,* 477–485.

Scarr, S. (1985). Constructing psychology: Making facts and fables for our times. *American Psychologist, 40,* 499–512.

Simpson, R.G. & Eaves, R.C. (1985). Do we need more qualitative research or more good research? A reaction to Stainback and Stainback. *Exceptional Children, 51,* 325–329.

Skipper, J.K., Guenther, A.L., & Nass, G. (1967). The sacredness of .05; A note concerning the uses of statistical levels of significance in social science. *The American Sociologist, 2,* 16–18.

Smart, J.C. & Elton, C.F. (1981). Structural characteristics and citation rates of education journals. *American Educational Research Journal, 18,* 399–414.

Smith, D.D., Deshler, D.D., Hallahan, D.P., Lovitt, T., Robinson, S., Voress, J., & Ysseldyke, J. (1984). Minimum standards for the description of subjects in learning disability research reports. *Learning Disability Quarterly, 7,* 221–225.

Smith, J.K. & Heshusius, L. (1986). Closing down the conversation: The end of the quantitative-qualitative debate among educational researchers. *Educational Researcher, 15,* 4–12.

Soltis, J. (1984). On the nature of educational research. *Educational Researcher, 13,* 5–10.

Stainback, S. & Stainback, W. (1984). Broadening the research perspective in special education. *Exceptional Children, 50,* 400–408.

Sterling, T.D. (1959). Publication decisions and their possible effects on inferences drawn from tests of significance—or vice versa. *Journal of the American Statistical Association, 54,* 30–34.

Strauss, A. (1987). *Qualitative analysis for social scientists.* Cambridge, MA: Harvard University Press.

Summers, E.G. (1986). The information flood in learning disabilities: A bibliometric analysis of the journal literature. *Remedial and Special Education, 7,* 49–60.

Swanson, H.L. (1988). Toward a metatheory of learning disabilities. *Journal of Learning Disabilities, 21,* 196–209.

Swanson, H.L. & Alford, L. (1987). An analysis of the current status of special education research and journal outlets. *Remedial and Special Education, 8,* 8–18.

Taylor, C. (1977). Interpretation and the sciences of man. In F.R. Dallamyr & T.A. McCarthy (Eds.), *Understanding and social inquiry* (pp. 98–126). Notre Dame, IN: University of Notre Dame Press.

Toulmin, S. (1972). *Human understanding.* Princeton, NJ: Princeton University Press.

Toulmin, S. & Leary, D.E. (1985). The cult of empiricism in psychology, and beyond. In S. Koch & D. Leary (Eds.), *A century of psychology as science* (pp. 594–617). New York: McGraw-Hill.

Tryon, W.W. (1979). The test-trait fallacy. *American Psychologist, 34,* 402–406.

Tyler, R.W. (1931). What is statistical significance? *Educational Research Bulletin, 10,* 115–118.

Ullman, J.D. & Rosenberg, M.S. (1986). Science and superstition in special education. *Exceptional Children, 52,* 459–460.

Wachtel, P.L. (1980). Investigation and its discontents: Some constraints on progress in psychological research. *American Psychologist, 35,* 399–408.

Walberg, H.J. (1984). Quantification reconsidered. *Review of Research in Education, 2,* 369–402.

Warner, M.M. & Bull, K.S. (1986). Grounding LD definitions and practices in systems of educational thought. *Journal of Learning Disabilities, 19,* 139–144.

Weener, P. (1981). On comparing learning disabled and regular classroom children. *Journal of Learning Disabilities, 14,* 227–232.

Wicker, A.W. (1985). Getting out of our conceptual ruts: Strategies for expanding conceptual frameworks. *American Psychologist, 40,* 1094–1103.

Wong, B.Y.L. (1988). Basic research in learning disabilities: An introduction to the special series. *Journal of Learning Disabilities*, *21*, 195.

Yoels, W. (1974). The structure of scientific fields and the allocation of editorship on scientific journals: Some observations on the politics of knowledge. *Sociological Quarterly*, *15*, 164–176.

Ziman, J.M. (1968). *Public knowledge: An essay concerning the social dimension of science*. Cambridge, England: Cambridge University Press.

Part II
Methodological Issues: Descriptive Research

4
The Role of Classification in Learning Disabilities

DEBORAH L. SPEECE

This is an exciting time for research in the field of learning disabilities. A diverse group of investigators is tackling the very thorny issues of learning difficulties from a variety of vantage points including biological (e.g., Duane & Gray, 1991), psychological (e.g., Torgesen, 1991), and ecological (e.g., Speece, 1993) perspectives. This diversity of research provides a wealth of information on the children we seek to understand, but it also produces a bewildering array of findings that are difficult to comprehend in a systematic manner. Accordingly, one of the more challenging issues facing the field is how to organize this knowledge.

We know that, as a group however defined, children who experience learning problems are heterogeneous on virtually any variable we can measure. We also know that almost every variable has been used in the plethora of group difference, univariate investigations that have populated the literature. Scholarly reflections on this history conclude that research in learning disabilities has been "chaotic" (Kavale, 1987) for many reasons, including but not limited to lack of theory (Kavale, 1987), the absence of research predicated on explanatory rather than descriptive goals (McKinney, 1987), and confusion on the multiple purposes of research that leads to muddied methodology (Keogh, 1987a). Searching for order is difficult because the research has, for the most part, not proceeded in an orderly fashion.

It may seem premature to discuss how we might classify children who fail to learn, given a history of research with little direction and its share of conceptual and methodological flaws. Without a firm empirical base it is difficult to know where to start. However, it is for precisely these reasons that taxonomies are needed. It is generally understood that classification is fundamental to all branches of science as it promotes organization and understanding of the phenomena of interest (Aldenderfer & Blashfield, 1984; Jain & Dubes, 1988). The field of learning disabilities, until recently, has not devoted a great deal of interest to this activity, perhaps due to the assumption that a learning disability represented a single entity and/or a univariate cause could be identified. That is, if there was one etiological factor and one powerful treatment that needed to be discovered then there would be little reason to pursue classification. Confronted with overwhelming evidence that a multivariate perspective was needed, classification of learning disabilities has become a frequently discussed if not universally embraced topic of research and thought (e.g., Fletcher & Morris, 1986; Kavale & Forness, 1987; Keogh, 1990; Lyon & Risucci, 1988; Speece & Cooper, 1991).

From this backdrop emerges a need to analyze the role of classification in the study of learning disabilities. This task will be approached from conceptual and methodological perspectives and will attempt to place classification research into the broader realm of investigations in learning disabilities.

Conceptual Issues in Classification

The inclusion of conceptual underpinnings in the analysis of classification research represents an advance in the development of this line of inquiry in learning disabilities. It is not unreasonable to conclude from the past decade of literature that the topic has been fueled more by the statistical potential of classification techniques than from a clear vision of how the results of such manipulations may promote understanding. Up to this point in the chapter, the connection between classification and statistical methods used to classify (i.e., cluster analysis) has been intentionally avoided to emphasize that classification, defined as the process of forming groups, is independent of the method used to form groups (Jain & Dubes, 1988; Keogh, 1987b). This distinction has often been blurred by some observers through equating classification and cluster analysis either implicitly or explicitly. Groupings may be formed logically, intuitively, or statistically. The point under consideration is whether classification, divorced from method, should be done at all. To organize this discussion the following questions will be addressed: Why classify?, how to classify?, and what to classify?

Why Classify?

As mentioned earlier, classification is basic to any scientific field as it organizes information and provides a basis for furthering understanding. Gould (1989) put a finer point on its importance: Taxonomy (the science of classification) is often undervalued as a glorified form of filing . . . but taxonomy is a fundamental and dynamic science, dedicated to exploring the causes of relationships and similarities among organisms. Classifications are theories about the basis of natural order, not dull catalogues compiled only to avoid chaos (p. 98).

While the work in the field of learning disabilities still has much to accomplish with respect to capturing the dynamic and theoretical aspects of classification, this perspective should be central to future studies. To elaborate, there is a sense that classifications that are derived are absolute and not subject to modification (Speece, 1990a). This rigidity in interpretation of results will greatly reduce the value of these studies and will limit the design of further investigations by unnecessarily placing restrictions on problems to be addressed.

In addition to capturing the dynamic aspects of order and relationships, classification also provides a vehicle for communication and prediction (Blashfield & Draguns, 1976). Blashfield and his colleagues (Blashfield & Draguns, 1976; Cromwell, Blashfield, & Strauss, 1975; Skinner & Blashfield, 1982) have defined the communicative value of classification as usefulness for clinical practice. Prediction furthers scientific understanding. They identified a fundamental tension between these goals as communication necessitates simplicity, whereas prediction necessitates complexity. While the cited articles pertained to psychiatric classification, the themes are also germane to learning disabilities, given shared clinical and scientific goals. Classification research in learning disabilities has had almost an exclusive focus on scientific goals of prediction, broadly defined. If classification research is to have a significant impact on practice, the communicative value of results will need elaboration. This comment, of course, does not diminish the importance of promoting scientific goals. There is often confusion on this distinction with respect to the worthiness of classification activities (Speece & Cooper, 1991). The point to be made is that investigators need to clarify the goal of any classification activity. Both communication and prediction are difficult to accomplish.

The most frequently cited reason for pursuing classification in learning disabilities is the heterogeneity of child characteristics. The rationale is to develop groupings of children that are more homogeneous on criteria of interest for further study. While the logic is intuitively obvious and sensible, homogeneity carries the requirement of defining similarity; in other words, homogeneous on what basis? For example, special education has a history of using intelligence test scores as the criterion to distinguish mental retardation and learning disabilities and within mental retardation, differing levels of impairment. The usefulness of this definition of similarity can be debated but it serves to reduce some variability and, thus, increase homogeneity.

The subject of similarity will be taken up in a later section but it should be noted that homogeneity, however defined, is not necessarily accepted as an important goal (Speece, 1993). Deno (1990), for example, argued that "this emphasis on classification actually contradicts the assertion of individual uniqueness; it suggests that different individuals can be placed together in a group where their individual uniqueness does not interact with different sets of learning experiences" (p. 161). This argument seems to promote individual instruction in all educational settings since it would be impossible to catalogue all nuances of individual differences. However, not all differences are relevant for learning and our task is to identify those that further scientific aims of communication and prediction (Meehl, 1954). D.H. Cooper (personal communication, February, 1991) noted that raising the specter of individual differences as an argument against classification is an invitation to chaos and provided an apt analogy: We can assert that no two snowflakes are alike (individual uniqueness) but what matters is how deep, how wet, how powdery (categories) the snow is. If individual instruction is the best we can do, classification would likely be unnecessary; however, if we are interested in more specific treatments, etiology, and prediction, then classification is necessary to further those aims (Doris, 1986).

How to Classify?

Three approaches to classification have the most currency in learning disabilities: rational, dimensional, and empirical. Rational methods draw upon clinical, data-based, and/or theoretical tenets to identify the variables to define subgroups or types of children (Torgesen, 1982). The number of variables considered is small and decisions must be made as to criteria for membership. Torgesen has developed a well-designed program of research using this approach in which short-term memory is the variable of interest for studying the cognitive processes underlying school failure (e.g., Torgesen & Houck, 1980; Torgesen, Rashotte, Greenstein, & Portes, 1991).

As applied by Torgesen, two subgroups are identified within a sample of children with learning disabilities (those with and without a specific deficit), but rational grouping does not preclude multiple groups (e.g., Boder, 1973; Bradley & Bryant, 1983). The advantages of rational groupings include dealing with sample heterogeneity via well-defined samples that enhance possibilities for replication, experimentation, and application as few variables are considered. This is also a drawback as there is likely a host of variables contributing to academic failure other than the ones selected for study and the rational approach does not provide a means for estimating prevalence of the disorder in the population (Torgesen, 1982). The rational approach is a monothetic model of classification that defines the necessary and sufficient features for membership that are considered sequentially (Jain & Dubes, 1988). A difficulty with this model is that absolute homogeneity of features is required which is difficult to accomplish (Blashfield, 1993).

A related approach is the dimensional model of classification in which the focus is on the continuous distribution of variables. This model does not require the assumption of clusters of individuals (Blashfield, 1993).

This perspective has been favored by those who believe it is not reasonable to expect natural, nonoverlapping clusters of children and who emphasize that within a cluster there will be important variation (Ellis, 1985; Stanovich, 1989; Torgesen, 1991). The arguments for dimensions as opposed to clusters may be fueled by cluster analysis investigations in the social sciences that attempt to mirror the findings of studies in the natural sciences (e.g., botany, zoology). That is, there has been a search for discrete clusters of children that are compact with well-defined boundaries. This type of clarity is rarely achieved in practice and it has been suggested that these requirements be relaxed in the face of our current knowledge of clustering results (Speece, 1993). While the dimensional model has much to offer as a general research approach it does not serve well as a model for classification. The dimensional approach does not result in the formation of categories; it thus inhibits communication and does not assist with the organization of scientific knowledge (Blashfield, 1993).

Empirical approaches to classification use statistical methods to define subgroups or clusters of persons based on their performance on a multivariate data set. Cluster analysis is an umbrella term for a large number of methods that statistically divide entities into different subtypes or clusters. After selecting the variables to be used, it must be decided on what basis two entities will be judged as similar. Essentially, cluster analysis methods will group persons who are similar, however defined, and then the usefulness of the clusters must be determined. This account is overly simplistic, but provides a point of comparison with rational methods. Both must draw on logic and theory for definition of subjects and variables. Rational methods use a monothetic model and few variables, whereas empirical methods resemble a polythetic model of classification and can handle many variables. In this model, compared with the monothetic approach, no single characteristic is necessary for membership; rather, subsets from a list of features are necessary and considered simultaneously (Blashfield, 1993; Jain & Dubes, 1988). Blashfield (in press) also noted that polythetic classifications do not require absolute homogeneity of characteristics, a condition that is less difficult to meet. It is also assumed that clusters of persons exist that have similar symptom patterns. It should be emphasized that empirical classification research in learning disabilities has yet to accomplish the identification of a true polythetic classification system. The advantages of an empirical approach are the ability to analyze many variables simultaneously, the opportunity to assess the prevalence of a particular cluster of persons, and the possibility of identifying previously unrecognized groupings that were not predicted. The drawbacks include a need for large samples, intense data collection efforts, and statistical methods that are incredibly diverse and not necessarily derived from statistical theory. Although it would seem that there is a fundamental conflict between rational and empirical methods of classification, there is some agreement that both are necessary and are actually complementary (Speece & Cooper, 1991; Torgesen, 1991). Rational methods do not have the potential for identifying a true classification scheme because the focus is on only a small corner of the landscape known as learning disabilities. However, these methods allow examination of more specific properties of learning failure, thus providing an avenue of investigation while more broad-based classification efforts are pursued (Torgesen, 1982). Empirical methods provide a method of surveying the heterogeneity of children from a wide angle lens and result in categories that may enhance understanding via further description and experimentation. Both approaches, as stated, assume methodological rigor. From a conceptual perspective, one could predict interaction of both methods to promote the description and explanation of learning disabilities.

What to Classify?

This discussion is potentially as endless as the number of professionals interested in learning disabilities. However, it is not pointless to at least consider possible means of organization. Research on learning generally and learning disabilities specifically has not produced a well-articulated perspective on the learning process. This is so despite Doris' (1986) observation that "we may suspect that the range and pattern of individual differences have not undergone significant change since before the least retreat of the polar ice cap" (p. 5).

Cromwell et al., (1975) suggested that classes of data should be recognized in classification for their value in defining categories and assessing the utility of the categories. Classes of data for definition include historical/etiological characteristics and current child characteristics derived from assessment data. Four classes of data were identified to judge utility and included treatment, prognosis, prevention, and treatment outcome (Cromwell et al., 1975). Different combinations of definitional and utility classes provide different categorical systems. For example, classification efforts that include the two definitional classes and the prognosis class is a valid approach but it useful only for prognosis. Other arrangements are possible and produce classification schemes with different emphases. This approach is a viable method of structuring our thinking about variable selection and may serve as a means of disengaging ourselves from automatically selecting a favorite set of variables for classification.

Although not necessarily supportive of a categorical approach to the study of learning disabilities, Hagen and his colleagues (Hagen & Kamberlis, 1990; Hagen, Kamberlis, & Segal, 1991) promote a multilevel analysis incorporating neurological, psychological, developmental, and environmental levels of variables. They note that research tends to favor a single level of analysis and seldom is consideration given to moving up or down the scale. Of particular importance is the emphasis on environmental variables that is noticeably absent from most considerations of learning disabilities (Hagen et al., 1991). It has been argued elsewhere that failure to consider ecological issues, specifically the instructional environment, will ultimately limit our understanding and description of learning disabilities (Speece, 1990b; 1993). Initial work in this area indicates that this emphasis has the potential to expand our thinking about the correlates of learning failure (e.g., Cooper & Speece, 1990; Cross & Paris, 1988; Speece & Cooper, 1990). Classification efforts in learning disabilities have centered primarily on the psychological level without appropriate attention to biological and ecological variables.

In summary, the perspective offered here is that classification is necessary in the study of learning disabilities. Whether rational or empirical, monothetic or polythetic, there is much to gain theoretically and practically by providing organization to our observations. We need not be dismayed that results of past classification research may have been narrowly conceived and that we are far from consensus on the levels and types of variables that may be most illuminating. The goal of every classification effort does not need to be the development of the ultimate taxonomy. Careful work within levels and within the separate domains that define levels, in addition to more ambitious investigations across levels, will lead to classification schemes that serve scientific and/or clinical aims. It is unlikely that the field will experience the "big bang" with respect to classification. Instead, slow and steady progress is a more reasonable goal.

Methodological Issues in Cluster Analysis

As stated, cluster analysis is a generic term for a group of statistical methods used to form homogeneous clusters of entities from a heterogeneous population. Statistically speaking, clusters should be compact and well-separated. The purpose of this section is to provide an overview of the more important considerations on conducting an empirical classification study. Details regarding application of techniques and associated studies in learning disabilities were provided by Speece (1990a) and will be only summarized here.

Stepping from the conceptual level of discussion on classification to the methodological level of empirical issues is much like wading in a cool, refreshing lake and encountering a severe drop-off. What seemed to be a reasonable, if not enjoyable activity is suddenly questioned and beating a hasty retreat looms as the only sensible option. This is because there are several steps in conducting a cluster analysis and, within each step, a variety of methods from which to choose. The interested researcher must be willing to accept a degree of uncertainty that is not typical in the use of most statistical techniques. If one can gain some level of comfort with the knowledge that results will not be in the form of a single significance test, then "taking the plunge" may be a satisfying experience.

At the outset, it is important to emphasize that clustering methods are not sterile tools to be applied blindly to a data set. One does not park theory and clinical insight at the cluster analysis door. As elaborated by DeLuca, Adams, and Rourke (1991), "what is required is the formulation of classification models based on the union or interrelationship of clinical insight and empirical method" (p. 46). For example, in a longitudinal analysis of behavioral subtypes of children with learning disabilities, McKinney and Speece (1986) combined clusters identified at year 1 of the study that appeared to have similar patterns of performance (problem behavior), but kept distinct the clusters that were clinically meaningful (e.g., attentional problems, pattern of withdrawn behavior). This interplay between rational and empirical perspectives on classification should promote both communication and predictive goals.

With some modifications, Skinner's (1981) delineation of theoretical framework, internal validity, and external validity as essential elements of a cluster analysis study remains a useful organizational device for discussion of method. Skinner (1981) included subject and variable selection and generation of hypotheses under theory formulation. Selection of an algorithm (how subjects are joined) and similarity measure (why subjects are joined) were added by Speece (1990a) as part of the theoretical framework. Internal validity (reliability) refers to procedures by which to judge the replicability of a cluster solution. External validity represents procedures designed to assess the meaningfulness of a reliable solution. Validity efforts operationalize the earlier discussion of the communicative and predictive value of a classification. That is, well-conceived validity studies assess the clinical or scientific importance of the clusters derived from the two preceding stages of theory formulation and reliability procedures.

Theory Formulation

Because a theory of learning disabilities does not exist at present, selection of subjects and variables in classification studies have not been theory-driven but rather guided by the results of previous research generally in single domains such as neuropsychological functioning (Lyon, Stewart, & Freedman, 1982), classroom behavior (Speece, McKinney, & Appelbaum, 1985), language (Feagans & Appelbaum, 1986), and reading (Morris, Blashfield, & Satz, 1986). The selection of variables in these investigations reflects an implicit theory that learning disabilities are primarily a within-child difficulty. The importance of viewing learning disabilities and classification in a broader context that includes environmental variables is gaining emphasis (Ellis, 1985; Kavale, 1990; Keogh, 1987b; Speece, 1993) and relevant investigations are beginning to appear (e.g., Cooper & Speece, 1990; Cross & Paris, 1988). This expansion of variables should add to the description of learning disabilities and provide necessary data from which a theory may evolve. Thus, there appears to be agreement among some researchers that cataloging child characteristics to the exclusion of recognizing contextual influences will result in a limited view of classification in learning disabilities. How to handle this complexity is another matter but it should become a more important ingredient in contemporary efforts to forge classification schemes.

The focus on within-child problems in past classification efforts has been accompanied by the use of school-defined samples of children with learning disabilities. The lack of uniformity in criteria for identification is well known and greatly limits the generalizability of any resulting classification. This is a methodological issue for all research purporting to study learning disabilities. Without more careful thought to the implications of subject selection and the design of strategies to overcome current limitations, the efforts that take place after subject selection will have little value.

In the formulation of a cluster analysis investigation, one must also make informed decisions regarding the similarity index for how clusters will be formed and the algorithm for defining why mergers are made. This discussion will focus only on hierarchical, agglomerative methods as they are the most widely used. Iterative techniques such as K means are also useful (see Aldenderfer & Blashfield, 1984; Jain & Dubes, 1988).

The issues surrounding decisions about algorithm and similarity measures have been discussed by Speece (1990a). Briefly, the choice in similarity measures is between a correlational metric that will judge entities as similar based on the shape of the multivariate profile, and a distance metric in which similarity is influenced not only by the shape but also the scatter (variance) and elevation (severity) of the profile (Skinner, 1978). Thus, a correlational index of similarity will likely cluster together children exhibiting learning disabilities and normal performance as it is not affected by levels of performance, only shape. This choice has implications for the type of classification system derived which should be based on one's perspective of the relationship between learning disabled and normal performance (Speece, 1990a).

There is even a wider array of algorithms to choose among (e.g., average linkage, complete linkage, Ward's method). The statistical literature provides guidance with respect to the joint performance of algorithms and similarity measures where "performance" is defined as the ability to recover true cluster structure (see Speece, 1990a for references). The point to be made here is that the user of cluster analysis techniques must make the methodological decisions by knowing the implications for the resulting cluster structure. Fisher, Anglin, Weisman, and Pulliam (1989) provided a convincing illustration of the problems associated with simply using default selections available on statistical packages.

Reliability

Reliability in a cluster analysis investigation is perhaps the most critical and most difficult to achieve. The task is to demonstrate that the clusters derived from the application of the algorithm and similarity measure are not random partitions. Unfortunately, there is not a straightforward method of testing the null hypothesis that no clusters exist. Jain and Dubes (1988) reviewed statistical methods of assessing nonrandom structure and provided some evaluation of effectiveness while Speece (1990a) provided a description of heuristic methods used to assess reliability of cluster structure.

An issue for consideration was previewed in the section on conceptual issues: Should clusters of children be conceived as discrete with clear boundaries in multivariate space or are clusters better viewed as overlapping with some shared characteristics? The latter view contains elements of both classical clustering (i.e., discrete groups) and a dimensional model (i.e., continuous distribution of variables). Some attempts at defining a "hybrid" approach to classification have been made and may be appropriate in learning disabilities (e.g., Fletcher, Morris, & Francis, 1991; Skinner, 1979). Relatedly, Jain and Dubes (1988) described fuzzy clustering in which entities can belong to more than one cluster and possess a grade of membership ranging from 0 to 1. They noted that fuzzy clustering has not been widely used in practical applications and it is not clear if there are any advantages over classical clustering. While these approaches possess some appeal in resolving the clusters versus continua debate, further articulation is needed with respect to assessing reliability. Current approaches are based on the assumption that clusters are compact and may not be applicable to other definitions of clusters.

Validity

At this stage of analysis the usefulness of the classification is examined. Procedures and variables selected are independent of the variables used for the cluster analysis and should be tied to the theoretical framework guiding the study. Earlier classification studies were notably short on validity information and it was not unusual to find studies that provided only a description of clusters without any validation evidence. Current efforts in learning disabilities are more sophisticated. Validation efforts are largely in the area of prediction (i.e., discerning cluster differences on external data sets such as achievement, observed classroom behavior) and not communication (i.e., assessing differential response to treatment by cluster). Future investigators must more carefully define the relationships between classification variables and validation procedures to avoid the post hoc flavor of past validation efforts (Speece, 1990a).

Conclusions

Classification in learning disabilities is a complex research agenda that demands a confluence of rational and empirical methods. Each contributes different information and serves, essentially, to keep the other approach "honest." How best to use the strengths of each approach to classification has yet to be determined but it appears indisputable that an organizational system is required and cannot be relegated to the back burner. Classification efforts in learning disabilities should continue to widen the scope of important variables to include biological and environmental domains. A particularly difficult issue is meeting the needs of both the scientific and applied communities. Both are valuable and it seems short-sighted to argue for the preeminence of one over the other. Instead, it may be useful to recognize that we are some distance from a classification scheme that serves either purpose. Following Keogh's advice (1987a), what is called for is careful explication of purpose and design of methods that best serve the stated purpose.

References

Aldenderfer, M.S. & Blashfield, R.K. (1984). *Cluster analysis*. Beverly Hills, CA: Sage Publications.

Blashfield, R.K. (1993). Taxonomic models for psychiatric classification. In G.R. Lyon, D.B. Gray, J.F. Kavanagh, & N.A. Krasnegor (Eds.), Better understanding learning disabilities: New views from research and their implications for education and public policies (pp. 17–26). Baltimore: Brooks. New York: Springer-Verlag.

Blashfield, R.K. & Aldenderfer, M.S. (1988). The methods and problems of cluster analysis. In J.R. Nesselroade & R.B. Cattell (Eds.), *Handbook of environmental psychology*, Vol. 1 (pp. 7–40). New York: Wiley.

Blashfield, R.K. & Draguns, J.G. (1976). Evaluative criteria for psychiatric classification. *Journal of Abnormal Psychology*, 85, 140–150.

Boder, E. (1973). Developmental dyslexia: A diagnostic approach based on three atypical reading-spelling patterns. *Developmental Medicine and Child Neurology*, 15, 663–687.

Bradley, L. & Bryant, P. (1983). Categorizing sounds and learning to read-A causal connection. *Nature*, 301, 419–421.

Cooper, D.H. & Speece, D.L. (1990). Maintaining at-risk children in regular education settings: Initial effects of individual differences and classroom environments. *Exceptional Children*, 57, 117–126.

Cromwell, R.L., Blashfield, R.K., & Strauss, J.S. (1975). Criteria for classification systems. In N. Hobbs (Ed.), *Issues in the classification of children*, Vol. 1 (pp. 4–25). San Francisco: Jossey-Bass.

Cross, D.R. & Paris, S.G. (1988). Developmental and instructional analyses of children's metacognition and reading comprehension. *Journal of Educational Psychology*, *80*, 131–142.

DeLuca, J.W., Adams, K.M., & Rourke, B.P. (1991). Methodological and statistical issues in cluster analysis. In B.P. Rourke (Ed.), *Neuropsychological validation of learning disability subtypes* (pp. 45–54). New York: Guilford.

Deno, S.L. (1990). Individual differences and individual difference: The essential difference of special education. *The Journal of Special Education*, *24*, 160–173.

Doris, J. (1986). Learning disabilities. In S.J. Ceci (Ed.), *Handbook of cognitive, social, and neuropsychological aspects of learning disabilities* (Vol. 1, pp. 3–53). Hillsdale, NJ: Erlbaum.

Duane, D.D. & Gray, D.B. (Eds.). (1991). *The reading brain: The biological basis of dyslexia*. Parkton, MD: York Press.

Ellis, A.W. (1985). The cognitive neurospychology of developmental (and acquired) dyslexia: A critical survey. *Cognitive Neuropsychology*, *2*, 169–205.

Feagans, L. & Appelbaum, M.I. (1986). Validation of language subtypes in learning disabled children. *Journal of Educational Psychology*, *78*, 358–364.

Fisher, D.G., Anglin, M.D., Weisman, C.P., & Pulliam, L. (1989). Replication problems of substance abuser MMPI cluster types. *Multivariate Behavioral Research*, *24*, 335–352.

Fletcher, J.M. & Morris, R. (1986). Classification of disabled learners: Beyond exclusionary definitions. In S.J. Ceci (Ed.), *Handbook of cognitive, social, and neuropsychological aspects of learning disabilities* (pp. 55–80). Hillsdale, NJ: Erlbaum.

Fletcher, J.M., Morris, R.D., & Francis, D.J. (1991). Methodological issues in the classification of attention-related disorders. *Journal of Learning Disabilities*, *24*, 72–77.

Forness, S.R. (1990). Subtyping in learning disabilities: Introduction to the issues. In H.L. Swanson & B.K. Keogh (Eds.), *Learning disabilities: Theoretical and research issues* (pp. 195–200). Hillsdale, NJ: Erlbaum.

Gould, S.J. (1989). *Wonderful life: The Burgess Shale and the nature of history*. New York: W.W. Norton.

Hagen, J.W. & Kamberelis, G. (1990). Cognition and academic performance in children with learning disabilities, low academic achievement, diabetes mellitus, and seizure disorders. In H.L. Swanson & B.K. Keogh (Eds.), *Learning disabilities: Theoretical and research issues* (pp. 299–314). Hillsdale, NJ: Erlbaum.

Hagen, J.W., Kamberelis, G., & Segal, S. (1991). A dimensional approach to cognition and academic performance in children with medical problems or learning difficulties. In L.V. Feagans, E.J. Short, & L.J. Meltzer (Eds.), *Subtypes of learning disabilities: Theoretical perspectives and research* (pp. 53–82). Hillsdale, NJ: Erlbaum.

Jain, A.K. & Dubes, R.C. (1988). *Algorithms for clustering data*. Englewood Cliffs, NJ: Prentice Hall.

Kavale, K.A. (1987). Theoretical quandaries in learning disabilities. In S. Vaughn & C.S. Bos (Eds.), *Research in learning disabilities: Issues and future directions* (pp. 19–33). Boston: College-Hill Press.

Kavale, K.A. (1990). A critical appraisal of empirical subtyping research in learning disabilities. In H.L. Swanson & B.K. Keogh (Eds.), *Learning disabilities: Theoretical and research issues* (pp. 215–230). Hillsdale, NJ: Erlbaum.

Kavale, K.A. & Forness, S.R. (1987). The far side of heterogeneity: A critical analysis of empirical subtyping research in learning disabilities. *Journal of Learning Disabilities, 20*, 374–382.

Keogh, B.K. (1987a). A shared attribute model of learning disabilities. In S. Vaughn & C.S. Bos (Eds.), *Research in learning disabilities* (pp. 3–18). Boston: College-Hill Press.

Keogh, B.K. (1987b). Learning disabilities: In defense of a construct. *Learning Disabilities Research, 3*, 4–9.

Keogh, B.K. (1990). Definitional assumptions and research issues. In H.L. Swanson & B.K. Keogh (Eds.), *Learning disabilities: Theoretical and research issues* (pp. 13–19). Hillsdale, NJ: Erlbaum.

Lyon, G.R., Stewart, N., & Freedman, D. (1982). Neuropsychological characteristics of empirically derived subgroups of learning disabled readers. *Journal of Clinical Neuropsychology, 4*, 343–365.

Lyon, G.R. & Risucci, D. (1988). Classification of learning disabilities. In K. Kavale (Ed.), *Learning disabilities: State of the art and practice* (pp. 44–70). San Diego: College-Hill Press.

McKinney, J.D. (1987). Response. In S. Vaughn & C.S. Bos (Eds.), *Research in learning disabilities* (pp. 64–66). Boston: College-Hill Press.

McKinney, J.D. & Speece, D.L. (1986). Academic consequences and longitudinal stability of behavioral subtypes of learning disabled children. *Journal of Educational Psychology, 78*, 365–372.

Meehl, P.E. (1954). *Clinical versus statistical prediction.* Minneapolis: University of Minnesota Press.

Morris, R., Blashfield, R.K., & Satz, P. (1986). Developmental classification of learning disabled children. *Journal of Clinical and Experimental Neuropsychology, 8*, 371–392.

Skinner, H.A. (1978). Differentiating the contribution of elevation, scatter, and shape in profile similarity. *Educational and Psychological Measurement, 38*, 297–308.

Skinner, H.A. (1979). Dimensions and clusters: A hybrid approach to classification. *Applied Psychological Measurement, 3*, 327–341.

Skinner, H.A. (1981). Toward the integration of classification theory and methods. *Journal of Abnormal Psychology, 20*, 68–87.

Skinner, H.A. & Blashfield, R.K. (1982). Increasing the impact of cluster analysis research: The case of psychiatric classification. *Journal of Consulting and Clinical Psychology, 50*, 727–735.

Speece, D.L. (1990a). Methodological issues in cluster analysis: How clusters become real. In H.L. Swanson & B.K. Keogh (Eds.), *Learning disabilities: Theoretical and research issues* (pp. 201–213). Hillsdale, NJ: Erlbaum.

Speece, D.L. (1990b). Aptitude-treatment interaction: Bad rap or bad idea? *The Journal of Special Education, 24*, 139–149.

Speece, D.L. (1993). Broadening the scope of classification research: Conceptual and ecological perspectives. In G.R. Lyon, D.B. Gray, J.F. Kavanagh, & N.A. Krasnegor (Eds.), Better understanding learning disabilities: New views from research and their implications for education and public policies (pp. 57–72). Baltimore: Brooks.

Speece, D.L. & Cooper, D.H. (1990). Ontogeny of school failure: Classification of first grade children. *American Educational Research Journal, 27*, 119–140.

Speece, D.L. & Cooper, D.H. (1991). Retreat, regroup or advance? An agenda for empirical classification research in learning disabilities. In L.V. Feagans, E.J. Short, & L.J. Meltzer (Eds.), *Subtypes of learning disabilities: Theoretical perspectives and research* (pp. 33–52). Hillsdale, NJ: Erlbaum.

Speece, D.L., McKinney, J.D., & Appelbaum, M.I. (1985). Classification and validation of behavioral subtypes of learning-disabled children. *Journal of Educational Psychology*, *77*, 67–77.

Stanovich, K.E. (1989). Various varying views on variation. *Journal of Learning Disabilities*, *22*, 366–369.

Torgesen, J.K. (1982). The use of rationally defined subgroups in research on learning disabilities. In J.P. Das, R.F. Mulcahy, & A.E. wall (Eds.), *Theory and research in learning disabilities* (pp. 111–131). New York: Plenum Press.

Torgesen, J.K. (1991). Subtypes as prototypes: Extended studies of rationally defined extreme groups. In L.V. Feagans, E.J. Short, & L.J. Meltzer (Eds.), *Subtypes of learning disabilities: Theoretical perspectives and research* (pp. 229–246). Hillsdale, NJ: Erlbaum.

Torgesen, J.K. & Houck, D.G. (1980). Processing deficiencies in learning disabled children who perform poorly on the digit span task. *Journal of Educational Psychology*, *72*, 141–160.

Torgesen, J.K., Rashotte, C.A., Greenstein, J., & Portes, P. (1991). Further studies of learning disabled children with severe performance problems on the digit span test. *Learning Disabilities Research & Practice*, *6*, 134–144.

5
A Screening Test Built of Cognitive Bricks: Identification of Young LD Children

MARCIA STRONG SCOTT AND RUTH PEROU

Introduction

The need for early identification of children with learning disabilities (LD) is being driven by two factors. The first is Public Law 99-457, The Education of the Handicapped Act Amendments of 1986. The passage of this act changed the status of the states' position with respect to the provision of special educational services for preschool handicapped children. Under P.L. 94-142, the states were encouraged to offer those services under enabling legislation. P.L. 99-457 changed that component of the law from enabling to mandated legislation; the states were now legally obliged to provide educational services to all handicapped preschoolers.

The second factor is the documented belief that the educational outcome of children with learning disabilities is enhanced if an intervention is begun earlier rather than later (e.g., Muehl & Forell, 1973; Strag, 1972). In a recent publication (The Infant Health and Development Program, 1990), results were reported from the most methodologically rigorous clinical trial of the impact of an early intervention program on infants "at risk" for a poor outcome because of their low birth-weight and prematurity. Since Carran and Scott (1989) have shown that low-birth-weight infants are at elevated risk for being classified as learning disabled in grade school, these results are relevant for evaluating the potential impact of early intervention on the prevalence of learning disabilities. A positive effect of the educational intervention begun at age 1, on the cognitive performance of those children at age 3, was clearly demonstrated. Also documented was the presence of significantly fewer behavior problems in the intervention group as assessed by the Child Behavior Checklist for ages 2 to 3 years (Achenbach, Edelbrock, & Howell, 1987). In another study of the same sample (Scott, Hogan, & Bauer, 1991), the intervention group also demonstrated less disruptive behavior and more positive social skills when these were assessed with a new measure of social behavior, the Adaptive Social Behavior Inventory (Hogan, Scott, & Bauer, 1991). Lazar and Darlington (1982) reported the results of analyses on pooled data from 12 early childhood education programs for low-income children, a condition that would put those children at elevated risk for poor educational outcomes, compared to children from financially more advantageous families. The data showed that children who had participated in the interventions were half as likely as control children to be assigned to special education classes. Positive effects on educational measures, as well as on child and maternal attitudes toward schooling, were also observed.

Conceptually, the generality of the positive effects of early intervention on both cognitive and social measures to young children with learning disabilities is self-evident. By definition, LD children must have specific cognitive impairments, and many also demonstrate social deficiencies and/or inappropriate behavior (see Vaughn & Hogan, 1990 for a recent review). Recently, Morrison, Mantzicopoulos and Carte (1989) reported data on a sample of kindergarten children considered to be "at risk" for developing learning difficulties based on scores below the 33rd percentile on at least four of the nine valid SEARCH subtests (Silver & Hagin, 1981). That subset of "at-risk" children who showed inadequate preacademic reading skills were also rated as having more behavior problems. Vaughn, Hogan, Kouzekanani and Shapiro (1990) have also reported that a sample of children who were subsequently identified as learning disabled demonstrated social difficulties prior to identification. It is reasonable to conclude that data on the positive impact of early intervention on both the cognitive and social behavior of young at-risk children has high relevance for assessing the potential remediational effect of an early intervention program on the subsequent prevalence of children with learning disabilities, and/or the breadth of their academic difficulties.

Although the impact of these data support the conclusion cited more than 10 years ago by Reynolds and Clark (1983), that compensatory education will have the greatest possibility of success if provided during the early years of life, "most children with reading and learning problems are not referred for diagnostic evaluations until approximately 10 years of age, when they are maturationally less ready and have already been exposed to years of academic failure" (Satz & Fletcher, 1988). In a recent publication of national data covering the 1986–1987 school year, reported in the *Tenth Annual Report to Congress on the Implementation of The Education of the Handicapped Act* (cited in Gerber & Levine-Donnerstein, 1989), it was reported that of all the children between 3 and 21 who received special education services as LD students under the Education of the Handicapped Act during that school year, only about 1% were served during the preschool years. This data is particularly damning since there appears to be a great deal of support for providing preschool programs. Data collected at approximately the same time (Esterly & Griffin, 1987), through a survey sent to learning disabilities consultants in the 50 state departments of education, indicated that a majority (68%) of the states responding (44%) did provide services for preschool children with learning disabilities. Yet, the late identification of most LD children precludes their exposure to the remediating effects of an early intervention program. Even when data reflect students living in a major urban city, where extensive preschool screening is carried out and a large preschool educational program is in place, the late identification of LD children is still being reported (Scott, Urbano, & Boussy, 1991).

The implementation of P.L. 99-457 is being hindered by the limitations of current screening tests. Many questions have been raised about the psychometric properties of early screening instruments (e.g., Bracken, 1987; Lichtenstein & Ireton, 1984; Lindsay & Wedell, 1982; Meisels, 1987) and when Meisels (1989) reviewed the literature evaluating the Denver Developmental Screening Test, he concluded that this most widely used of all screening instruments failed to identify large numbers of mildly impaired at-risk children. That is, the test's sensitivity, the proportion of all risk children identified as children "at risk" by their test scores, was too low. These documented deficiencies in the basic psychometric properties of many of the screening tests currently in use is particularly disturbing since an implication of P.L. 99-457 is that "as services for preschoolers with handicaps increase, legal challenges to the validity of early childhood measures are also likely to increase" (Sheehan, 1989). Screening tests used to identify children as needing early intervention must pass rigorous psychometric investigations if they are to be used with confidence by those agencies charged with identifying young handicapped children.

Development of a Cognitive Screening Test: Initial Results

An obvious implication of (a) the availability of services, (b) the demonstrated and implied impact of early intervention for LD children, and (c) the psychometric deficiencies of many available screening tests, is the need to develop a new screening test that is psychometrically sound and more effective than those in current use. Preliminary data on the development of a cognitive screening test, designed to improve upon the detection rate of young LD children, will be presented in this chapter.[1] The rationale for using a cognitive approach is discussed in detail in Greenfield and Scott (1985).

---

[1] The aim of the screening test is to detect young children who will later be identified as either learning disabled or mildly retarded. Only data pertaining to detection of learning disabilities will be reported here even though some studies cited include a mildly retarded group.

Scott and Greenfield began this project by deciding that selecting test components through empirical evaluations of their ability to discriminate between normally achieving students and those already classified as learning disabled, as well as a few other characteristics, would increase the probability that any screening test that included these preselected and evaluated tasks would identify young children with learning disabilities more effectively than currently available screening tests. Demonstrated predictive validity for the test components should result in predictive validity for the total test, and as Jones and Appelbaum (1989) have pointed out, "it is unlikely that a test, no matter how firm its construct validity, will go unchallenged if it cannot also be shown to predict to a desired outcome." Based on preliminary data collected over several years, Scott (PI) and Greenfield (Co PI) were awarded a 5-year grant from the National Institute of Child Health and Human Development (July 1, 1987 to June 30, 1992). A number of cognitive tasks which assessed informational areas or processes reported to be impaired in children with learning disabilities have been evaluated. The children in the studies were 6, 7, or 8 years of age, with a few exceptions. Both males and females were included in each study, although there were always more males, and all three major ethnic groups residing in Miami were represented, that is, Black/non-Hispanic (non-Latin Black), White/non-Hispanic (non-Latin White), and White/Hispanic (Latin White). Each student with learning disabilities was matched to a normally achieving (NA) student on age, sex and ethnicity. The NA match nearly always came from the same school the exceptional student was attending.

Multiple Oddity Variations Task

The first NA versus LD contrast data was reported in Scott, Greenfield, and Partridge (1991), in which the two groups were compared on their ability to detect the odd stimulus when the oddity relation was defined in a number of different ways. Following training on standard oddity problems, in which three pictures (two identical and one different) made up each oddity array, the students' accuracy in selecting the odd picture in eight different oddity variations was assessed. Each variation was represented by six cards. The odd picture in each of the variations: was a different type of object; was identical to two other line drawings except that one element was missing; was a different cartoon character or the same cartoon character in a different pose; was a different color and/or form and/or size; was placed in a different orientation than the other two pictures; was not related to the other two pictures which formed an association; had a different number of components; or was from a different taxonomic category than the other two pictures. Both groups showed very high accuracy levels based on the number of correct oddity selections out of six. The slight, albeit consistent, performance differences favoring the NA group were significant for five of the eight oddity types.

The presence of group differences does not allow one to infer how well the task might serve to identify LD children. The best way to evaluate the potential utility of any of the tasks to detect LD children, is to see how well the task does when the students' task performance is used to make individual student classificational decisions (e.g., Lichtenstein, 1981; Lichtenstein & Ireton, 1984; Meisels, 1989; Satz & Fletcher, 1988). Not surprisingly, given the small differences in accuracy observed, when performance on the two oddity types, selected by a discriminant function analysis as best separating the two groups (taxonomic and missing element), was used to predict school classification, only 49% of the LD children were correctly identified as such. This value represents the sensitivity (SN) of the task. In contrast, the percentage of NA children who were correctly identified as NA based on their oddity performance was high (81%). This value represents the specificity (SP) of the task. Both SN and SP were first described by Yerushalmy (1947) and are common measures for examining the utility of tests. Since even the two oddity types that best segregated the NA and LD groups identified so few of the LD students as LD, we inferred from these data that the oddity types evaluated in this study would not contribute towards the accurate differentiation of young LD from normal children and, therefore, should not be included in the screening test.

Taxonomic Information Task

Since the near ceiling-level of performance might well have obscured potential group differences, we decided that the next task examined should not have a predetermined limit on the number of correct responses. The task selected for evaluation was one we called the taxonomic information task. It assessed the students' ability to identify categories and exemplars, and contrast exemplars from those categories in terms of their similarities and differences (Scott & Greenfield, 1991). It was on the latter measures, where no external limit existed on the number of correct responses possible, that we believed group differences would be most apparent. Thirty-four pairs of NA and LD students were pretrained by using object class stimuli (telephones and purses), a task deemed easy enough to both illustrate, and evoke responses appropriate to, the task demands. The 12 categories probed were: animals, body parts, fruit, furniture, people, tools, musical instruments, vegetables, clothing, jewelry, vehicles, and toys. Although many descriptors were generated, the NA and LD groups did not differ significantly on either the number of same descriptors generated (means = 14.1 vs. 10.6) or the number of different descriptors generated (means = 20.2 vs. 15.6). However, since the greatest group separation occurred for the number of differences measure, that was used to predict educational classification using a discriminant function analysis. Once again, however, more than half of the LD students were incorrectly identified as NA. The SN was only 47% and the SP was only 59%. The overlap between the two groups was too great to permit accurate individual student classification. Even when selecting the best of the categories within this measure, values for SN (65%) and SP (53%) were still inadequate. Evaluating this task's potential contribution to the screening test by using a discriminant function analysis to classify the students on a student-by-student basis, leads to the same conclusion as was made for the oddity variations task; do not include as a component in the test because the SN and SP are too low. What was present in these data, however, was the finding that 8 of the 34 LD students, which represented 24% of the sample tested, generated fewer different descriptors than any of the NA students. At that time, we offered the tentative conclusion that this task might be sensitive to a subgroup of LD students. However, nothing further was made of this finding.

Reflections and Implications

The results of these two studies were consistent with a position taken by Ceci and Baker (1989), who have argued that deficiencies in cognitive processing skills are not the major impairment of most LD students. That is, while the cognitive processing skills of many LD students may not be as good as those of their NA peers, these children are not sufficiently impaired to account for the severe academic difficulties they experience. Rather, it is deficiencies of some informational domains that create the major problem for this group. In the authors' words, many LD children may have "poorly elaborated knowledge representations in the pertinent domains." How well cognitive processes can be used will interact with the quality of the knowledge domain. When operating on well-organized, elaborated domains these less efficient cognitive processes will work at their maximum level, but when operating on less well-structured domains they will be even less efficient (Ceci, 1989).

This position was explored post hoc by Scott and Greenfield (1992), who concluded that the data from the taxonomic information task supported the Ceci and Baker (1989) position generally, but that the taxonomic knowledge base did not differentiate between the NA and LD group in this study because the categories could be shown to be adequately represented in normal preschoolers. The depth of information generated was not sufficiently demanding to discriminate between the two groups. The poor-performing LD outliers were considered to be an exception to this conclusion.

Our next step was to explore this position systematically in an a priori fashion. Discovering the limits of the Ceci and Baker position would assist us in discovering those tasks that might best identify young LD children. In addition, another factor had come to our attention regarding when to expect group differences: specifically, the interactive theory of learning disabilities (e.g., Lipson & Wixson, 1986), which alerted us to the mediating effects of such variables as task, materials, teacher or experimenter, and setting (Mosenthal, 1982; Simmons & Kameenui, 1990). Highly structured tasks, for example, where the responses are provided and the responders need only make an identification, are predicted to be associated with minimal NA versus LD group differences. In contrast, if little external support is provided, as when students are asked to produce responses, then the groups should be more discrepant. Clearly, other things being equal, we should not expect significant group differences if we use tasks that provide choices, but group differences should be present if we use tasks where the students have to generate responses. However, this must be added to what we know from the Ceci and Baker (1989) position. When we do that, we can say that reduced group differences should be associated with identification tasks; tasks where there are only few choices and these are provided, tasks making no demands on informational domains, and tasks where the informational domain or modality tapped is not impaired in LD students. On the other hand, a production task, which requires knowledge in a domain known to be deficient in many LD children, should result in large group differences. The impact of these variables was examined systematically in a series of studies.

Letter-Group Oddity Task

In the first study of the impact of mediating variables on NA and LD group differences, we compared the performance of these two groups on an oddity task that was highly structured and required systematic stimulus processing skills, but did not require information from any semantic domain. Under these conditions, no or minimal group differences were predicted. Additionally, the possibility of a ceiling effect was again present because there was an externally set limit on the number of correct selections.

The students were required to select the odd letter-group. For the first oddity problems presented, the stimulus arrays consisted of three letters; two were identical and one was different. For the other problems, the oddity arrays consisted of groups of two, three, four, five, six, or seven letters where the odd letter-group differed from the two identical letter-groups by only one letter. The number of letters per group was designated as the *level* and there were six cards at each level. An example of one of the six cards from Level 1 is *i* versus *r* versus *r*, from Level 3 is *yjt* versus *ijt* versus *ijt*, and from Level 7 is *ytsaonx* versus *ytsaoux* versus *ytsaoux*. The cards were presented in the order of Level 1 through 7. At the first level where more than one error was committed, the game was stopped. This was called the failure level and was the major dependent measure. The details are presented in Scott, Perou, Greenfield, Partridge, and Swanson (1993).

It should be noted that we thought this task would provide a strong test of the potential importance of processing skills when evaluating potential NA and LD group differences. Towards the latter part of the series, if not before, correct choices demanded very systematic, orderly comparisons on a letter-by-letter or some other grouping basis. The utilization of careful scanning and comparisons would represent the voluntary application of one or more strategic processing skills. Accurate performance could not occur if strategic processing skills were not being used. If LD children did have significantly impaired processing skills, contrary to the position of Ceci and Baker (1989), then group differences should be observed. Frankly, looking at the stimuli for the higher levels, we could not imagine that anyone could maintain a high accuracy level unless they attended very carefully to the stimuli and systematically compared the three arrays. This is not a statement that one expects to use to describe the behavior of LD children.

The groups were compared on two dependent measures. These were the failure level and the level at which the first error was committed. As predicted, the groups were very similar in their oddity performance. The means for the 33 pairs making up the NA and LD groups on the failure level measure were 7.2 ($SD = 1.6$) versus 6.7 ($SD = 1.8$), and on the level of first error measure the means were 5.2 ($SD = 1.8$) versus 4.6 ($SD = 2.1$). Not unexpectedly, given the similarity in performance, an overall MANOVA of groups was not significant, $p > .40$. Although about twice as many LD as NA students failed the task (42% vs. 24%), more than half of the students in both groups never failed, never made more than 1 out of 6 errors. It was amazing to us that most of the LD group were able to maintain near-perfect performance on the latter levels of this task.

The children's failure level score was used in a discriminant function analysis to categorize the students into an NA or LD classification. As was expected, given the extent of the overlap between the groups, individual classification was not very accurate for either group although the SP (76%) was much better than the SN (36%). About two-thirds of the LD sample was misclassified as NA based on the failure level measure.

For this chapter we examined the accuracy with which the students could be classified on an individual basis. The children's failure level score etc.

When analyzing the data from the taxonomic information task, we found that there were some low-performing LD outlyers, whose scores were worse than all of the NA students. Since ultimately we want to be able to detect low-performing children on the screening test, that is, children achieving scores below a specified cutoff score, we decided to introduce a systematic exploration of all our data in terms of a frequency distribution of the number of LD and NA students achieving each of the scores obtained on a given task.[2] In this manner, if there were a subgroup of low-performing students they would be detected. Such a group would not necessarily come to light if linear models were the only type of analyses applied to the data. In this particular instance, no low-performing LD outliers were identified. The first outlier students failed at Level 2 (1 LD and 1 NA), the next at Level 3 (1 LD and 1 NA) and then 2 LD students failed at Level 4.

In general, these results support the minimal role Ceci and Baker (1989) have assigned to cognitive processing skills as a causal factor in the impaired, albeit specifically impaired, learning performance typically associated with LD students. Also supported is the expectation that there will be a reduction or minimizing of group differences associated with highly structured tasks that require only identification responses. With respect to the potential of this task to contribute towards more effective identification of LD children, results from the distribution of students by failure level lead to the conclusion that this task will not help to identify LD children and should not, therefore, be included as a component of the screening test.

Dot Matrix Oddity and Rhyme Oddity Tasks

The role of these mediating variables was further tested using two different oddity tasks. Both were highly structured, requiring only the identification of the appropriate stimulus from three choices available. However, one of them made no demands on any knowledge base while for the second, identification of the odd stimulus required knowledge of phonological similarities and differences, an informational domain known to be deficient among many LD students (e.g., Kamhi & Catts, 1896; Kamhi, Catts, Mauer, Apel, & Gentry, 1988; Siegel & Ryan, 1984). Basically, these two studies looked at the impact of an impaired informational domain within a highly structured task.

Thirty-four matched LD and NA pairs were pretrained on standard oddity problems displayed on nine, 5 in. × 13¼ in. black posterboard cards, consisting of two identical and one different picture. They were subsequently presented two different oddity tasks. This pair of oddity tasks was presented in one session and a different set of paired tasks was presented in a second session. The "no informational demand" oddity task consisted of three types of dot matrix oddity problems, each represented by seven, 5 in. × 13 in. black cards. The first set of 7 dot matrix

---

[2] Hereafter, when the data are examined using the distribution of the number of students obtaining each of the observed values of the dependent measure, we will simply refer to this as using a frequency distribution technique.

problems were the first 7 cards presented in the 21-card series. Displayed on these cards were 3 in. × 3 in. matrices, divided into nine 1 in. squares in which the odd matrix had *two* more, or fewer, red dots. The contrasts on the seven cards were 1 versus 3 dots, 2 versus 4 dots, . . . up to 7 versus 9 dots. Shown in Table 5.1 is an example of the 1 versus 3 dots contrast. The particular squares in which the dots were placed were the same across the three matrices, except that for the larger pattern, two additional squares were filled. Cards 8 through 14 in the dot matrix series were similarly constructed except that the number of dots in the smaller and larger dot patterns differed by only *one*. The contrasts were 1 versus 2, 2 versus 3, . . . up to 7 versus 8. The 6 versus 7 contrast is illustrated in Table 5.1.

TABLE 5.1. Examples of stimulus cards for the dot matrix and rhyme oddity tasks.

Cards	Dot matrix oddity		

Card	Rhyme oddity		
2	fox	*tank*	box
6	carrot	parrot	*ladder*
12	*watch*	house	mouse

For the final seven cards presented, 15–21, all three matrices had the *same number of dots*, that is, 2, 3, 4, . . . 8, but they were placed in a *different pattern*. Once the squares-to-be-filled for one pattern on a card was determined, the squares-to-be-filled for the second pattern were selected from those not used in the first pattern. When the number of squares filled reached five, then the squares-to-be-filled for the second pattern were selected so as to minimize the overlap of specific squares filled. The 5-dot pattern difference card is shown in Table 5.1.

For the rhyme oddity task, the children were shown twelve, 12¼ in. × 4 in. light-blue cards. On each card, three meaningful pictures were displayed. Two of them had names which rhymed while the third did not. The odd stimulus was the nonrhyming picture. Three examples are shown in Table 5.1. The experimenter named each of the pictures before the student made his/her selection.

As the first dot matrix card was presented, the experimenter pointed out the three matrices and asked the student to point to the different one. As the first rhyme oddity card was presented, the experimenter named each of the pictures and said, "I will name each of these pictures for you. Listen carefully and point to the picture whose name does not sound the same as the other two." The experimenter probed with, "Point to the one that doesn't sound the same, the one that has the different sounding name."

As predicted, there were minimal differences between the NA and LD groups on the dot matrixoddity task, means = 19.6 correct versus 19.1 correct choices, and the group effect was not reliable, $p > .05$. A discriminant function analysis using the same dependent measure resulted in correctly identifying only 38% of the LD sample (SN) and 65% of the NA group (SP). These values would imply exclusion of this task from the screening test. However, shown in Table 5.2 are the data organized using a frequency distribution technique. Using a cutoff score of ≤ 14, 3 LD students and 1 NA student could be described as low-performing outliers. The 3 LD children averaged 57% correct choices (range = 48% to 67%) and the NA student was correct only 62% of the time. The next lowest score was 17 (81% correct), a score achieved by 4 NA and 4 LD students. With these 3 LD students excluded from the LD group, the remaining 31 students averaged 94% correct choices as did the 33 NA students when the single NA outlier was excluded. When evaluated this way, the dot matrix task is selecting a small number of low-performing LD students who perform differently than 97% of the NA sample. Consistent with predictions, this highly structured task with no informational demands was associated with minimal group differences. Although we would reject this task as a component of the screening test based on the results of the discriminant function analysis, using the frequency technique, 3 low-performing LD outliers were identified. Perhaps this task will contribute towards more effective identification of LD children. Different ways of evaluating the task may lead to different conclusions.

TABLE 5.2. Frequency distribution of the number of students obtaining each of the observed scores as a function of task and group.

	Dot matrix oddity			Rhyme oddity	
	NA	LD		NA	LD
10	0	1	4	0	3
12	0	1	6	0	1
13	1	0	7	1	1
14	0	1	8	1	4
17	4	4	9	1	0
18	3	0	10	2	3
19	4	6	11	7	6
20	8	10	12	22	16
21	14	11		34	34
	34	34			

When knowledge from an informational base known to be impaired in many LD students was grafted onto this highly structured task in the rhyme oddity problems, the NA group averaged 11 out of 12 correct choices and the LD group 10 out of 12 correct selections. This was associated with a significant effect of group, $F(1, 66) = 5.80; p < .02$. This significant group effect, however, was not associated with very accurate classification of the LD students, SN = 35%, although few NA students were misclassified, SP = 85%. Again, these results would lead one to exclude this task from further consideration as a test component. However, when using a frequency distribution method of evaluation (see Table 5.2), 26% of this LD sample and only 6% of the NA sample had 8 or fewer correct selections. The mean percent correct for these 9 LD students was 53%, and the mean for the 2 NA students was a similar 62%. With these students excluded, both the remaining NA students (mean = 96%) and the remaining LD students (mean = 96%) averaged near-perfect performance. Using this method of task evaluation, we would tentatively conclude that this task should be included in the test. Again, different methods of evaluation have yielded different conclusions.

Since the same students were administered both tasks, we examined the specific students classified as low-performing outliers to see if the same children were identified on both tasks. Two of the 3 LD students identified as low performing on the dot matrix task were also identified as low performing on the rhyme oddity task. These two had scores on the rhyme oddity task of 4 and 6, two of the lowest scores included in the cutoff which was set at ≤ 8. Perhaps these represent students whose rhyme oddity performance is also impaired by significantly deficient cognitive processing skills.

Collectively, these data support the position described by Ceci and Baker (1989) who emphasized knowledge domains as the more critical variable to explain the academic performance of most LD children. The data from the dot matrix oddity task indicate that there may well be some LD children who show significant deficiencies in processing skills, at least when applied to perceptually similar stimuli. The fact that low-performing outliers were not evident in the letter-group oddity task, which was also a perceptually based oddity task, suggests that it is difficult to pick these few students out when compared to their NA peers.

Rhyme Generation Task

On this next task, we examined group separation when high performance demanded knowledge in a domain known to be impaired in many LD children. This time, however, phonological knowledge was not embedded in a highly structured task, as was true for the rhyme oddity task, but was accessed using a production task. This should allow for greater group differences to emerge.

The 33 NA and LD pairs who were administered the letter-group oddity task were also presented three other tasks. The oddity task was paired with a rhyme generation task, which we will report at this time. The other paired tasks were a taxonomic generation task and a picture recall task. They will be discussed after this.

The details of this comparison are presented in Scott, Perou Greenfield, and Swanson (in press). Essentially, the children were asked to generate as many real and/or fake words as they could that rhymed with each of four probes (*fan*, *hat*, *mouse*, and *steam*), following pretraining on the word *book*. Appropriate examples of both types of rhymes were provided by the experimenter during the pretraining. The children were required to generate rhymes to the next word in the four-probe series only after indicating that no more rhymes could be generated to the current probe. The NA students' performance was compared in terms of the number of real rhymes generated, the number of fake rhymes generated, the number of errors (nonrhyming words) generated, and a penalty measure which was computed by deducting the number of error made to a given probe from the number of real rhymes generated to that probe. Although the greatest group separation was achieved with this last measure, NA mean = 10.9, LD mean = 3.6, the NA group also generated more real words (13.5 vs. 8.8) and more fake words (9.8 vs. 5.5), while making fewer errors (2.6 vs. 5.2) than the LD group.

Some additional analyses were computed for this chapter. The penalty measure was associated with the greatest group separation and it incorporates two aspects of good rhyming skills, namely the generation of phonologically correct rhymes and the generation of few or no phonologically inaccurate responses. Therefore, it was this measure for all four probes that was used in a stepwise discriminant function. Only *hat* was selected for inclusion in the discriminant function analysis. The resulting classifications were the most accurate we have seen to this point. The SN was 70% and the SP was 73%. While these values are not as high as is desirable for a test, when reflecting the potential contribution from one of several components they would seem to be acceptable. Thus, for the first time when evaluating a task using a discriminant function analysis, we would conclude that this task should be part of the screening test. A similar conclusion was reached when using the frequency method. After looking at each of the probes on an individual basis, it was determined that combining the penalty scores for two probes, *hat* and *mouse*, resulted in the best differentiation of low-performing LD outliers. Twelve LD students (36% of the sample) demonstrated poorer rhyming skills than *all* of the NA students.

These data strongly support the Ceci and Baker (1989) position about the importance of knowledge domain in understanding the variable performance of LD children, and the role of task as a mediating variable from an interactionist perspective. When an impaired knowledge domain (phonological knowledge) was combined with a production task with no externally imposed limitations on the number of responses, the groups were quite discrepant.

Taxonomic Generation Task

For this task, we combined a production task, which should tend to increase group separation, with a varied array of information domains. By using many different semantic categories, it was expected that for some categories, deficiencies in some of the students would be present and lead to reduced performance levels when compared to their NA peers. It was deemed possible that different students might have impaired knowledge domains for different semantic categories.

The 33 pairs of NA and LD students were presented a series of 10 cards, on each of which appeared two exemplars from a given taxonomic category, e.g. *elephant* and *giraffe*. The 10 categories probed were: *animals*, fruit, *clothing*, *toys*, *vegetables*, *tools*, *sports*, *furniture*, *people*, and *transportation*. The students were pretrained using the categories *body parts* and *jewelry* and the experimenter provided or added correct examples. As each category card was presented, the student was asked to name the two pictures and the experimenter corrected any responses that were not categorically accurate. If, for example, a child gave the name "hippo" to the stimulus "elephant" it was not corrected, although it was scored as an incorrect identification, because as long as it was a legitimate category exemplar, the sense of the task demand was maintained without having to tell the child that his/her response was wrong. After the exemplars on each card were identified, the experimenter said, "Tell me as many things as you can that belong to the same family as the (first exemplar) and the (second exemplar)." The NA and LD groups did not differ significantly on the total number of taxonomic exemplars generated (means = 23.2 vs. 20.9), or the number of incorrect items generated (means = 3.9 vs. 4.2). When these two measures were combined into a penalty score for each category, the LD and NA groups were still not significantly different (means = 16.8 vs. 19.2 respectively). When the groups were compared on separate MANOVAs for each of the three dependent measures, with scores on each of the 10 categories serving as 10 correlated dependent measures for each analysis, there were no significant effects. Apparently, the performance of the students in the two groups overlap considerably on each of the categories, precluding the detection of significant group differences. It might, however, be possible to predict individual student classification by combining several categories. We computed a stepwise discriminant function analysis using the students' penalty measure for each of the 10 categories. The penalty measure was used because it reflected both accurate generation of within-category exemplars and the nongeneration of inappropriate responses. Using just four categories, *transportation*, *people*, *fruit*, and *tools*, 70% of the LD sample (SN) and 73% of the NA group (SP) were correctly identified. As one of several task components, these values suggest that we should include this task in the screening test.

A similar conclusion was reached when using the frequency technique. It was determined that combining penalty scores on *clothing*, *transportation*, and *furniture*, and using a cutoff score of ≤ +3, resulted in the isolation of 11-low performing LD children (33% of the sample) and only 2 NA students (6% of the NA sample). These data are shown in Table 5.3. Even when there were no significant group differences, individual student scores enabled sufficiently accurate classification (discriminate function analysis) and permitted the isolation of a number of low-performing LD students (frequency method) to support its inclusion in a screening test. As was found for the rhyme generation task, the two methods of task evaluation led to the same conclusion. The use of a production task in this instance was not associated with increased group differences. When there is the potential for a great deal of individual student variability, for example, student differences in strengths and weaknesses for particular categories, perhaps the same variables that foster group differences will maximize within-group individual differences that may swamp overall mean differences between the groups. If no or only a few students have impaired informational bases on any given category, then on a category-by-category basis, group differences will also be absent. If such is the case, then methods that compare groups within an individual student framework (discriminant function, frequency technique) will be better suited for determining potential group differences.

TABLE 5.3. Frequency distribution of the number of students obtaining each of the observed scores as a function of task and group. (Categories = clothing, transportation, and furniture).

	Taxonomic generation				Picture recall	
	NA	LD			NA	LD
−1	0	1		3	0	1
0	0	1		4	1	6
+1	1	2		5	16	20
+2	1	3		6	15	5
+3	0	4		7	1	1
+4	5	2			33	33
+5	6	2				
+6	7	7				
+7	2	5				
+8	5	2				
+9	1	1				
+10	3	1				
+11	2	0				
+12	0	1				
+13	0	1				
	33	33				

Picture Recall Task

This free recall task was the fourth in the four-task battery. The students were presented a series of cards on which were displayed from 1 to 8 unrelated meaningful pictures. The number of pictures on a card was called the level. Each level was represented by two cards. The cards were presented sequentially starting with Level 1 and continuing until the student failed to recall one or more of the just-seen pictures on both cards representing a given level. At that time, no further cards were presented. This level was called the failure level. The pictures were displayed in one or two rows of no more than four pictures. As each card was presented, the experimenter named each at a rate of 1 per second in a sequence that went from left to right and from top to bottom. After the last picture was named, the card was turned down and the student was asked to recall as many of the pictures as he or she could. Time for the free recall of the pictures on a given card was ended after a probe, "Can you remember any more," elicited no further responses over the next 30 seconds or when the student said that he/she could not remember any more.

There are many studies that report poorer memory performance for LD children and this is typically related to deficiencies in one or more of several memory processing skills (e.g., Bauer, 1982; Ceci, 1984; Howe, O'Sullivan, Brainerd, & Kingma, 1989; Simpson & Lorsbach, 1983;

Swanson, 1990). If lower memory performance is related to memory processing variables, then according to Ceci and Baker (1989), minimal group differences would be expected because processing skills are purported to be of less importance in understanding the dramatically varied academic performance of LD children, perhaps because they reach levels where they produce significant impairment in only a small proportion of LD students. The to-be-remembered material consisted of simple meaningful items. These object class exemplars should be in the long-term memory base of children at this age. This fact should also tend to reduce group differences. Although the number of responses are limited, they must be produced, not merely identified, as would occur with a recognition task, and they must be only those that appeared on the "just seen" card. Considering the dependency on processing skills and the simplicity of the stimulus material, we would predict small group differences. The production component of the task, however, should allow for individual differences in memory processing skills to be expressed. If significantly impaired processing skills are less prevalent than, for example, impaired phonological knowledge in a heterogeneous sample of LD students, then perhaps fewer low-performing outliers will be identified. This subset of students might not be enough in number, or produce sufficiently large absolute differences, to be reflected in significant mean differences between the groups.

The mean failure level for the NA group was only slightly higher than that for the LD group (means = 5.5 vs. 5.0). This slight difference is consistent with expectation. However, it was a significant difference. When failure level was entered into a discriminant function, a high level of SN was observed (82%) but the SP was poor (48%). Based on the extremely poor SP, we would exclude this task from further consideration. However, using a frequency technique (see Table 5.3), it can be seen that 7 out of 33 (21%) of the LD sample and only 1 NA student (3%) would be described as low-performing outliers using as a cutoff of a failure level ≤4.

Classification Using Multiple Tasks

Since our aim is to pool the best components from the tasks evaluated, we wanted to see how well we could discriminate those children requiring services from those not requiring services if the four tasks presented together, two at each sessim, served as a mini-cognitive battery. While the results would not reflect the best we hope to do, they would indicate if this method for test development was providing useful data. These four tasks were: letter group oddity; rhyme generation; taxonomic generation; and picture recall.

We derived a total battery score by adding up the children's scores on the four tasks, or the best components of those tasks, this is, for

TABLE 5.4. Frequency distribution of the number of students obtaining each of the observed total scores as a function of group and tasks included.

Total score Summed over All four tasks			Total score excluding Oddity task		
	LD	NA		LD	NA
4	1	0	−2	1	0
6	1	0	+1	2	0
7	1	0	+4	2	0
10	1	0	+7	1	0
12	2	0	+8	4	0
14	1	0	+9	1	0
15	1	0	+10	2	0
16	3	0	+11	1	0
17	2	0	. . . .		
. . . .			+12	1	1
18	3	1	+13	3	2
19	2	2	+14	3	1
20	1	1	. . . .		
21	0	1	+15	2	4
22	3	0	+16	3	4
. . . .			+17	1	4
23	3	4	+18	0	2
24	2	5	+19	0	2
25	0	6	+20	0	4
26	0	1	+21	2	3
27	1	2	+22	1	3
28	2	2	+23	3	1
29	1	3	+25	0	1
30	1	3	+28	0	1
31	1	0		33	33
33	0	1			
36	0	1			
	33	33			

taxonomic and rhyme generation. The results are shown in Table 5.4. It can be seen that the cutoff associated with the most accurate identification of low performing, to be referred students, would be at a total score of ≤17. At this cutoff, all 13 students referred would be LD. This represents 39% of all the LD students tested. We would miss 20 out of 33 or 61% of the LD sample. Using a cutoff of ≤22, 27 students would be referred. Of these, 22 out of 27 (82%) would be LD. This represents 67% of the LD group. We would fail to refer 11 out of 33 or 33% of the LD sample and of those referred, 18% would not be LD.

Using only those three tasks in which outliers were identified, similar results were found. At a cutoff of ≤ +11, 14 out of 33 or 42% of the LD sample are referred and all of the referred are LD. We would fail to identify 58% of the LD students. At a cutoff of ≤ +14, 64% of the LD students are correctly referred, missing only 36% of the LD sample, and 12% of the NA group are referred in error. Of the children referred, 21 out of 25 or 84% should be referred.

These data, we believe, are encouraging. They indicate that this process of task evaluation may well lead to more effective identification of young LD children. Even using the more conservative criterion where no NA students are referred, the correct referral of 39% to 42% of 4- and 5-year-old LD children would result in many more LD children receiving early intervention in preschool classrooms than are currently being served.

One might ask if there are any data contrasting the performance of preschool-aged normally achieving and LD children, the actual age of the target group for screening. The answer to this question is *yes*. The accuracy with which normal 4- and 5-year-old children could be differentiated from same-age school-identified LD or mildly retarded children by their performance on a mini-cognitive battery was reported by Scott et al. (1991). We will report only the results related to identification of LD children.

Contrasting Normal and LD Preschool-Aged Children

Twenty-four normal and 24 LD preschool-aged children matched on age, sex and ethnicity were presented a cognitive battery consisting of seven different tasks. These tasks/components were selected using a combination of discriminant function analyses and frequency distributions. In both groups, there were 17 males and 7 females of whom 4 were black/non-Hispanic, 12 were white/Hispanic and 8 were white/ non-Hispanic. Following a series of analyses, we were able to show that the students' total score, summed over just three selected tasks, was associated with the correct identification of 21 out of 24 LD students (SN = 88%) and 18 out of 24 NA students (SP = 75%). The three tasks consisted of: five taxonomic generation cards, five taxonomic information cards using number of different descriptors generated as the dependent measure, and a word-meaning task.

Summary and Implications for Future Research

The evaluation of potential test components using school-identified LD children has resulted in preliminary data that support the contention that this approach will result in the development of a more effective screening test to identify young LD children. In the next year we will be evaluating additional tasks using 4- and 5-year-old LD children as a criterion reference group. This should provide us with the best information about the discriminatory value of additional cognitive tasks in the limited time remaining to us to complete the task evaluations. Then we must fix the components for the initial version of the screening test so that we may evaluate its predictive, as well as its concurrent, validity. In addition, an estimate will be made of the stability of the test. "Streamlining" or "tailoring" the test to maximize the accuracy of prediction will be done on one sample of children, while a second will serve as a cross-validation sample. If the results indicate that the test is working effectively, then the standardization of the test would be undertaken. We do, however, have miles to go before that decision is upon us.

Acknowledgments. The authors would like to express their thanks to the Dade County Public School System for allowing us access to their students and to the participating staff for cooperating so generously with us. We would also like to thank Ms. Olga Laffita and Ms. Leslie Swanson for all the work they did to gather and enter the data. Dr. Daryl B. Greenfield's contribution to the project must also be recognized. This research was supported in part by HD 22952 from the National Institute of Child Health and Human Development and by FDLRS/Mailman, a specialized university center of the Florida Diagnositc and Learning Resources System, funded through State General Revenue appropriations to provide multidisciplinary evaluation services in exceptional student programs.

References

Achenbach, T.M., Edelbrock, C.S., & Howell, C.T. (1987). Empirically based assessment of the behavioral/emotional problems of 2- and 3-year-old children. *Journal of Abnormal Child Psychology*, *15*, 629–650.

Bauer, R.H. (1982). Information processing as a way of understanding and diagnosing learning disabilities. *Topics in learning and learning disabilities*, *2*, 33–45.

Bracken, B.A. (1987). Limitations of preschool instruments and standards for minimal levels of technical adequacy. *Journal of Psychoeducational Assessment*, *4*, 313–326.

Carran, D.T. & Scott, K.G. (1989). The relative risk of educational handicaps in two birth cohorts of normal and low birthweight disadvantaged children. *Topics in Early Childhood Special Education*, *9*(1), 14–31.

Ceci, S.J. (1984). A developmental study of memory and learning disabilities. *Journal of Experimental Child Psychology*, *38*, 352–371.

Ceci, S.J. (1989). On domain specificity ... more or less general and specific constraints on cognitive development. *Merril-Palmer Quarterly*, *35*(1), 131–142.

Ceci, S.J. & Baker, J.G. (1989). On learning ... more or less: A knowledge × process × context view of learning disabilities. *Journal of Learning Disabilities*, *22* (2), 90–99.

Esterly, D.L. & Griffin, H.C. (1987). Preschool programs for children with learning disabilities. *Journal of Learning Disabilities*, *20*(9), 571–573.

Gerber, M.M. & Levine-Donnerstein, D. (1989). Educating all children: Ten years later. *Exceptional Children*, *56* (1), 17–27.

Greenfield, D.B. & Scott, M.S. (1985). A cognitive approach to preschool screening. *Learning Disabilities Research, 1* (1), 42–49.

Hogan, A.E., Scott, K., & Bauer, C. (1991). *A new measure of adaptive social behavior.* Manuscript submitted for publication.

Howe, M.L., O'Sullivan, J.T., Brainerd, C.J., & Kingma, J. (1989). Localizing the development of ability differences in organized memory. *Contemporary Educational Psychology, 14* (4), 336–356.

Infant Health and Development Program. (INDP). (1990). Enhancing the outcomes of low-birth-weight, premature infants. *Journal of the American Medical Association, 263*(22), 3035–3042.

Jones, L.V. & Appelbaum, M.I. (1989). Psychometric methods. *Annual Review of Psychology, 40,* 23–43.

Kamhi, A.G. & Catts, H.W. (1986). Toward an understanding of developmental language and reading disorders. *Journal of Speech and Hearing Disorders, 51,* 337–347.

Kamhi, A.G., Catts, H.W., Mauer, D., Apel, K., & Gentry, B.F. (1988). Phonological and spatial processing abilities in language-and reading-impaired children. *Journal of Speech and Hearing Disorders, 53,* 316–327.

Lazar, I. & Darlington, R. (1982). Lasting effects of early education: A report from the consortium for longitudinal studies. *Monographs of the Society for Research in Child Development, 47*(2–3, Serial No. 195).

Lichtenstein, R. (1981). Comparative validity of two preschool tests: Correlational and classificational approaches. *Journal of Learning Disabilities, 14,* 68–72.

Lichtenstein, R. & Ireton, H. (1984). *Preschool screening: Identifying young children with developmental and educational problems.* Orlando, FL: Grune & Stratton.

Lindsay, G.A. & Wedell, K. (1982). The early identification of educationally "at risk" children revisited. *Journal of Learning Disabilities, 15,* 212–217.

Lipson, M.Y. & Wixson, K.K. (1986). Reading disability research: An interactionist perspective. *Review of Educational Research, 56,* 111–136.

Meisels, S.J. (1987). Uses and abuses of developmental screening and school readiness testing. *Young Children, 42* (4–6), 68–73.

Meisels, S.J. (1989). Can developmental screening tests identify children who are developmentally at risk? *Pediatrics, 83*(4), 578–585.

Morrison, D., Mantzicopoulos, P., & Carte, E. (1989). Preacademic screening for learning and behavior problems. *Journal of the American Academy of Child and Adolescent Psychiatry, 28*(1), 101–106.

Mosenthal, P. (1982). Designing training programs for learning disabled children: An ideological perspective. *Topics in Learning and Learning Disabilities, 2* (1), 97–107.

Muehl, S. & Forell, E.R. (1973). A followup study of disabled readers: Variables related to high school reading performance. *Reading Research Quarterly, 9,* 110–123.

Reynolds, C.R. & Clark, J.H. (1983). Assessment of cognitive abilities. In K.D. Paget & B.A. Bracken (Eds.), *The psychoeducational assessment of preschool children* (pp. 163–189). New York: Grune & Stratton.

Satz, P. & Fletcher, J.M. (1988). Early identification of learning disabled children: An old problem revisited. *Journal of Consulting and Clinical Psychology, 56* (6), 824–829.

Scott, K.G., Hogan, A.E., & Bauer, C. (1991, April). *The effects of early intervention on the Adaptive Social Behavior Inventory: A new measure of prosocial behavior.* Paper presented at the biennial meeting of the Society for Research in Child Development, Seattle, WA.

Scott, K.G., Urbano, J., & Boussy, C. (1991). Longterm psychoeducational outcome of prenatal substance exposure. *Seminars in Perinatology, 15*(4), 317–323.

Scott, M.S. & Greenfield, D.B. (1991). The screening potential of a taxonomic information task for the detection of learning disabled and mildly retarded children. *Journal of Applied Developmental Psychology, 12*, 429–446.

Scott, M.S. & Greenfield, D.B. (1992). A comparison of normally achieving, learning disabled and mildly retarded students on a taxonomic information task. *Learning Disabilities Research & Practice, 7*, 59–67.

Scott, M.S., Greenfield, D.B., & Partridge, M.F. (1991). Differentiating between two groups that fail in school: Performance of learning disabled and mildly retarded students on oddity problems. *Learning Disabilities Research & Practice, 6*, 3–11.

Scott, M.S., Perou, R., Greenfield, D.B., & Swanson, L.J. (in press). *Rhyming skills: Differentiating among mildly restarded, learning disabled and normally achieving students, Learning Disabilities Research & Practice.*

Scott, M.S., Perou, R., Greenfield, D.B., Lafitta, O., Swanson, L.J., & Sutton, M. (1991, May). *Classifying four-and five-year-old children as normal or mildly impaired using a mini battery of cognitive tasks.* Paper presented at the Gatlinberg Conference on Research and Theory in Mental Retardation and Developmental Disabilities, Key Biscayne, FL.

Scott, M.S., Perou, R., Greenfield, D.B., Partridge, M.F., & Swanson, L.J. (1993). A comparison of normally achieving, mildly retarded, and learning disabled students on a perceptually based oddity task. *Journal of Developmental and Physical Disabilities, 5*(2), 129–150.

Sheehan, R. (1989). Implications of P.L. 99-457 for assessment. *Topics in Early Childhood Special Education, 8*(4), 103–115.

Siegel, L.S. & Ryan, E.B. (1984). Reading disability as a language disorder. *Remedial and Special Education, 5*(3), 28–33.

Silver, A. & Hagin, R. (1981). *SEARCH Manual.* New York: Walker Educational Book Corporation.

Simmons, D.C. & Kameenui, E.J. (1990). The effect of task alternatives on vocabulary knowledge: A comparison of students with and without learning disabilities. *Journal of Learning Disabilities, 23*(5), 291–297, 316.

Simpson, G. & Lorsbach, T. (1983). The development of automatic and conscious components of contextual facilitation. *Child Development, 54*, 760–772.

Strag, G.A. (1972). Comparative behavioral ratings of parents with severe mentally retarded, special learning disability, and normal children. *Journal of Learning Disabilities, 5*, 52–56.

Swanson, H.L. (1990). Executive processing differences between learning-disabled, mildly retarded, and normal achieving children. *Journal of Abnormal Child Psychology, 18*(5), 549–563.

Vaughn, S. & Hogan, A. (1990). Social competence and learning disabilities: A prospective study. In H.L. Swanson & B. Keogh (Eds.), *Learning disabilities: Theoretical and research issues* (pp. 175–191). Hillsdale, NJ: Erlbaum.

Vaughn, S., Hogan, A., Kouzekanani, K., & Shapiro, S. (1990). Peer acceptance, self-perceptions, and social skills of learning disabled students prior to identification. *Journal of Educational Psychology*, *82*(1), 101–106.

Yerushalmy, J. (1947). Statistical problems in assessing methods of medical diagnosis, with special reference to X-Ray techniques. *Public Health Reports*, *62*, 1432–1449.

Part III
Methodological Issues: Intervention Research

6
Instructional Issues in Conducting Intervention Research at the Elementary Level

CAROL SUE ENGLERT

The focus of this chapter is on issues that relate to effectively conducting and interpreting intervention research in learning disabilities. Intervention research involves "scientifically based efforts to document specific techniques whose intention is to improve, in some socially acceptable way, the functioning of individuals characterized as learning disabled" (Scruggs, 1990, pp. 66–67). However, intervention research cannot be expected to produce educational programs similar to a pill or injection that will cure students (Shavelson & Berliner, 1988). In fact, several scholars argue that simple mechanistic concepts from engineering and medicine are incorrectly applied to the field of psychology and education (Danziger, 1990; Shavelson & Berliner, 1988). Instead, these authors suggest that learning is a social event and knowledge is socially constructed by members of the learning community. "With learning both socially mediated and individually constructed . . . prescriptions for educational policy or practice are impossible" (Shavelson & Berliner, 1988, p. 10). Research needs to focus on the long-term development of knowledge as well as on short-term "fixes" (Shavelson & Berliner, 1988).

In this chapter, the general characteristics of efficacious intervention research will be examined. In the first part, some of the limitations and problems that have typified special education intervention research will be related. Second, the implications and trends of the sociocultural perspective will be discussed to provide another set of principles that can broaden and enrich the nature and quality of intervention research. Third, empirical issues related to this perspective will be briefly discussed with attention to the guiding research questions and assessment measures that might inform the intervention literature.

Conceptual Paradigms for Conducting Intervention Research

One of the first tasks of a researcher is to clearly articulate a theoretical paradigm that underlies the intervention research. Theory involves the belief system that a researcher brings to the work. It provides the guiding force that helps the researcher identify the intervention method and procedures, dependent measures, data collection methods, analysis and interpretations, and conclusions. The separation of theory from research and practice in educational research does considerable damage, inasmuch as the researcher lacks the conceptual lenses for designing effective interventions (Kavale, this volume).

In special education, conceptual paradigms that have driven much of the intervention research have been based on behavioral notions of teaching and learning, as well as on educational models such as direct instruction and cognitive behavior modification. Methodologically, the teacher (or experimenter) in these models is seen as one who has particular knowledge about the strategies or skills to be instructed, and his/ her role is to inform students of this knowledge (Poplin, 1988; Reid, in press; Winn, 1991). Typically, only a few strategies are introduced at a time, with the introduction of new strategies extending over a long period of time (Pressley, Goodchild, Fleet, Zajchowski, & Evans, 1989). Furthermore, individuals master only a small set of prerequisite, sequentialized components before they use them holistically to engage in complex problem solving and learning for real purposes (Heshius, 1991).

Instructionally, intervention researchers in these models envision the teacher's role as that of one who engages in didactic instruction as he/she defines each strategy step, models its use, and guides students in verbally rehearsing and practicing each step until they attain mastery. Feedback on errors is immediate and direct. Once students demonstrate mastery of a particular strategy step or skill, the next step is presented. Formative evaluation in these models is based upon whether or not the students are following the identified steps, whether they can accurately verbalize the strategy self-instructions, and whether they have attained the mastery criterion (Palincsar, David, Winn, & Stevens, 1990).

Interventions based on direct instruction and cognitive behavior modification principles indicate that they are successful paradigms for teaching academic skills (Adams, Carnine, & Gersten, 1982; Baumann, 1984; Schumaker, Deshler, Alley, Warner, & Denton, 1982). Furthermore, a series of studies using cognitive behavior modification principles indicate that students can generalize to content area materials when instructional procedures include conditions in which students are prompted to apply and practice implementing strategies in grade-level texts and curriculum (Ellis, Lenz, & Sabornie, 1987a, Ellis, Lenz, & Sabornie, 1987b). Thus, the techniques are successful in promoting academic learning and transfer.

Nevertheless, there are several limitations of this research that warrant a broadening of the methodology and techniques used in experimental research. First, strategy instruction in these paradigms tends to focus on the transmission of discrete strategies (e.g., strategies that are sequentially introduced and in the context of subjects or specific stimulus materials). This, however, assumes that the component skills or strategies have an independent reality apart from other strategies, goal-embedded tasks, and learning for intrinsically relevant purposes (Heshius, 1991). Further, it is assumed that students will come to understand the complexity of the entire cognitive process from its parts, as well as understand the relationship of individual strategies to the whole even though they have only experienced the process as components (Michaels & O'Connor, 1990). An equally imposing problem occurs because the skills curriculum in special education is often distinct and separate from the content-driven curriculum that students encounter in mainstream classes (Ellis, in press), leaving to students the difficult task of figuring out what strategies to use and when.

Second, the detailed and explicit specification of the sequence of behaviors renders the task into the execution of a sequence of verbal and nonverbal behaviors (Poplin, 1988; Stone, 1989). Students are generally expected to use the exact words, language, and questions provided by the instructor, resulting in a product that looks exactly like the instructor's. The preciseness of the teaching scripts and curriculum suggests that children are required to learn in a prescribed way, without emphasis on their own personal views, experiences, or content knowledge (Heshius, 1991; Poplin, 1988). Under these conditions, students with learning disabilities may come to distrust their own knowledge and natural problem-solving abilities, and instead, respond to cognitive tasks as though they are discrete, isolated skills to be performed for teacher approval (Rueda, 1990).

Third, instruction in this tradition tends to focus on the transmission of facts and strategies rather than on higher-order thinking and problem-solving processes. The step-by-step instructional procedures and materials are designed to obtain a high number of correct responses and ensure the procedural fidelity that will produce predictable outcomes and unambiguous empirical results. At the same time, there is a tendency to view students' errors as problems that are a threat to the stimulus control procedures and intervention's effectiveness. The goal seems to be the enculturation of learners as students, rather than as thinkers and problem solvers (Brandt, 1990). In this way, what seems to "count" as efficacious instructional interventions are those that get students to accurately reproduce what the instructor has presented rather than those that present tasks that model the real world of problem solving, involve multiple correct solutions, and guide students in generating multiple strategies as part of their self-organizing and self-regulating activities (Heshius, 1991).

Fourth, interventions based on these models tend to ignore the social and constructive activities important in learning. Intervention research has been treated as though experimentation was a purely cognitive activity

(Danziger, 1990). However, this perspective ignores its social character, in which the social arrangements of the classroom community determine how phenomena are produced and witnessed. Teachers and students are active participants in constructing new knowledge during strategy instruction (Pressley et al., 1991), and attention to these issues can positively influence classroom learning and the quality of intervention research.

Finally, the emphasis on validating and maintaining control of instructional procedures has resulted in a proliferation of vocabulary that focuses on experimental control such as "measurement, efficiency, programming, components, task analysis, mastery, objective, data, graphs." At the same time, there is a less apparent concern for understanding the teaching/ learning process or the personal and social nature of learning, as might be reflected by vocabulary such as "teaching, learning, holistic, motivation, interaction, reciprocity, ownership, transformation, history, culture, zones of proximal development, and constructivism" (Heshius, 1991). Furthermore, while the special education literature has relied on quantitative or applied behavior analyses nearly exclusively in arriving at conclusions (usually using outcome measures that do not directly examine the teaching effects or the developmental course of students' learning), there is less attention to other research tools that might provide a richer description of strategy instruction as it occurs in schools (Pressley et al., 1991). More diverse research methods and experimental curricula are warranted, with particular attention to the teaching-learning process, the instructional tools that might better represent the complexity of the cognitive processes being taught, and the social and constructive processes that enhance students' learning of higher-order processes.

Dimensions of Intervention Research

Several conceptions of teaching/learning can provide intervention researchers with new conceptual lenses to design experimental curricula and studies that will yield useful information about the teaching of higher-order thinking, and shed light on the nature of teaching and learning in classrooms. These conceptions, based on the social constructivist perspective, are not intended to supplant current intervention research, but can expand the repertoire of methodology and conceptual tools that researchers have available in their experimental research. These principles include assumptions that (a) learning must be for authentic purposes, (b) learning is dialogic and socially mediated, and (c) learning reflects the broader learning and social community of the classroom. In this section, these three principles are explicated with examples from the experimental literature to represent how these principles might be applied in intervention research in special education.

The Use of Authentic Purposes and Goals

One of the first principles emanating from the social constructivist perspective that can be usefully incorporated into intervention research involves the growing recognition that students need to absorb not only the facts and fundamentals of a particular subject matter, they need to be taught the methods of inquiry and habits of thought that scientists, historians, mathematicians, and writers use (Finn, 1988). The fact that lower-achieving students in a classroom profit more from an emphasis on higher-order thinking than an emphasis on academic engagement suggests that task engagment and factual learning are insufficient conditions for improving conceptual abilities (Peterson, 1988; Peterson, Fennema, Carpenter, & Loef, 1989). Factual learning must be at the service of efforts to develop students' higher-order thinking and problem-solving abilities.

Intervention research, therefore, needs to be designed and conducted with a view that strategies are tools for learning and knowledge. As such, a repertoire of strategies needs to be presented to students in order for them to flexibly respond to different tasks and contextual demands (Palincsar et al., 1990). Strategies must be designed to develop students' fundamental understandings and control of the cognitive process.

There are several characteristics of interventions that highlight the role of strategy instruction at the service of developing higher-order thinking. These interventions are likely to emphasize that: (a) higher-order thinking and learning occur through the mental activity of the learner as they interpret, elaborate upon, and represent information rather than through the direct transfer of knowledge from teacher to students (Wertsch, 1991); (b) tasks are viewed as problems to be solved rather than as stimuli for the recall of specific information and the use of specific strategies; further, these task goals change as the problem and the cognitive abilities of the learner change (Anderson, 1989); (c) questions have many correct answers rather than one, and explanations of thinking are as valued as the answers (Anderson, 1989); (d) multiple representations of a concept rather than a single correct model are presented to promote long-term understanding and knowledge use (Lampert, 1989); (e) strategies and skills are presented in holistic contexts, involving authentic purposes and goals; and (f) instruction is integrated across the curriculum rather than taught in discrete contexts and conditions.

Several pilot studies illustrate of these principles were conducted by Palincsar and her associates (Palincsar et al., 1990; Winn, 1991). These researchers developed a collaborative problem solving procedure to provide students with control over their comprehension learning by selecting and evaluating strategy use in relation to tasks and contextual demands (Winn, 1991). In the collaborative problem-solving procedure, students were first asked to examine different hypothetical children's comprehension strategies, label the strategies, and evaluate the effectiveness of the strategies. They then suggested the strategies they would like to use, tried to employ them as a group, and evaluated their helpfulness. They also developed procedures for using the various strategies in concert. Thus, students were actually involved in selecting, interpreting, elaborating upon, and representing strategies for the comprehension of texts, and measuring their comprehension of passages to evaluate the effectiveness of various strategies. Within this paradigm, texts were presented as problems to be solved through the use of various strategies rather than as stimuli for the recall of specific information, and students' explanations of their thinking were as valued by teachers as their answers. Furthermore, students were actively involved in seeing how strategy goals changed in relation to particular tasks, problems, and contexts, and their discussions focused on the employment and evaluation of several strategies rather than one.

The results of a study with children from third grade classes revealed several trends (Palincsar et al., 1990). First, for heterogeneous student populations, collaborative problem solving was more effective than a direct instruction condition on a criterion test of reading comprehension. In fact, whereas none of the lowest-achieving children in the directed learning condition achieved criterion levels of performance (e.g., 70% accuracy), 60% of the lowest-achieving students in the collaborative problem-solving condition achieved criterion levels. Furthermore, on a test of strategy knowledge and use, the direct instruction condition was not as effective as the collaborative problem-solving condition for high-achieving students (no significant differences among conditions were found for the strategy knowledge of low-achieving students). The authors concluded that collaborative problem solving tended to be more effective for heterogeneous groups of learners. This result by itself was considered of importance, given the tendency to assume that lower-achieving students require direct instruction in order to make academic gains (Palincsar et al., 1990).

Learning is Dialogic and Socially Mediated by the Instructor

A second principle emanating from the social constructivist perspective that can enhance intervention research involves the role of dialogue, language, and social mediation in the classroom. Vygotsky (1978) proposed that learning is socially mediated by a more knowledgeable person (e.g., teacher or peer). At first, the teacher models the language and actions of the problem-solving process. However, this modeling soon gives way to a joint process in which the teacher and learner mutually perform the process. At this point, the problem-solving process exists on the interpsychological plane (between people) as the participants jointly share the cognitive work and engage in a joint or social dialogue. The learner becomes responsible for whatever actions and dialogue he or she is able, while the instructor assists students when their performance falters, or helps students to construct new knowledge at the points where their confusion becomes apparent. Finally, the problem-solving process is performed by the individual alone on the intrapsychological plane, as the processes that were once performed on the social plane become internalized as dialogue with oneself. However, the process remains quasi-social as the social dialogue that once was performed collaboratively is performed in the private sphere, retaining much of the cognitive, social, and regulatory functions of the social interaction (Vygostky, 1978).

There are several facets of this second principle that need to be considered and reflected in the design of instructional interventions. These facets, or assumptions, embody three fundamental principles concerning the nature of dialogic instruction (e.g., instruction in advance of learning, the role of language and dialogue, and teachers' roles in mediating students' performance in the zones of proximal development).

Instruction in Advance of Learning and the Nature of Errors

First, inherent in the dialogic approach is the assumption that instruction needs to lead development in awakening cognitive problem-solving approaches and strategies that the learner is not capable of devising alone (Gallimore, Tharp, & Rueda, 1989). Instruction, therefore, occurs in advance of the students' independent level (Stone, 1989). This means that students are invited to participate at cognitive levels where mistakes are inevitable (Reid, in press). Correspondingly, mistakes and errors are viewed as important sources of knowledge construction and meaning; that is, students are viewed as "meaning-makers" and their mistakes the substance of making new meanings rather than viewed as problems that should be avoided (Lampert, 1989).

The Role of Language and Dialogue

A second assumption pertains to the important role of language in mediating cognitive performance. That is, language is viewed as an important symbolic tool that mediates one's own and other people's performances. To become enculturated into a subject matter or discipline means that learners must be enculturated into its particular discourse.

The development of a language or shared conceptual vocabulary within a literacy community represents an important instructional aim of educators and researchers (Edwards & Mercer, 1987, 1989). Just as children acquire a new vocabulary to "speak a new language," they must acquire and participate in a scientific vocabulary associated with "talking physics" or a literacy vocabulary for "talking writing" or "talking reading" (Lemke, 1989). In fact, some have proposed that students who fail may be students who not only do not simply learn enough facts or strategies, but who also do not gain access to school-based discourses (Michaels & O'Connor, 1990). This is particularly problematic for students with learning disabilities given the instructional focus in special education on basic facts and basic skills. Teachers and researchers must move beyond facts and skills to conventionalize a disciplinary knowledge and a discourse for thinking.

Heath (1983) even suggests a practical sequence of classroom activities that might be used to apprentice students in new social discourses and ways of thinking. She suggests that teachers: (a) start with familiar content and familiar kinds of talk about that content, (b) go on to new kinds of talk and provide models of control over these discourse forms (e.g., the teacher makes and asks students to make explicit metacognitive and metadiscursive talk about their cognitive strategies and activities), (c) provide opportunities for the children to practice the new kinds of talk (in public and in private), and (d) talk with the children about the thinking and talk itself. In this way, educators can make cognitive processes explicit and help students talk their way to new ways of thinking. Moreover, by entering into a dialogue with others and taking over their voices, children are, as it were, "importing" basic forms of mediation as they begin to experience, practice, master, and eventually internalize the voices of more experienced problem solvers (Bakhtin, 1986; Wertsch, 1991). The ways in which these classroom dialogues about higher-order cognitive processes can be constructed, the nature of children's participation in these discourses, factors that influence children's appropriation of the social discourse of the classroom, and the effects of the acquisition of these social discourses on cognitive performance represent important empirical questions that need to be addressed in intervention research.

Zones of Proximal Development

A third assumption important in the design of classroom discourse involves teachers' abilities to transact with students in their learning zones to construct more complex cognitive structures from the simpler structures that students bring to the learning task. The zone of proximal development is the distance between the level at which the child can perform independently and the level obtained by the child in cooperation with a more knowledgeable problem solver (Vygotsky, 1978). There are four traits that are likely to typify the design of effective teacher interactions with students in their zones of proximal development.

First, interventions that are sensitive to students' zones of proximal development are likely to instruct students in new procedures in response to actual problem-solving needs rather than defer to the dictates of the formal curriculum. Within these interactions, it is recognized that not all students will have the same notion of the instructional episode and what is going to happen. Inevitably, interventions must "start with where the child is" to find ways to enlist all children of different ability levels and knowledge to participate in the activity rather than begin at prescribed points where the formal curriculum starts (Newman, Griffin, & Cole, 1989). In fact, a great variety of systems of cognitive functioning and response may be entry points into a given learning zone (Newman et al., 1989), and different students will have their own entry points where new knowledge can be constructed.

Second, it is recognized that lessons need to be adjusted on a moment-to-moment basis, given what the students say and know, as well as what they need to know. It is impossible to entirely construct a predetermined set of activities, strategies, and teaching scripts in advance of instruction. Teachers must move within students' learning and knowledge zones to push them upward to expert performance by modeling and prompting at precisely those points where students begin to show cognitive confusion (Englert, in press). The incorporation of students' actions and language into the teacher's discourse and system of activity (e.g., using students' ideas and linking these to new knowledge), and the elevation of students' actions and thoughts into more expert levels of performance enables students' participation in a more complex activity than they are able to perform alone (see Palincsar, 1986). Bos and Anders (1990), for example, describe an instructional intervention in which the background knowledge of students became an important instructional framework upon which new textual ideas from content area texts was then linked. In this way, teachers' acknowledgement and appropriation of students' ideas was a critical feature of their interactions with students in the zones of proximal development (Newman et al., 1989). Furthermore, students' background knowledge, their "living knowledge," became the entry point that gave rise to new understandings of content knowledge and learning-to-learn strategies.

Third, teachers mediate performance in students' learning zones using a variety of discursive moves. Teachers mediate and scaffold performance by modeling thinking strategies, prompting students to lead or carry out tasks, and using reinforcing strategies (Palincsar, 1986). Primary in these interactions are teachers' relinquishing strategies. Teachers increasingly "up the ante" by using relinquishing strategies that increase students' self-control of a cognitive process, prompt self-regulation of the strategy and move control of the lesson discourse from teacher to student (see Diaz, Neal, & Amaya-Williams, 1990; Englert, in press).

Finally, the discourse created by teachers and students has a participation structure that is distinguishable from recitation structures. Whereas, the turn-taking pattern in recitation formats goes from student to teacher, and back again; in constructivist environments teachers intentionally exert less control over whose turn it is to talk (Winn, 1991). Students are as likely to interact with one another as the teacher, and students are involved in frequent requests of one another for expansions, elaborations, justifications, and evaluations (see interventions of Bos & Anders, 1990; Palincsar & Brown, 1984; Winn, 1991). Furthermore, in these constructive environments, students literally assume the voices of the teacher as the social discourse becomes their own, and as they participate in the dialogue in the roles of questioner, critic, and expert. In the process, students take over more and more of the teachers' regulative responsibilities (Wertsch, 1991), and provide their own set of answering words for each word or utterance they hear (Voloshinov, 1973). This contrasts with traditional learning environments where such requests and the control of thinking typically come from the teacher. Since meaning comes into existence only when two or more voices come into contact (Bakhtin, 1986) and the abilities of students to assume the social language of the teacher and community is important to their development (Wertsch, 1991), the incorporation of these new types of participant structures by researchers could have a profound impact on the development of students' cognitive and thinking abilities.

There are several intervention studies in the special education literature that have illustrated the role of dialogue in strategy instruction (Bos & Anders, 1990; Englert, Raphael, Anderson, Anthony, & Stevens, 1991; Palincsar & Brown, 1984; Winn, 1991; Wong, Wong, Darlington, & Jones, 1991). However, two studies specifically emphasized and focused on the nature of teachers' dialogue in instruction. Reciprocal Teaching (Palincsar, 1986; Palincsar & Brown, 1984) was a comprehension procedure that used four strategies as a language in the form of tools to solve problems of understanding expository texts (Palincsar & Brown, 1984; Palincsar & David, 1990). In reciprocal teaching, participants took turns assuming the role of teacher in leading the group dialogue about a text's meaning using the four strategies to summarize a section of text, ask questions, clarify misleading sections of the text, and predict what the next section of text will be about. Initially, teachers had to provide a great deal of support to help students use the four strategies (Palincsar & Brown, 1984). Gradually, however, students assumed increasing responsibility for leading the dialogue in their role as discussion leaders, and monitoring the group's performance.

There were four principles that guided the development and implementation of reciprocal teaching, including: (a) explicit theories and comprehension strategies were taught, and the need for particular strategies and their limits were made public; (b) teaching was embedded in real, meaningful tasks of interpreting expository text; (c) adults' scaffolding was responsive to the student's contribution, and although adults played many roles (e.g., modeling expert behavior, monitoring group's understanding, pushing for deeper understanding), a primary goal was to gradually "up the ante" so that students were called upon to adopt the self-regulative role of the teacher fully and independently; and (d) students had to explicitly appropriate and demonstrate the voice of the more experienced problem solver as their roles were switched from having to respond to teachers' utterances to making decisions themselves as the leaders who controlled and monitored the classroom discourse.

The results of studies with remedial and special education students indicated that students made significant gains in their reading comprehension (Palincsar, 1987; Palincsar & Brown, 1984). Furthermore, when teachers' dialogue was examined more closely, several features emerged which was associated with students' level of independence in using the strategies and their performance on a transfer test. These features included the extent to which teachers: (a) supported students' contributions at the idea versus word level (e.g., producing the precise word the teacher sought to answer a question); (b) used students' ideas and linked these ideas to new knowledge; (c) developed dialogues with focus and direction; (d) made the purposes and focus of dialogue explicit to students; (e) constructed new meanings from errors by changing the complexion of a students' incorrect response to form a conceptually correct response (Palincsar, 1986). In sum, teachers' management of the instructional dialogue and their ability to scaffold students' thinking was an important facet that influenced students' comprehension.

Cognitive Strategy Instruction in Writing (CSIW) was a program that was developed to emphasize teachers' and students' dialogic interactions in writing instruction (Englert, in press; Englert & Raphael, 1989; Englert et al., 1991). In CSIW, students were instructed in the use of writing strategies related to planning (considering audience, purpose, background knowledge), organizing (using expository text structure genres), drafting (implementing the writing plans), editing (monitoring text for audience, purpose, meaning, text structure), and revising (using revision strategies). However, these strategies were introduced simultaneously in the context of guiding students through the writing process rather than being introduced consecutively and sequentially as part of a task analyzed curriculum.

To model strategies, teachers carried on classroom-wide dialogues about the writing process, as they made visible their own inner thinking and the thinking of their students. In these classroom dialogues, students' own background knowledge was activated as they were asked to contribute their respective viewpoints and experiences. These experiences were then used by teachers to model writing strategies, discuss problem-solving responses, present multiple representations of concepts, and to transform students' living knowledge into a new vocabulary for thinking that was practiced in the actual context of planning, organizing, drafting, editing, and revising a class story (see Englert, 1990; Englert, 1992). Throughout the process, teachers modeled an inner dialogue for thinking, prompted students to assume control of the vocabulary and dialogue for thinking, and prompted their participation in both the collaborative and social dialogue of the lessons as well as in peer editing and collaborative writing sessions (Englert, 1990, 1992). Students' writing performances were further scaffolded as teachers presented think-sheets that prompted the students to use the inner dialogue and strategies of CSIW.

The results of several studies showed that CSIW students significantly surpassed control students in writing ability (Englert et al., 1991), and that they made significant gains in their knowledge and ability to talk about expository writing processes (Englert, Raphael, & Anderson, in press). As with reciprocal teaching, however, the dialogic skill of teachers had a significant impact on writing performance. When teachers' implementation of CSIW instructional principles was examined more closely, differences among teachers emerged (Anderson, Raphael, Englert, & Stevens, 1991; Englert, 1992). Whereas all teachers implemented the curriculum, some teachers rotely adhered to the CSIW curriculum, as they rigidly presented strategies and think-sheets to students. In contrast, more effective teachers clearly took conceptual leadership and ownership of the strategies of the CSIW program. These latter teachers made strategies accessible to students as they emphasized writing as a cognitive and communicative process, made visible the cognitive strategies and the inner language that directed writing, encouraged flexible rather than rote application of strategies, and encouraged peer interactions around writing. Englert (1992) illustrated how one of the more effective special education teachers successfully scaffolded students' performances by using their knowledge and errors as a basis for constructing new knowledge about strategies, and by dynamically interacting with students at the point of their confusion to bridge the gap between what they knew and what they needed to know. Data analyses further revealed that, whereas all CSIW children progressed in their acquisition of writing strategies for trained text structures, only students in the classrooms of more effective teachers successfully transferred their knowledge to self-regulate in generating their own text structures to write about self-selected topics (Anderson et al., 1991). Thus, teachers' interactions with students in the construction of a classroom dialogue about strategies affected writing performance in a durable and transformative way.

Taken together, these two studies highlight some of the features of dialogic instruction essential for the design of effective instructional interventions in classrooms. These features include emphases on: (a) the creation of classroom discourses where divergent viewpoints, experiences, ways of speaking, and the methods of inquiry related to a particular subject matter come into contact with a teacher-orchestrated dialogue (Michaels & O'Connor, 1990); (b) mastery of content, concepts, strategies, and ways of thinking and knowing through classroom dialogues where students discuss, debate, question, and participate (Michaels & O'Connor, 1990); (c) the use of students' ideas and knowledge as anchoring points to link up to new knowledge and strategies, and the treatment of students' errors as critical cognitive junctures for the construction of new knowledge, awarenesses, and strategies; (d) enculturation of students as thinkers and inquirers, as typified by the representation of tasks as problems to be solved rather than as stimuli for the recall of specific information; and (e) the successful mediation by teachers of students' learning within their zones of proximal development (e.g., adjusting the difficulty of any task on the spot, sharing the cognitive burden of problem solving with students, dynamically interacting with students to bridge the gap between what they know and what they need to know, appropriating students' language and actions) is critical to the development of students' cognitive abilities.

Building Learning Communities: The Social Nature of Learning

Finally, the third principle of the social constructivist perspective important in the design of interventions relates to the important contribution that students make to the learning process as well as to the nature of social interactions within that process (Winn, 1991). Student-student interactions may have as much impact on social and cognitive development as teacher-student interactions (Reid, in press). Thus, experts do not simply give cognition away. Knowledge that is formed in interactive social and constructive environments with other members of the learning community is more powerfully and richly formed than the knowledge and interactions created by the teacher alone (Anderson, 1989).

In conceiving of the interactive nature of knowledge, it is known that students actively construct meanings, with the multitude of voices, experiences, knowledge that make up individual students' background knowledge and the learning community of the classroom. Through mutual sense-making activities that involve classroom negotiation about meanings and experiences, all members of the literacy community offer their experiences, and begin to modify and shape their perspectives to reach intersubjectivity about the meanings of particular processes; that is, some shared understandings of learning events or concepts. In the process, teachers and students alike negotiate, calibrate, and adjust their language and meaning registers to incorporate and be sensitive to the perspectives of others. Everyone in the community stretches to understand and incorporate the interpretations of others in their understanding of new concepts.

At the same time, as teachers find occasions to make students' responses public and create collaborative learning environments, they provide students with public access to the knowledge of individual students and the social discourse. Social conversations make accessible the knowledge, perspectives, and discourses of others, creating a bank of shared meanings, experiences, and vocabulary that help make learning possible (Rowe, 1989). As a result, students can begin to appropriate the content, processes, strategies, and purposes demonstrated by other students as the beginning points for their own thinking; as well as to use their interactions with others to clear up doubts and confusions, and request information of one another as they revise their academic hypotheses (Englert & Palincsar, 1991; Rowe, 1989). Students' oral and written texts also demonstrate the quality of intertextuality: they have a social history that goes beyond a single text and that predates the current academic episode, they are formed and embedded in the larger history of the social structures, interactions, and communications in the classroom. For example, one student's written text may begin where another student's ended, retaining the same main character and genre in a new story context (Englert, 1992; Rowe, 1989). For these reasons, the shared knowledge of the classroom is far greater and richer than the contributions of individual students, and even greater than that provided by the teacher alone in communicative interactions with individual students.

Finally, the joint construction of meanings and strategies in collaborative environments involves a social discourse that inherently moves from teacher-to-student to student-to-student. As members of the community begin to share responsibility for defining the task, stragegies, and problem-solving processes, there is a realignment of the thinking load that redistributes it from the teacher to all the members of the community (Winn, 1991). Research suggests that students working in dyads outperform students working alone, suggesting that the level of performance attained in collaboration exceeds the level attained independently (Daiute, 1986; Winn, 1991). Even for higher-ability students, students learn more by explaining and by helping others arrive at correct answers, perhaps explaining why small-group cooperative learning interactions are most productive in groups with students differing in ability levels and expertise (Reid, in press). Furthermore, it is likely that new strategies and ways of thinking don't belong to students until they can run the instructional group without the teacher (Jacobs, 1990). Thus, the creation of collaborative problem-solving groups provides an effective means to transfer control of the dialogue from the teacher to students, as well as apprentice students in the cognitive work of academic learning, and provide exposure to a multitude of voices that the student can appropriate to direct his or her own cognitive activity.

An example of an intervention study in which the social and constructive nature of learning was emphasized was conducted by Zaragoza and Vaughn (Zaragoza, 1987; Zaragoza & Vaughn, 1992). In this study, process writing instruction was implemented in a general education classroom with mainstreamed special education students. Authors in the classroom collaborated with peers in writing about their own selected topics, and editing their own papers. The teacher provided public access to children's stories by publishing their stories and asking students to read their stories aloud in an author's chair. During Author's Chair, students used a response strategy called the TAG strategy to respond to other students' stories: They *T*old what they liked, *A*sked Questions, and *G*ave ideas.

There were several features notable in this intervention research. First, the teacher specifically empowered students to take over the curriculum by selecting examples of students' strategies as a basis for constructing a classroom discourse about particular skills or strategies in writing. Thus, students' own strategies, voices, and processes had authority over the prescribed curriculum. Second, students frequently borrowed ideas from other students, and other students became experts known for their use of particular strategies. For example, one student with learning disabilities became known as the classroom expert in how to write clever endings, and other students sought out this student to help them compose their own story endings. In this way, students in the community became recognized as "knowledgeable others" who could inform others about particular writing strategies, and they actually apprenticed their peers in the use of these strategies. In a similiar way, students' use of particular genres (poetry, diaries, adventure stories) and literary voices entered the public domain as they shared their stories with others in author's chair. Once in the public domain, other students began to appropriate these genres to fuel their own writing activities, as they "imported" the voices and strategies of their more knowledgeable peers. Third, the teacher situated her own instruction within students' learning zones, as she actively used students' own writing activities and knowledge as anchoring points to link up students' ideas to new knowledge and advance their writing performances. Skill lessons were situated in response to what her students knew and what they needed to know, and were adjusted on a moment-to-moment basis rather than in response to some predetermined writing curricula. Fourth, the teacher emphasized that the goal of instruction was the enculturation of students as thinkers and inquirers, as typified by her emphasis on student-generated topics, peer collaboration, empowerment of students, and problem-solving responses to writing events. In this way, she valued the teaching-learning process and demonstrated a sensitivity to students' cognitive needs that took precedence over any concern that students needed to accurately reproduce a specific product, genre, or strategy.

The results of the intervention study showed that students made large gains in performance on the Woodcock Johnson Achievement Test in diction, writing, language, proofreading, and mechanical skills (punctuation, spelling, usage). Furthermore, on a county-wide test, students in the process-writing classroom outperformed other students in reading and writing (Zaragoza, unpublished data). Although there were no control groups or statistical analyses conducted on the experimental data, the results point to the fact that instruction in higher-order thinking goals and writing strategies need not adversely affect the development of basic writing skills (e.g., mechanics).

Changing the Character of Intervention Rearch:
A Personal Case Study

As one who is interested in conducting intervention research, I personally have found myself drawn to the social constructivist perspective in my attempts to document and explain instructional processes in intervention research. Specifically, this literature has helped me focus on the dynamic interaction of teachers and students, as I have attempted to unpack how learning has occurred with the implementation of particular interventions (see Englert, Raphael, & Mariage, in press; Englert, Tarrant, Mariage, & Oxer, 1993). In addition, the social constructivist literature has provided new directions in selecting and constructing assessment measures. Rather than rely solely on achievement tests, the nature of the group's dialogue and the group's performance on collaborative tasks are other important outcome measures to be considered. Thus, my conception of the unit of analysis has expanded beyond individual cases and group data to include the broader social context and discourse of learning communities of which members are a part, as well as the collective thinking and knowledge of dyads, groups, and classrooms (Englert & Palincsar, 1991). If the origins of cognitive activity are truly embedded in social activity, then people interacting in that activity represent critical instructional and experimental outcomes, and changes in the group process itself should be the subject of investigations (Englert & Palincsar, 1991). These assessment notions and the instructional principles discussed in this chapter are being examined in intervention research we are conducting with primary grade students in special education (Englert, Raphael, & Mariage, in press). As we conduct this research, however, several key empirical questions and issues related to conducting intervention research within a social constructivist framework have arisen.

First, it is apparent that intervention research and methods must be designed in ways that involve children in holistic and situated activities. Researchers must conceive of intervention methods that abet children in using their natural astuteness as problem solvers (e.g., encourage, as well as recognize and employ, children's own hypotheses about subject matter content). Intervention studies that address the nature and effects of such instruction are clearly needed, particularly those designed for young students with learning disabilities who lack basic literacy skills that teachers often consider fundamental to students' participation in higher-order thinking.

Second, information concerning the ways in which teachers apprentice students in cognitive processes, and the effectiveness of their various relinquishing strategies would provide critical information concerning the nature of teachers' interactions with students in their zones of proximal development. Such intervention research should examine how teachers support students in the acquisition, internalization, and transformation of higher-order thinking strategies to achieve competent levels of academic performance. Simultaneously, research needs to examine the ways in which students appropriate and transform the knowledge, process, structure, and functions in the pursuit of achieving their learning goals, and the teacher activities that support students' appropriation of strategies and talk. This latter research will likely involve ethnographic research and case studies of both teachers and students.

Third, researchers need to investigate ways to develop discourse communities in classrooms, the patterns of teacher-student interactions that support the development of such a learning community, the effects of such communities on students' knowledge, the reciprocal influences of various discursive practices on teachers and students, and the ways in which dialogic instruction evolves and changes as teachers move from public (modeling) to student internalization of strategies. Further, in designing the intervention research, teachers' roles need to be expanded from that of conducting recitation to creating occasions for "shared talk" in which the classroom discourse is interactive, social, and jointly created.

Fourth, research methods must incorporate a broader array of dependent measures. Traditional emphases on normative and criterion-referenced tests must be expanded to include dynamic assessment (assessment in supported and instructional conditions), portfolio assessment, and classroom talk. In addition, since the social constructivist perspective emphasizes the performance of the individual in collaboration with the group, we need to reexamine the legitimacy of relying solely on individual's performance as the unit of analysis in evaluating instructional interventions. The effects of peer collaboration on individuals' (group's) knowledge, performance, and dialogue, needs to be examined over time to determine how students' interactions, communications, and group communications within the discourse community change over time. Such a study might also provide valuable information about the development of intersubjectivity, and the intertextual nature of children's communications. In this way, effective experimental methodology must account for the fact that children's oral and written texts are historically situated and informed by the larger literacy community.

Fifth, intervention research needs to be conducted that acknowledges that experts do not "own" the process; instead, meanings and processes are consensually constructed in the social environment. Attention to the ways in which strategy instruction looks different across classrooms, and the classroom or social processes that shape these differences represent important junctures for examining teacher effects, teacher beliefs, and the factors that influence conceptual change in teachers. In this vein, intervention research needs to address the collaborative roles of teachers and students (Englert, Tarrant, & Rocerdal, 1993). It is becoming apparent that the research agenda cannot be entirely predetermined (e.g., where teacher and learner follow expert's agenda and where questions essentially belong to the researcher rather than owned by the teacher and child). Teachers and researchers must foster a more collaborative, contextualized, embedded, evolving program of intervention research that is sensitive to the social context of the classroom. In the end, such collaborative arrangements can only enhance the quality of intervention research, by supporting the appropriation and transformation of teaching activities and strategies by teachers and researchers, and situating the intervention activities within teachers' and students' learning zones.

References

Adams, A., Carnine, D., & Gersten, R. (1982). Instructional strategies for studying content area texts in the middle grades. *Reading Research Quarterly, 18*, 27–55.

Anderson, L.M. (1989). Implementing instructional programs to promote meaningful, self-regulated learning. In J.E. Brophy (Ed.), *Advances in Research on Teaching* (Vol. 1, pp. 311–341). Greenwich, CT: JAI Press.

Anderson, L.M., Raphael, T.E., Englert, C.S., & Stevens, D.D. (1991, April). *Teaching writing with a new instructional model: Variations in teachers' practices and students' performances*. Paper presented at the annual meeting of the American Educational Research Association, Chicago.

Bakhtin, M.M. (1986). *Speech genres and other late essays* (C. Emerson & M. Holquist, Eds.; V.W. McGee, Trans.). Austin: University of Texas Press.

Baumann, J.F. (1984). The effectiveness of a direct instruction paradigm for teaching main idea comprehension. *Reading Research Quarterly, 21*, 70–90.

Bos, C.S. & Anders, P.L. (1990). Interactive teaching and learning: Instructional practices for teaching content and strategic knowledge. In T.E. Scruggs & B.Y.L. Wong (Eds.), *Intervention research in learning disabilities* (pp. 166–185). New York: Springer-Verlag.

Brandt, M. (1990). Getting social about critical thinking: Power and constraints of apprenticeship. *Quarterly Newsletter of the Laboratory of Comparative Human Cognition, 12*, 56–63.

Daiute, C. (1986). Do 1 and 1 make 2? *Written Communication, 3*, 283–408.

Danziger, K. (1990). *Constructing the subject: Historical origins of psychological research*. New York: Cambridge University Press.

Diaz, R.M., Neal, C.J., & Amaya-Williams, M. (1990). The social origins of self-regulation. In L.C. Moll (Ed.), *Vygotsky and education: The instructional implications and applications of sociohistorical psychology* (pp. 127–154). New York: Cambridge University Press.

Edwards, D. & Mercer, N. (1987). *Common knowledge: The development of understanding in the classroom*. New York: Methuen.

Edwards, D. & Mercer, N. (1989). Reconstructing context: The conventionalization of classroom knowledge. *Discourse Processes, 12*, 91–104.

Ellis, E.S. (in press). Integrating explicit and implicit teaching models when integrating content-area instruction with cognitive strategy instruction. *Reading and Writing Quarterly*.

Ellis, E.S., Lenz, B.K., & Sabornie, E.J. (1987a). Generalization and adaptation of learning strategies to natural environments: Part 1: Critical agents. *Remedial and Special Education*, *8*(1), 6–20.

Ellis, E.S., Lenz, B.K., & Sabornie, E.J. (1987b). Generalization and adaptation of learning strategies to natural environmenta: Part 2: Research into practice. *Remedial and Special Education*, *8*(2), 6–24.

Englert, C.S. (1990). Unraveling the mysteries of writing through strategy instruction. In T.E. Scruggs & B.Y.L. Wong (Eds.), *Intervention research in learning disabilities* (pp. 186–223). New York: Springer-Verlag.

Englert, C.S. (1992). Writing instruction from a sociocultural perspective: The holistic, dialogic and social enterprise of writing. *Journal of Learning Disabilities*, *25*, 153–172.

Englert, C.S. & Mariage, T.V. (1991). Shared understandings: Structuring the writing experience through dialogue. *Journal of Learning Disabilities*, *24*, 330–342.

Englert, C.S. & Palincsar, A.S. (1991). Reconsidering instructional research in literacy from a sococultural perspective. *Learning Disabilities Research and Practice*, *6*, 225–229.

Englert, C.S. & Raphael, T.E. (1989). Developing successful writers through cognitive strategy instruction. In J.E. Brophy (Ed.), *Advances in research on teaching* (Vol. 1, pp. 105–151). Greenwich, CT: JAI Press.

Englert, C.S., Raphael, T.E., & Anderson, L.M. (in press). Socially-mediated instruction: Improving students' knowledge and talk about writing. *Elementary School Journal*.

Englert, C.S., Raphael, T.E., Anderson, L.M., Anthony, H.M., & Stevens, D.D. (1991). Making writing strategies and self-talk visible: Cognitive strategy instruction in writing in regular and special education classrooms. *American Educational Research Journal*, *28*, 337–372.

Englert, C.S., Raphael, T.E., & Mariage, T.V. (in press). Developing a school-based discourse for literacy learning: a principled search for understanding. *Learning Disability Quarterly*.

Englert, C.S., Tarrant, K.L., Mariage, T.V., & Oxer, T. (1991, April). *Lesson talk as the work of reading groups: The effectiveness of two interventions*. Paper presented at the national meeting of Council for Exceptional Children, Atlanta.

Englert, C.S., Tarrant, K.L., & Rozendal, M.S. (1993). *Educational innovations: Achieving long-lasting curricular change through extended collaboration and reflective practice*. Manuscript submitted for publication.

Finn, C.E., Jr. (1988). What ails education research. *Educational Researcher*, *17*, 5–8.

Gallimore, R., Tharp, R., & Rueda, R. (1989). The social context of cognitive functioning in the lives of mildly handicapped persons. In D. Sugden (Ed.), *Cognitive approaches in special education* (pp. 51–81). London: Falmer Press.

Heath, S.B. (1983). *Waves with words: Language, life, and work in communities and classrooms*. New York: Cambridge University Press.

Heshius, L. (1991). Curriculum-based assessment and direct instruction: Critical reflections on fundamental assumptions. *Exceptional Children*, *57*, 315–328.

Jacobs, S.E. (1990). Scaffolding children's consciousness as thinkers. *The Quarterly Newsletter of the Laboratory of Comparative Human Cognition*, *12*, 70–75.

Lampert, M. (1989). Choosing and using mathematical tools in classroom discourse. In J.E. Brophy (Ed.), *Advances in research on teaching* (Vol. 1, pp. 223–261). Greenwich, CT: JAI Press.

Lemke, J.L. (1989). Making text talk. *Theory into Practice, 28*(2), 136–141.

Michaels, S. & O'Connor, M.C. (1990). *Literacy as reasoning within multiple discourses: Implications for policy and educational reform.* Paper Presented at the Summer Institute for the Council of Chief State School Officers. Newton, MA: Clark University.

Newman, D., Griffin, P., & Cole, M. (1989). *The construction zone: Working for cognitive change in school.* New York: Cambridge University Press.

Palincsar, A.S. (1986). The role of dialogue in promoting scaffolded isntruction. *Educational Psychologist, 21,* 73–98.

Palincsar, A.S. (1987). *Collaborating for collaborative learning of text comprehension.* Paper presented at the annual meeting of the American Educational Research Association. Washington, DC.

Palincsar, A.S. & Brown, A.L. (1984). Reciprocal teaching of comprehension-fostering and comprehension-monitoring activities. *Cognition and Instruction, 1,* 117–175.

Palincsar, A.S. & David, Y.M. (1990). *Learning dialogues for comprehension and knowledge acquisition.* Paper presented at the Annual Meeting of the Council for Exceptional Children, Toronto, Canada.

Palincsar, A.S., David, Y.M., Winn, J.A., & Stevens, D. (1990). *Examining the differential effects of teacher- versus student-controlled activity in comprehension instruction.* Paper presented at the annual meeting of the American Educational Research Association, Boston.

Peterson, P.L. (1988). Selecting students and services for compensatory education: Lessons from aptitude-treatment interaction research. *Educational Psychologist, 23,* 313–352.

Peterson, P.L., Fennema, E., Carpenter, T.P., & Loef, M. (1989). Teachers' pedagogical content beliefs in mathematics. *Cognition and Instruction, 6,* 1–40.

Poplin, M.S. (1988). The reductionistic fallacy in learning disabilities: Replicating the past by reducing the present. *Journal of Learning Disabilities, 21,* 389–400.

Pressley, M., Ed-Dinary, P.B., Gasins, I., Schuder, T., Bergman, J.L., Almasi, J., & Brown, R. (1991). *Direct explanation done well: Transactional instruction of reading comprehension strategies.* Unpublished paper. University of Maryland, College Park, MO.

Pressley, M., Goodchild, F., Fleet, J., & Zajchowski, R., & Evans, E.D. (1989). The challenges of classroom strategy instruction. *Elementary School Journal, 89,* 301–342.

Reid, D.K. (1991). Learning disabilities in an educational context. In D.K. Reid, W.P. Hresko, & H.L. Swanson (Eds.), *A cognitive approach to learning disabilities* (2nd ed.). Austin, TX: PRO-ED.

Rowe, D.W. (1989). Author/audience interaction in the preschool: The role of social interaction in literacy learning. *Journal of Reading Behavior, 21,* 311–349.

Rueda, R. (1990). Assisted performance in writing instruction with learning-disabled students. In L.C. Moll (Ed.), *Vygotsky and education: The instructional implications and applications of sociohistorical psychology* (pp. 403–426). New York: Cambridge University Press.

Schumaker, J.B., Deshler, D.D., Alley, G.R., Warner, M.M., & Denton, P.H. (1982). Multipass: A learning strategy for improving reading comprehension. *Learning Disability Quarterly*, *5*, 295–304.

Scruggs, T.E. (1990). Foundations of intervention research. In T.E. Scruggs, & B.Y.L. Wong (Eds.), *Intervention research in learning disabilities* (pp. 66–77). New York: Springer-Verlag.

Shavelson, R.J. & Berliner, D.C. (1988). Erosion of the education research infrastructure. *Educational Researcher*, *17*, 9–11.

Stone, C.A. (1989). Improving the effectiveness of strategy training for learning disabled students: The role of communicational dynamics. *Remedial and Special Education*, *10*(1), 35–42.

Voloshinov, B.N. (1973). *Marxism and the philosophy of language* (L. Matejka & I.R. Tutunik Trans.). New York: Seminar Press.

Vygotsky, L.S. (1978). *Mind in society*. Cambridge, MA: Harvard University Press.

Wertsch, J.V. (1991). *Voices of the mind: A sociocultural approach to mediated action*. Cambridge, MA: Harvard University Press.

Winn, J.A. (1991). *An investigation of the implementation and student outcomes of instruction for self-regulation through mediated collaborative problem solving*. Dissertation. Michigan State University, East Lansing, MI.

Wong, B.Y.L., Wong, R., Darlington, D., & Jones, W. (1991). Interactive teaching: An effective way to teach revision skills to adolescents with learning disabilities. *Learning Disabilities Research and Practice*, *6*, 117–127.

Zaragoza, N. (1987). Process writing for high-risk and learning disabled studets. *Reading Research and Instruction*, *26*, 290–301.

Zaragoza, N. & Vaughn, S. (1992). *The effects of process writing instruction on three second grade students with different achievement profiles*. Learning Disabilities Research & Practice, *7*, 184–193.

7
Issues in Conducting Intervention Research: Secondary Students

THOMAS E. SCRUGGS AND MARGO A. MASTROPIERI

When considering intervention research with students with learning disabilities, one is initially struck by the paucity of such research relative to other types of research in learning disabilities. In a recent evaluation of major special education journals, Lessen, Dudzinski, Karsh, and Van Acker (1989) were able to identify only 119 academic intervention studies with students with learning disabilities, from a pool of 3,106 articles published since 1978. Only 35 of these articles involved secondary students. In contrast, Kavale and Nye (1985–1986) located over 1,000 descriptive studies that compared learning disabled and normally achieving students on any number of measures of social or academic functioning. This relative shortage of intervention research in special education in favor of a plethora of comparative research has previously been noted by Forness and Kavale (1985) and by Scruggs and Mastropieri (1985). Although one may not agree with Lovitt's (1989) declaration that "we don't need any more comparison studies in the field of learning disabilities" (p. 480), there nevertheless does appear to be far too little research intended to identify methods for improving the social or academic functioning of students with learning disabilities.

Why does this relative scarcity of intervention research exist? Several possibilities have been suggested. Forness and Kavale (1985) argued that early special education research was conducted by psychologists who were more comfortable evaluating psychological characteristics of exceptional populations than evaluating the effectiveness of classroom interventions. As a result of this, "special education interventions did not evolve as completely as they should" (Forness & Kavale, 1985, p. 7). Swanson (1988a, 1988b), speaking for many basic researchers, has argued that theoretically oriented comparative research is necessary to provide structure and foundation for the field of learning disabilities, before more meaningful intervention research can be conducted. Since a comprehensive and generally agreed-upon theory of learning disabilities does not exist at present, researchers may serve the field better by making more contributions in this area, so that intervention research can proceed more systematically and meaningfully.

It is also possible that fewer intervention research studies are conducted because such studies are simply more difficult to design and execute and more costly in terms of necessary resources. This may be especially true when classroom teaching of curriculum units, rather than individual teaching of lessons, is undertaken. Because of the obstacles to the systematic design and execution of intervention research, much important work is not completed, or when completed, suffers from validity threats that make the outcomes difficult or impossible to interpret. This results in fewer intervention studies being completed successfully, and as a consequence, fewer follow-up studies being contemplated. In this chapter, we described what we think are the most common design flaws in intervention research, and then describe our position on conducting systematic applied research in learning disabilities at the secondary level.

Problematic Designs

A major problem in conducting intervention research stems from the understandable desire of researchers to conduct the research in "real" classroom settings. Findings from such settings, it could be argued, will be more valid because they will more closely resemble the settings in which they are intended to be used. Unfortunately, researchers commonly have very limited control in classroom settings. Ideally, researchers should assign students to classrooms at random, have a sufficient sample size of classrooms, ensure against attrition, and ensure complete fidelity of treatment implementation. Given that such ideal conditions are probably never met, virtually all intervention research designs that exist represent some degree of departure from this model. Such considerations, problematic in any classroom research, presents special problems in research with students with learning disabilities, who may be represented in only one or two classrooms per school. Following are descriptions of some designs which, we feel, may sacrifice experimental validity in the interest of ensuring "ecological validity" of the treatment.

Pre-Post Designs

Researchers who have found themselves with access to only one group of students, or a desire not to withhold what they consider to be a valuable treatment from a control group (see Vaughn, this volume), have sometimes elected to employ pre-post designs. Such designs involve administration of a pretest, followed by an intervention, which is in turn followed by a posttest. Any observed gain on posttest scores is then attributed to the effectiveness of the treatment. If the instrument used is a standardized, norm-referenced test, a "control" group is implied by the norming sample of the test, and any increase in standard scores is interpreted as an increase over this sample. This design has been commonly seen in the early intervention literature (Casto & Mastropieri, 1986), and in "process" interventions such as psycholinguistic training (Hammill & Larsen, 1974).

The potential problems with pre-post designs are primarily that (a) the observed gain score could be attributed to factors other than the intervention in question, and (b) any gain score reported can say little about the *relative* efficacy of a given intervention. In the latter case, even if a strong argument for treatment can be advanced (in that, for example, the treatment bears a strong, obvious relation to the outcome measure, and that other possible influences can be logically eliminated), whether such a treatment is better than other possible treatments is simply unknown.

Finally, there can be unanticipated measurement problems which can seriously compromise pre-post outcome measurements of a particular intervention. Mastropieri and Scruggs (1990a), for example, found that developmental index scores of handicapped and at-risk infants may tend to decline over the first few years of life, as test items sample an increasingly varied and complex population of behavioral responses. And although early intervention efforts can be shown to reduce this level of decline, pre-post evidence can appear to indicate that intervention has a negative effect on development! Although measurement problems may not be so dramatic with secondary-age populations, they are still likely to be manifest in pre-post, no-control-group designs.

A variation of this design was reported by Polloway, Epstein, Polloway, Patton, and Ball (1986), in an evaluation of the effectiveness of the Corrective Reading Program (CRP) with middle and secondary school learning disabled and educably mentally retarded (EMR) students. Polloway et al. compared gain scores obtained over the year the CRP was used with gain scores achieved by the same students over the year prior to the introduction of the CRP, when a traditional basal reading program was employed. Since the differences in gain scores (favoring CRP) were relatively large, the authors concluded that gains were very likely to have been due to the reading program differences. It should be noted here that the use of two year-long gain scores per student provided a good deal more information than, for example, a reading pretest followed by treatment followed in turn by a reading posttest. The authors acknowledged that several validity threats were manifest in their design; nevertheless, it should also be acknowledged that this study remains one of our few accessible sources of information about the effectiveness of published direct instruction materials on secondary-age mildly handicapped students.

Classroom by Treatment Confounding

A common design found in curriculum comparisons is the "random" assignment of classrooms, rather then individuals, to treatment. This problem is at its greatest when each treatment condition is implemented in only one classroom. For example, a researcher may wish to compare a traditional textbook-based curriculum with two alternate curricula programs. Permission is obtained to use three classrooms; by some random or nonsystematic procedure, each classroom is assigned to a different treatment. After the intervention, an achievement measure is given to all students and a statistical test is employed to determine whether any differences in test scores are "significant." Any obtained differences are then attributed to the curriculum materials or instructional techniques that were the focus of the investigation.

Although some interesting descriptive information can be derived, assessment of relative treatment efficacy is extremely difficult from a design that essentially confounds treatments with classrooms. Many important variables that can potentially impact on learning and are not related to the putative independent variable may be present in such a design. Teacher enthusiasm, for example, has been shown to exhibit a profound impact on both learning and social behavior, even when the same curriculum materials are being used (Brigham, Scruggs, & Mastropieri, 1992). If only one teacher (and one classroom) is employed for each experimental treatment, any obtained classroom differences after treatment could be a result of different levels of teacher enthusiasm, rather than the independent variable being studied. Even if the same teacher teaches all three classes, factors such as time of day, student interpersonal relations, or classroom atmosphere can compromise the independent variable. Additionally, students attending different classes can be functioning at different ability levels, even though all groups can be similarly characterized as learning disabled. In this case, obtained differences among groups may have been due to the fact that one class of students was more able, or had more prior knowledge, than the other classes. Some researchers have used analysis of covariance, with a pretest or ability measure as the covariate, to offset any pre-existing differences among classes. However, this will be of little use if the covariate is not highly sensitive to any real differences among classrooms.

The best and most workable way to address the problem of classroom-by-treatment confounding is simply to assign more than one treatment per classroom. Although treating each classroom as an experimental "unit," in which classroom mean scores replace individual scores, may not be feasible, it is possible to treat individual students nested within classrooms as the units of analysis (Hopkins, 1982). In this way, an estimate of the effect of classrooms can be obtained and separated from the effect of treatment. And although such a design may still fall somewhat short of the "ideal," it may be practical enough to be used, and still be rigorous enough for interpretation.

Programmatic Intervention Research

We (Mastropieri & Scruggs, 1991; Scruggs & Mastropieri, 1990a, 1990b) recently described a method for conducting intervention research, and described our research on mnemonic (memory enhancing) instruction with middle school and secondary-level students as an example. We argued that intervention research should first be established on a strong theoretical foundation (i.e., there are empirical as well as rational reasons to believe the intervention in question may be effective). Research should then be conducted as a series of interdependent investigations, and the design of such research should evolve as information is gathered and research questions become increasingly applied. As with all scientific inquiry, researchers in special education interventions should base their work on what is known, and be careful not to advance too rapidly by addressing too many research questions in the same investigation.

Some researchers have argued that intervention research should be "ecologically valid," in that interventions should be conducted in existing classrooms under "real" classroom conditions (e.g., Shepherd & Gelzheiser, 1987). However, if it is not known whether a particular teaching or learning strategy is effective *at all*, the classroom may not be the best first test of strategy effectiveness (Pressley, Scruggs, & Mastropieri, 1989). We argued (Scruggs & Mastropieri, 1990a) that, in the very early stages of an intervention research program, it is important to maximize experimental power, so that any possible utility of the intervention can be documented.

Maximizing Experimental Power

Although classroom-based research can provide important advantages, enhancement of experimental power is not among them. If the researcher's question is whether a particular teaching routine or learning strategy is effective at all, the following considerations are important in maximizing experimental power, so that any evidence of treatment effectiveness is made apparent and important details of the intervention can be carefully examined (Scruggs & Mastropieri, 1990a, 1990b):

1. Assign individual students at random to experimental conditions and train them in one-to-one teaching and testing situations.
2. Keep the experimental sessions brief and intensive to avoid fatigue and/or inattentiveness.
3. Develop experimental materials that directly reflect the strategies being taught, and for which learners are likely to have little or no prior knowledge. Any information included in experimental materials already known by learners will not discriminate among experimental conditions, and will serve to weaken the experiment.

4. If possible, use treatments that are only one session in length. In this way, when students leave the session, they leave the experiment, and are not vulnerable to information or attitudes they may acquire between sessions. Additionally, attrition, and especially differential attrition due to an unpopular experimental condition, cannot occur under such circumstances.

5. Employ only two or three treatment conditions and use sufficient numbers of subjects to maximize statistical power. If the potential effect of a treatment is uncertain, use only two conditions and a large (25–30) sample size for each condition. As additional research questions arise, plan additional experiments, and plan the number of subjects and conditions based on the obtained effect size from the previous investigations.

Applications

In our first experiment with mnemonic instruction (Mastropieri, Scruggs, & Levin, 1985), we were unsure whether students with learning disabilities would be able to execute the complicated cognitive routines necessary for mnemonic encoding and retrieval. This being the case, we employed the procedures described above: one-to-one treatments, delivered in one brief (about 20 minutes) session, using only three conditions and 30 students to a group. For an experimental task, we taught the hardness levels, according to the Mohs' scale, of several North American minerals. These met the criteria above, in that students were expected to have little or no prior knowledge of the information (that, e.g., hornblende is number 5 on the hardness scale, wolframite is number 4, etc.). Any observed learning effect could then be attributed to relative treatment effectiveness. In addition, hardness of minerals (as a content area) provided us with a faithful test of the effectiveness of the strategy. Although criticized by Shepherd and Gelzheiser (1987) as unlikely to be needed in school learning, minerals and their hardness levels provided an excellent test of the utility of both the "keyword" and "pegword" mnemonic techniques (Mastropieri & Scruggs, 1990b). Using the keyword method, the learner reconstructs unfamiliar words to acoustically similar proxies (hornblende = *horn*; wolframite = *wolf*), to be elaborated with their referent hardness levels. Using the pegword method, numbers are recoded to acoustically similar proxies (four is *door*; five is *hive*). To remember, then, that hornblende is five, the learner is given a keyword for hornblende (horn), a pegword for five (hive), and shown an elaborative illustration (a *horn* with a *hive* in it). Since the strategies are tied so closely to the content to be learned, any treatment advantage would have to be due to the applied strategies.

To determine the ultimate efficacy of such strategies, we used a rehearsal-based control condition ("The hardness level of hornblende is

5. What is the hardness level of hornblende?"). To determine whether the mnemonic strategies were effective *at all*, we added a third, free-study condition. Had students in the mnemonic condition not outperformed free-study condition students, we would have needed to conclude that, for the present, mnemonic strategies did not appear to be useful for students with learning disabilities. If mnemonic condition students outperformed free-study controls but not students in an active rehearsal condition, we would have concluded that there was limited utility for mnemonic strategies, but more refinement and tests would be necessary to determine whether such strategies could ever be optimal. In fact, students in the mnemonic condition greatly outperformed students in both comparison conditions (Mastropieri, Scruggs, & Levin, 1985), and these results suggested that mnemonic techniques may be of great value in enhancing recall of students with learning disabilities.

Extensions

In spite of the success of mnemonic techniques in this one investigation, we felt that a number of additional experiments to examine the effectiveness of variations of this strategy were necessary before we could proceed with curriculum adaptations and classroom applications. This included investigations that addressed how much mnemonic information could be related in one picture, and whether symbols and colors could be included with keyword mnemonics (e.g., Mastropieri, Scruggs, McLoone, & Levin, 1985; Scruggs, Mastropieri, Levin, & Gaffney, 1985; Scruggs, Mastropieri, Levin, McLoone, Gaffney, & Prater, 1985), whether redundancy in experimental list information would cause confusion (Levin, Morrison, McGivern, Mastropieri, & Scruggs, 1986; Scruggs, Mastropieri, & Levin, 1985), whether pictorial and imaginal mnemonics could be used for vocabulary learning (Mastropieri, Scruggs, Levin, Gaffney, & McLoone, 1985), whether information learned mnemonically is comprehended as well as recalled (Mastropieri, Scruggs, & Fulk, 1990), whether students could learn mnemonically from prose passages (Scruggs, Mastropieri, McLoone, Levin, & Morrison, 1987), whether students could be trained to employ their own mnemonic strategies (Fulk, Mastropieri, & Scruggs, in press; McLoone, Scruggs, Mastropieri, & Zucker, 1986), and whether an entire corpus of text-based information could be adapted mnemonically (Scruggs & Mastropieri, 1989b). Since the results of all the above investigations favored mnemonic instruction as employed with individual students with learning disabilities in single sessions, we designed investigations that employed small-group instruction and that extended into several experimental sessions.

Small-Group Investigations

Mastropieri, Scruggs, and Levin (1986, Exp. 1) taught information about minerals, in a single experimental session, to small groups of students with learning disabilities. In such a situation, researchers may be tempted to use the total number of experimental and control students employed as the N for the experiment. However, student scores may not be independent due to events unique to the individual session that impact on the group as a whole. For example, during implementation, one small-group presentation may be disrupted by the behavior of one student in the group. Given that the disruption impacted negatively on scores of all students in the group, those individuals' scores cannot be said to be truly independent. Mastropieri, Scruggs, and Levin (1986) addressed this "unit of analysis" problem (Hopkins, 1982) by computing the mean score for each group and using the group as the statistical unit. Although the number of observations is much smaller, statistical power is maintained to a certain extent by the fact that sets of group mean scores will almost certainly contain substantially less variance than will individual scores, because extreme individual scores are subsumed within the group mean. One alternative to this model is to treat individual student scores as nested within instructional group (Hopkins, 1982). This method allows for an estimate of the variance contribution from instructional groups to be included in the statistical model.

In order to examine whether mnemonics become confusing to students with learning disabilities over several days of instruction, Veit, Scruggs, and Mastropieri (1986) taught three lessons about prehistoric reptiles over a 3-day period. Order of presentation was counterbalanced so that relative increase or decrease of content acquisition over time could be evaluated without the influence of relative lesson difficulty. For this study, 24 small (2–4 people) groups of students were randomly assigned to experimental and control conditions, and the small-group mean score constituted the statistical unit of analysis. Since instruction proceeded for a 3-day interval and an additional 4th day delayed-recall test, student attrition became a concern. In order to address this concern, any group that fell below 2 students for any given day of instruction or testing was excluded from the study, and was replaced by another group. As can be imagined, this investigation was very time-consuming to implement, taking nearly 3 months to deliver 4 days of instruction and testing to 24 small groups. By contrast, investigations that assign two classrooms to two experimental conditions could complete the same instructional treatment in less than 1 week; nevertheless, much would be lost in meaningful interpretation of results.

Classroom Applications

Laboratory investigations, including small-group implementations, to date had suggested that mnemonic strategies were highly effective for students with learning disabilities, were versatile enough to include substantial amounts of information and could be adapted to a variety of content domains. Further research had suggested that students could be taught in small groups to use mnemonic strategies, and they would not lose potency nor would they cause any interference over at least several days' instruction. At this point, it appeared that classroom implementations would be appropriate. Such research is subject to threats that can be avoided in laboratory experiments, in that in long-term investigations it is difficult to (a) precisely control teacher and student dialogue, (b) anticipate all possible student interaction effects, (c) prevent attrition, and (d) ensure that pace, questioning, and feedback variables are *exactly* the same across conditions (given that these are not independent variables). Therefore, in our view, virtually all classroom implementation studies are subject to at least some question. These issues can be addressed by the following design considerations (Scruggs & Mastropieri, 1990a):

1. Classroom research should resemble laboratory research as closely as possible. If outcomes of classroom research are supported by previous laboratory research, they can be more easily defended.
2. Minimize classroom effects by employing at least two classrooms per experimental condition.
3. Plan several replications and extensions for classroom applications. Replications lend strength to outcomes based on imperfect research designs.
4. Whenever possible, consider using within-subjects research designs to maximize statistical power and control for student attrition.

Between-Subject Designs

Between-subject designs are commonly used for intervention research. In an idealized between-subject research design, students are assigned at random, then a substantial number (e.g., 10–20) of *classrooms* are assigned at random to each experimental condition, and comparisons are made on outcome measures using the classroom mean as the experimental unit of analysis, or students treated as a nested factor within classrooms (Hopkins, 1982). However, not only are such numbers of special education classrooms virtually unobtainable, but problems arising from monitoring and ensuring fidelity of experimental treatments could easily become insurmountable. One realistic alternative is to match three or four pairs of classrooms by ability or achievement, and assign classrooms from each pair at random to experimental conditions. In the statistical analysis, students nested within classrooms are treated as the experimental unit; within-classroom variation is identified as a separate source of variance. Again, outcomes from such designs are more conclusive if they are based on theoretically sound models of intervention effectiveness, components of the intervention were validated in laboratory-type experiments, and replications of the classroom study are executed.

Another example of an effective between-subjects design was reported by Lovitt, Rudsit, Jenkins, Pious, and Benedetti (1985), who evaluated two methods for adapting a chapter from a seventh-grade text in physical science. One method emphasized vocabulary drill and timed worksheet activities utilizing cloze format, while the other method emphasized vocabulary acquisition within a "framed outline" study-guide format, in which students filled in important terms in their study guide as the instructor lectured, and answered study questions. Students from seven science classrooms were taught using either of these procedures, or a traditional control procedure in which teachers delivered instruction in a manner consistent with published materials and teachers' guides for that material. Within each of seven classrooms, students were matched on achievement level, and assigned at random to one of the two experimental conditions or a control condition. Each classroom was then divided in half, and taught separately.

In the section that follows, we discuss applications of within-subject research designs for classroom research.

Within-Subject Designs

Augmented Pre-Post Designs

Although pre-post designs are typically very difficult to interpret due to a variety of validity threats, there are circumstances when they may represent part of a larger intervention evaluation. For example, Mastropieri, Jenne, and Scruggs (1988) evaluated the effectiveness of a "level system" in managing adolescents with learning disabilities and behavior problems in a secondary classroom. In this investigation, a 1-week "baseline" condition was followed by teacher application of the level system for the next 3 weeks. It was found that students' classroom behavior, as assessed by number of talk-outs and out-of-seat behavior, was substantially and significantly better when the level system was employed. Since it was altogether possible that some other factor which coincided with the initiation of the level system was responsible for the improved behavior, two supplementary features of this design were conducted. For the first, students were asked to give their opinion of the reason for the observed change in their behavior. Twelve of the 15 students attributed their improved behavior to the initiation of the level system, a finding that lent further credibility to the value of the intervention. For the second instance, an additional analysis of the level system was conducted in a second experiment with a smaller sample using a reversal design, as described in the next section.

Group "Reversal" Designs

Long used by single-subject researchers to validate treatments (e.g., Tawney & Gast, 1986), reversal, or A-B-A-B designs, can be used to evaluate classroom instructional research. Mastropieri et al. (1988), as a follow-up to the pre-post evaluation of a level system described above, with a baseline (3 weeks), treatment (4 weeks), return to baseline (1 week), and treatment reinstatement (1 week). Analysis of results indicated that students performed significantly better when the level system was implemented. For another example, Scruggs and Mastropieri (1989a) reported use of such a design to evaluate the effects of classroom mnemonic instruction of adolescents with learning disabilities, conducted over an 8-week period. In that investigation, students were taught four 2-week units of American history. For the first and third units, (World War I and the Great Depression) students were taught via mnemonic pictures, lectures, and practice activities. For the second and fourth units (Roaring Twenties and World War II), students were taught from the same text using traditional pictures, lectures, and practice activities. Each student was given one score for mnemonic condition tests, and one score for control condition tests. Analysis of the results favored the mnemonic instructional units by a wide margin.

Similarly, Lovitt et al. (1986) used a "reversal" group design to evaluate the effectiveness of adapted (vocabulary exercises and "framed" outlines) curriculum on the academic performance of seventh-grade learning disabled and normally achieving students. Students were taught information based on six chapters of a textbook on physical science in the following order: chapters 2 and 3, nonadapted; chapters 4 and 5, adapted; chapter 6, nonadapted; chapter 7, adapted. Students' mean scores on weekly tests of adapted chapter content significantly exceeded their mean scores on nonadapted content. Furthermore, most individual adapted chapter test scores statistically exceeded most individual nonadapted chapter test scores.

The major concern for this design in this situation is that content or test difficulty varied as a function of experimental condition. That is, experimental condition content or tests of experimental condition content were easier than control content or tests. Although the "reversal" aspect of this design makes such an alternative explanation seem less likely, replication efforts can be helpful in validating treatments. And, in fact, the results reported by Mastropieri et al. (1988, Study 2) were employed as a replication of the first study; the findings of Lovitt et al. (1986) replicate those of Lovitt, Rudsit, Jenkins, Prous, & Benedetti (1985); and the results reported by Scruggs and Mastropieri (1989a) were replicated by Mastropieri and Scruggs (1988) in a crossover design, as described below.

Crossover Designs

A method for controlling for chapter or unit difficulty and time of presentation is by means of the crossover design. In this design, one classroom receives treatment conditions in the order A-B, while another receives treatment conditions in the order B-A (for an example of a three-treatment, within-subject design, see Vaughn, Schumm, & Gordon, 1991).

This configuration necessitates development of experimental and control materials for each unit of instruction, but addresses important validity threats, while also directly addressing potential attrition problems. Since each subject serves as his or her own control, any subject who leaves the investigation does not compromise either treatment differentially. Analysis of results can be conducted either by means of t tests for paired comparisons (experimental condition score vs. control condition score) across classrooms (Mastropieri & Scruggs, 1989), or as a classroom by unit (e.g., week 1 vs. week 2, regardless of condition) analysis of variance (Scruggs & Mastropieri, 1992). In the latter case, evidence of treatment effectiveness is provided by an obtained significant interaction between classroom and unit of instruction. In this design, the classroom factor is between subjects and not easily interpretable.

Crossover designs such as the one described above were also reported by Mastropieri, Scruggs, Bakken, and Brigham (1992) for mnemonic social studies instruction, and Scruggs and Mastropieri (1992) for mnemonic science instruction. Additionally, such designs have been employed to evaluate the effects of teacher enthusiasm (Brigham, Scruggs, & Mastropieri, in press) and activities-oriented science materials (Scruggs et al., 1991).

An extended version of the crossover design was reported by Mastropieri and Scruggs (1988). In that investigation, four classrooms of adolescents with learning disabilities were taught four 2-week units of American history in which the presence of mnemonic techniques was systematically varied. Classroom #1 received treatments in order A-B-A-B (where A = traditional and B = mnemonic); Classroom #2 received order B-A-B-A; Classroom #3 received order A-A-A-B; and Classroom #4 received order B-B-B-A. The configuration employed in Classroom #4 was designed to investigate any spontaneous (i.e., unprompted) transfer of mnemonic strategies to novel content after 6 weeks of instruction (none was observed).

Well-conceived crossover designs can control for major validity threats while addressing such practical concerns for special education researchers as attrition and relatively small sample sizes. In the latter case, enhanced statistical power of within-subject designs can also be beneficial in avoiding Type II errors. A major potential problem of crossover designs is that a technique or strategy trained in one condition with be spontaneously employed in a subsequent "control" condition. This problem is analogous to the problem of "behavioral trapping" in single-subject research, in which a skill, once trained, is found not to be reversible (e.g., Tawney & Gast, 1984). Such problems may emerge when academic skills are being trained, or when specific generalization training is being undertaken. However, crossover designs can be very effective for evaluating the effects of instructional manipulations on the type of academic learning that is characteristic of secondary school programs.

Summary

In this chapter, we described issues in conducting intervention research with students with learning disabilities on the secondary level. We maintained that interventions should be well-grounded in theories of learning as well as characterizations of learning disabilities (Pressley, Scruggs, & Mastropieri, 1989); that they should first be conducted in a series of highly controlled, laboratory-like experiments to carefully assess the potential utility of the intervention; and that, if the intervention is successful in highly controlled settings, it should then be evaluated in classroom applications. We maintained that research designs should evolve as the research questions become more applied, and that the results of laboratory research should be used to support the findings of classroom applications. Finally, we described several research designs that we have found useful in conducting classroom intervention research.

There is a great deal more to conducting intervention research, of course, than experimental or quasi-experimental design. Intervention strategies likely to be effective must be identified, relevant literature must be reviewed, experimental materials must be developed, and cooperative schools, teachers, parents, and students must be located. Nevertheless, inadequate research designs can invalidate the best and most successful efforts in all of these areas, while effective and practical research designs can do much to document the best practices and advance our knowledge of effective interventions with students with learning disabilities.

References

Brigham, F.J., Scruggs, T.E., & Mastropieri, M.A. (1992). The effect of teacher enthusiasm on the learning and behavior of learning disabled students. *Learning Disabilities Research and Practice, 7,* 68–73.

Casto, G. & Mastropieri, M.A. (1986). The efficacy of early intervention programs: A meta-analysis. *Exceptional Children, 52,* 417–424.

Forness, S. & Kavale, K.A. (1985). De-psychologizing special education. In R.B. Rutherford & C.M. Nelson (Eds.), *Severe behavior disorders of children and youth* (pp. 2–14). Boston: College-Hill Press.

Fulk, B.J.M., Mastropieri, M.A., & Scruggs, T.E. (in press). Mnemonic generalization training with learning disabled adolescents. *Learning Disabilities Research and Practice.*

Hammill, D.D. & Larsen, S.C. (1974). The effectiveness of psycholinguistic training. *Exceptional Children, 44,* 402–414.

Hopkins, K.D. (1982). The unit of analysis: Group means versus individual observations. *American Educational Research Journal, 19,* 5–18.

Kavale, K.A. & Nye, C. (1985–1986). Parameters of learning disabilities in achievement, linguistic, neuropsychological, and social/behavioral domains. *Journal of Special Education, 19,* 443–458.

Lessen, E., Dudzinski, M., Karsh, K., & Van Acker, R. (1989). A survey of ten years of academic intervention research with learning disabled students: Implications for research and practice. *Learning Disabilities Focus*, *4*, 106–122.

Levin, J.R., Morrison, C.R., McGivern, J.E., Mastropieri, M.A., & Scruggs, T.E. (1986). Mnemonic facilitation of text-embedded science facts. *American Educational Research Journal*, *23*, 489–506.

Lovitt, T. (1989). *Introduction to learning disabilities*. Boston: Allyn & Bacon.

Lovitt, T., Rudsit, J., Jenkins, J., Pious, C., & Benedetti, D. (1985). Two methods of adapting science materials for learning disabled and regular seventh graders. *Learning Disability Quarterly*, *8*, 275–285.

Lovitt, T., Rudsit, J., Jenkins, J., Pious, C., & Benedetti, D. (1986). Adapting science materials for regular and learning disabled seventh graders. *Remedial and Special Education*, *7*(1), 31–39.

Mastropieri, M.A., Jenne, T., & Scruggs, T.E. (1988). A level system for managing problem behaviors in a high school resource program. *Behavioral Disorders*, *13*, 202–208.

Mastropieri, M.A. & Scruggs, T.E. (1988). Increasing the content area learning of learning disabled students: Research implementation. *Learning Disabilities Research*, *4*, 17–25.

Mastropieri, M.A. & Scruggs, T.E. (1989). Mnemonic social studies instruction: Classroom applications. *Remedial and Special Education*, *10*, 40–46.

Mastropieri, M.A. & Scruggs, T.E. (1990a). An evaluation of early intervention effectiveness at increasing age levels for program initiation. *Early Education and Development*, *1*, 217–224.

Mastropieri, M.A. & Scruggs, T.E. (1990b). Memory and learning disabilities. *Learning Disability Quarterly*, *13*, 234–235.

Mastropieri, M.A. & Scruggs, T.E. (1991). *Teaching students ways to remember: Strategies for learning mnemonically*. Cambridge, MA: Brookline Books.

Mastropieri, M.A., Scruggs, T.E., Bakken, J., & Brigham, F. (1992). A complex mnemonic strategy for teaching states and their capitals: Comparing forward and backward associations. *Learning Disabilities Research and Practice*, *7*, 96–103.

Mastropieri, M.A., Scruggs, T.E., & Fulk, B.J.M. (1990). Teaching abstract vocabulary with the keyword method: Effects on recall and comprehension. *Journal of Learning Disabilities*, *23*, 92–96.

Mastropieri, M.A., Scruggs, T.E., & Levin, J.R. (1985). Mnemonic strategy instruction with learning disabled adolescents. *Journal of Learning Disabilities*, *18*, 94–100.

Mastropieri, M.A., Scruggs, T.E., & Levin, J.R. (1986). Direct vs. mnemonic instruction: Relative benefits for exceptional learners. *Journal of Special Education*, *20*, 299–308.

Mastropieri, M.A., Scruggs, T.E., Levin, J.R., Gaffney, J., & McLoone (1985). Mnemonic vocabulary instruction for learning disabled students. *Learning Disability Quarterly*, *8*, 57–83.

Mastropieri, M.A., Scruggs, T.E., McLoone, B.B., & Levin, J.R. (1985). Facilitating the acquisition of science classifications in learning-disabled students. *Learning Disability Quarterly*, *8*, 299–309.

McLoone, B.B., Scruggs, T.E., Mastropieri, M.A., & Zucker, S. (1986). Memory strategy instruction and training with LD adolescents. *Learning Disabilities Research*, *2*, 45–53.

Polloway, E.A., Epstein, M.H., Polloway, C.H., Patton, J.R., & Ball, D.W. (1986). Corrective reading program: An analysis of effectiveness with learning disabled and mentally retarded students. *Remedial and Special Education*, *7*(4), 41–47.

Pressley, M., Scruggs, T.E., & Mastropieri, M.A. (1989). Memory strategy instruction for learning disabilities: Present and future directions. *Learning Disabilities Research*, *4*, 68–77.

Scruggs, T.E. & Mastropieri, M.A. (1985). The first decade of the journal *Behavioral Disorders*: A quantitative evaluation. *Behavioral Disorders*, *11*, 52–59.

Scruggs, T.E. & Mastropieri, M.A. (1989a). Mnemonic instruction of learning disabled students: A field-based evaluation. *Learning Disability Quarterly*, *12*, 119–125.

Scruggs, T.E. & Mastropieri, M.A. (1989b). Reconstructive elaborations: A model for content area learning. *American Educational Research Journal*, *26*, 311–327.

Scruggs, T.E. & Mastropieri, M.A. (1990a). The case for mnemonic instruction: From laboratory investigations to classroom applications. *Journal of Special Education*, *23*, 7–29.

Scruggs, T.E. & Mastropieri, M.A. (1990b). Mnemonic instruction for students with learning disabilities: What it is and what it does. *Learning Disability Quarterly*, *13*, 271–282.

Scruggs, T.E. & Mastropieri, M.A. (1992). Classroom applications of mnemonic instruction: Acquisition, maintenance, and generalization. *Exceptional Children*, *58*, 219–229.

Scruggs, T.E., Mastropieri, M.A., Brigham, F.J., & Bakken, J. (1991). *The effectiveness of an activities-oriented science curriculum in special education settings*. West Lafayette, IN: Purdue University, Department of Educational Studies.

Scruggs, T.E., Mastropieri, M.A., & Levin, J.R. (1985). Can children effectively re-use the same mnemonic pictures? *Educational Communication and Technology Journal*, *34*, 83–88.

Scruggs, T.E., Mastropieri, M.A., Levin, J.R., & Gaffney, J.S. (1985). Facilitating the acquisition of science facts in learning disabled students. *American Educational Research Journal*, *22*, 575–586.

Scruggs, T.E., Mastropieri, M.A., Levin, J.R., McLoone, B.B., Gaffney, J.S., & Prater, M. (1985). Increasing content area learning: A comparison of mnemonic and visual-spatial direct instruction. *Learning Disabilities Research*, *1*, 18–31.

Scruggs, T.E., Mastropieri, M.A., McLoone, B.B., Levin, J.R., & Morrison, C.R. (1987). Mnemonic facilitation of learning disabled students' memory for expository prose. *Journal of Educational Psychology*, *79*, 27–34.

Shepherd, M.J. & Gelzheiser, L.M. (1987). Strategies and mnemonics go to school. In H.L. Swanson (Ed.), *Memory and learning disabilities: Advances in learning and behavioral disabilities* (pp. 245–262). Greenwich, CT: JAI Press.

Swanson, H.L. (1988a). Toward a metatheory of learning disabilities. *Journal of Learning Disabilities*, *21*, 196–209.

Swanson, H.L. (1988b). Comments, countercomments, and new thoughts. *Journal of Learning Disabilities*, *21*, 289–285.

Tawney, J.W. & Gast, D.L. (1984). *Single subject research in special education.* Columbus, OH: Merrill.

Vaughn, S., Schumm, J.S., & Gordon, J. (1991). *Writing, tracing, and computer: Which one is most effective for teaching spelling to nonlearning disabled and learning disabled students?* Coral Gables, FL: University of Miami, School of Education.

Veit, D.T., Scruggs, T.E., & Mastropieri, M.A. (1986). Extended mnemonic instruction with learning disabled students. *Journal of Educational Psychology*, *78*, 300–308.

8
Cognitive Strategy Instruction: Methodological Issues and Guidelines in Conducting Research

Steve Graham and Karen R. Harris

An important by-product of the cognitive revolution in education and psychology has been the application of cognitive instructional procedures to a wide range of problems experienced by children. These approaches have been used to help children deal with anger, aggression, anxiety, depression, hyperactivity, impulsivity, chronic illness, and interpersonal relations (see Hughes & Hall, 1989; Kendall, 1991). There has also been considerable interest in the role of cognitive strategy instruction in academic learning, particularly in terms of promoting the academic progress of students with severe learning problems. Entire issues of special education journals have been devoted to this topic (e.g., October, 1986 *Exceptional Children*; Winter, 1989 *Learning Disability Quarterly*), and studies on strategy instruction are common fare in journals within the field of learning disabilities (LD). Enough research has been undertaken so that at least one group of investigators has developed and marketed a strategy-based curriculum (cf. Deshler & Schumaker, 1986).

There is good reason for all this interest. As Pressley and his associates have aptly noted, "Many strategies improve academic performance and can be taught to students" (Pressley, Woloshyn, Lysynchuk, Martin, Wood, & Willoughby, 1990). This is especially important for students with LD because they often have difficulty with the cognitive processes and strategies underlying effective performance in reading, writing, and mathematics (Wong, Harris, & Graham, 1991). In an area such as writing, for example, the poor performance of students with LD is, in part, the result of difficulties with planning, revising, and managing the composing process (Graham & Harris, 1989a). Students with LD often apply immature or ineffective strategies for carrying out these processes. Their writing performance (and performance in other academic areas) may be further hindered by characteristics such as low motivation or impulsivity. Cognitive strategy instruction provides an appealing match to the needs of students with LD, since these approaches: (a) focus on helping students more effectively execute the processes necessary for accomplishing academic tasks, and (b) include methods for addressing ineffective or maladaptive learning characteristics (see Hughes & Hall, 1989).

The current interest in cognitive strategy instruction makes it likely that research and development will continue during the 1990s. This will be fueled by three factors (Pressley, Symons, Snyder, & Cariglia-Bull, 1989). First, realistic analyses explicitly specifying the processes needed to carry out academic tasks in writing, reading, and mathematics are underway. Second, recent models of fully mature, competent strategy use are more complete. Third, models for teaching strategies are richer and more complete than their predecessors.

These factors, and the growing sophistication of investigators involved in cognitive strategy research, should result not only in more research, but also in better research in this area. The purpose of the current chapter is to examine methodological issues in conducting cognitive strategy instruction research. In the process, we propose guidelines for conducting strategy research and offer suggestions for future research. The issues and guidelines presented should also be useful to practitioners interested in evaluating the applicability of cognitive strategy instruction to their classroom.

Issues

What Strategies Should Be Studied?

While the definition for the term *strategy* varies, it is generally agreed that strategies are goal-directed, cognitive operations used to facilitate performance (Bjorklund, 1990; Pressley, Harris, & Marks, 1992). Examples of strategies include: brainstorming ideas to use in a composition, verbally rehearsing information to be remembered, and generating and answering questions while reading text. Strategies can range from the use of a single process to the coordination of multiple strategies, each aimed at accomplishing subgoals related to a larger goal.

Somewhat surprisingly, the number of academic strategies that have been evaluated using scientific methods is quite small. For example, a recent review by Pressley, Johnson, Symons, McGoldrick, and Kurita (1989) identified only a handful of strategies that have been shown to boost comprehension and memory of text by elementary-age students, including summarization, representational imagery, and story grammar strategies. Similar observations in the area of writing have been made by Graham and Harris (1992). Consequently, identification and development of additional academic strategies, particularly for students with LD, need to be undertaken. There are at least three criteria that should guide researchers (and practitioners) in this task.

Do Students Need Strategy Instruction?

An important first step is to determine if there is a need for strategy instruction. Diagnosis of students' current strategy use is a critical prerequisite to strategy selection and development. There is little value in teaching a strategy if students already have an effective approach to the task. If their approach to the task is ineffective or immature, however, then the information gained by such a diagnosis provides a basis for making informed decisions about the eventual shape and structure of the strategy to be taught.

This process can be illustrated by examining a recent study involving strategy instruction in mathematics (Case, Harris, & Graham, 1992). In this study, we asked teachers to identify students with LD who had significant difficulties in solving word problems. We then asked the identified students to solve simple addition or subtraction word problems, read the words found in these problems, and complete a test on basic addition and subtraction facts. While the students were able to read most of the words in the word problems and answer correctly 80% or more of the basic addition and subtraction facts, they were able to answer only about half of the word problems correctly. An analysis of their papers showed that 95% of the problems missed were a result of executing the wrong operation; they subtracted when they should have added and vice versa. This information was subsequently used to develop a strategy that was responsive to students' needs. The strategy included procedures for helping students both to understand what the problem required, and to devise an appropriate plan of action.

There are a variety of different ways for assessing students' current strategy use (cf. Harris, 1982). In the above example, inferences about students' processing were drawn from performance patterns. Other techniques that have been commonly used to assess strategy use include: self-reports, formal observations, simulated recall, and think-aloud procedures. The most convincing evidence of strategy use comes from observations or data collected under naturalistic conditions, especially when the results from different measures converge.

Does the Strategy Promote More Mature Cognitive Processing?

In addition to developing an understanding of students' current strategy use, the cognitive processes necessary, or at least sufficient, for carrying out the task must be determined as well. Thorough understanding of both the learner and the task are essential to developing strategies that are responsive to students' needs, that build on their existing competence, and that promote a more mature or complex approach to the task (Harris & Graham, 1992a). In the word problem example above, current knowledge of problem solving (cf. Goldman, 1989) was used to determine what cognitive and metacognitive processes were needed to facilitate performance. This knowledge was meshed with knowledge of the students' current strategy use to develop a more mature approach to the target task.

A crucial goal in strategy instruction, therefore, is to help students carry out tasks or processes that are slightly beyond their current means. It must be emphasized, however, that strategies taught to students represent a "do-able" challenge, that is, one that they can accomplish given adequate instructional assistance and guidance.

Several guidelines that we have found helpful for insuring that a strategy is do-able include (Harris & Graham, 1992a):

1. When possible, refine or extend strategies that students already use on their own.
2. Design the strategy so that it can be scaled upward or downward. Thus, if the strategy is initially too difficult, it can be scaled downward; or as the student is exposed to more complex tasks, it can be scaled upward.
3. Involve students in the selection, adaptation, or development of the strategy.
4. Keep the number of steps in the strategy appropriate to the learner's capabilities.
5. The wording for each step should be brief and in the students' own language (the steps are only a verbal reminder to carry out a process).
6. Develop a mnemonic or label to aid memory.

Is the Strategy Educationally Relevant?

There is little reason or justification for testing the effectiveness of strategies that are poorly matched to the demands students face. For instance, teaching high-school students a strategy for writing poetry will have little impact on school performance if all of their writing assignments involve expository tasks such as book reports, essay tests, and the like. Thus, one important criteria in selecting or developing a strategy to be tested is the match between the strategy and curricular demands.

A related issue involves how widely the strategies of interest can be applied. One way of categorizing strategies is according to their generality (Pressley, Goodchild, Fleet, Zajchowski, & Evans, 1989). Some strategies are *task-limited* and can be applied only to very specific situations (e.g., remembering the notes on the treble staff by using the sentence, *E*very *G*ood *B*oy *D*oes *F*ine). Other strategies can be applied to a much wider array of circumstances and cut across domains. These include *goal-limited* strategies and *general* strategies. Goal-limited strategies are used to achieve specific goals, such as writing a convincing argument. Strategies used to accomplish this goal, however, could also be used to write a term paper in science, since both forms of writing benefit from the use of prewriting organizational strategies. General strategies such as goal setting and self-monitoring can be applied even more widely, across many domains, to aid in meeting a wide variety of goals.

We recommend that researchers consider the development of multiple strategy packages that combine both goal-limited and general strategies. For example, in our work, we frequently use general strategies such as goal setting, self-assessment, and self-recording to help students regulate the use of goal-limited strategies (cf. Graham, Harris, MacArthur, & Schwartz, 1991). In the work by Englert, Raphael, Anderson, Anthony, Steven, and Fear (1991), students are taught a variety of different strategies for various writing tasks that are applied within the framework of a general cycle for planning, writing, revising, and editing.

How Should Strategies Be Taught?

Theorists and researchers generally agree that cognitive strategy instruction in academic domains include three major components: skillful use of effective strategies, knowledge about the use and significance of those strategies (metastrategy information), and self-regulation of strategic performance (cf. Brown, Campione, & Day, 1981). Variations in the operationalization of these components have led to the development of several different strategy instruction models, which have been applied in school-based settings (cf. Deshler & Schumaker, 1986; Harris & Graham, 1992b; Palinscar, 1986).

In recent years, two different theoretical camps have provided important positions on cognitive strategy instruction (Pressley et al., 1990). One camp has assembled around Vygotsky's (1978) analysis of learning. According to this perspective, skilled thinking develops as a result of social interactions with more capable others. Instruction is scaffolded by a more capable other, who initially provides a lot of structure and guidance through instructional dialogue. This instructional support, like a scaffold, is progressively removed as the less capable other internalizes cognitive processes and the dialogue used to regulate them.

The other camp places greater emphasis on explicitly teaching strategies. Instructional approaches are characterized by detailed modeling and discussion on how to use the strategy, numerous opportunities for practice, monitoring of progress in applying the strategy, and feedback and reexplanation as needed (Harris & Pressley, 1991; Pressley et al., 1992).

Despite different conceptual foundations (and various claims by supporters), these approaches are not radically different from each other. Vygotskian and cognitive-behavioral descriptions of effective teaching, for example, are very similar (Meichenbaum, 1977; Pressley, Snyder, & Cariglia-Bull, 1987). Likewise, dialogue, scaffolding, interactive learning, collaboration, reflection, and meaningful learning activities and environments can be found in cognitive strategy approaches from both camps (cf. Brown & Campione, 1990; Englert et al., 1991; Harris & Graham, 1992a; Meichenbaum, 1977). In fact, a number of researchers have purposefully taken an integrated approach to strategy instruction, using multiple components and procedures to directly address affective, behavioral, cognitive, and social/ecological processes. Our approach to cognitive strategy instruction, self-regulated strategy development (Harris & Graham, 1992a, 1992b), is based on such a perspective.

Intervention Integrity

One challenge posed by the multicomponent nature of cognitive strategy instruction involves intervention integrity. The concept of intervention integrity subsumes and expands upon the concept of treatment integrity (Harris, 1990). First, it is similar to treatment integrity in that each and every component/characteristic/procedure of the intervention must be carried out as intended and as recommended. This is necessary in order to validly compare different instructional approaches, and in performing replication studies. For instance, in a study presented at a recent conference, three approaches to strategy instruction were compared. In a videotape of the three conditions, the teacher in one condition placed a great deal more distance between herself and her students and was markedly less warm, enthusiastic, and responsive than the teachers in the other two conditions. Unfortunately, any differential outcomes that may have been due to planned differences in the interventions were confounded by differences in the characteristics of instruction.

Intervention integrity expands on the concept of treatment integrity by requiring *assessment of the processes of change as related to both intentions and outcomes*. Specifying and assessing intervention processes is needed to determine if strategy interventions work for the reasons they are hypothesized to work. For example, the case in favor of scaffolding would be substantially strengthened by documentation across a number of experiments demonstrating that scaffolding actually did take place and contributed to competent performance. By establishing intervention integrity, researchers can test and expand the theoretical basis of strategy instruction. Component analysis is one way processes of change can be investigated.

Component Analyses

Determining the relative contributions of instructional components and the variables responsible for change represents a major challenge. Even the simplest strategy interventions involve multiple components and procedures; determining the relative contributions of each is a formidable task. While component analyses studies remain rare, we believe that such investigations need to be given greater emphasis for at least two reasons. First, we have noted a disturbing tendency for some researchers to highlight specific instructional processes (for example, instructional dialogue) over others, to explain the success of their instructional regime. While such claims may be accurate, they need to be validated. For instance, we have conducted a series of component analyses studies examining whether explicit self-regulation procedures included as part of a strategy instructional regime made an important contribution (as we claimed) to students' performance (Graham & Harris, 1989b; Sawyer, Graham, & Harris, 1992).

Second, component analyses can help us better gauge how much and what types of instruction different groups of students need to learn a strategy. While we know that some students require a great deal of instructional resources to learn a strategy, there is little evidence about what components/characteristics/ procedures best match different student characteristics. One area that has been investigated involves explicitness of instruction. Less capable students require detailed and explicit instruction to acquire a variety of cognitive and metacognitive strategies, and the more complex the strategy to be learned, the more explicit instruction needs to be, even for capable students (Brown & Campione, 1990).

Maintenance and Generalization

One of the most difficult challenges faced by strategy researchers involves the identification of more effective procedures for promoting maintenance and generalization. Durable and flexible strategy use does not occur in all studies with all students (Harris & Pressley, 1991). Much has been learned, however, about how to facilitate these outcomes. Validated procedures for promoting strategy transfer and maintenance include: practicing strategy execution until it is automatic; providing diverse practice in using the strategy; encouraging students to personalize the target strategy; making students aware of gains following strategy execution; encouraging students to believe they can do well by using the right strategy; teaching students to self-reinforce contingent on strategy use; fostering development of self-coping statements such as, "I can do this"; teaching other strategies in conjunction with the main strategy, such as self-assessment and goal setting; asking students to share with their teachers and parents what they are learning and where they have used the strategy; encouraging students to maintain and generalize the use of the strategy; directly prompting students to use the strategy; and informing students about the value of a strategy and when and where it can be used, as well as when and where it may be best not to use it (Brown et al., 1981; Harris, 1982; Pressley et al., 1990; Stokes & Osnes, 1989).

Our experience in teaching academic strategies to low-achieving students has convinced us that there is no "magic bullet" for promoting maintenance and generalization. For example, in a recent investigation (Sawyer et al., 1992), we found that generalization was more likely to occur when multiple instructional procedures were applied in tandem. This included: having the teacher describe and model how to use the strategy, providing ample opportunities for students to apply the strategy under practice conditions (providing assistance and feedback when needed), helping students to develop an internal dialogue for directing the use of the strategy, having students set goals for using the strategy, encouraging students to evaluate the effects of employing the strategy, and discussing with the student when, where, and how the strategy can best be used. An important challenge for researchers is to determine what combinations of instructional components promote durable and flexible strategy use.

Follow-Up Procedures

Follow-up procedures may be especially important (as part of the overall package) for promoting maintenance and generalization. There are several reasons why we believe this to be the case. First, in a study by Schmidt and colleagues (reported in Schumaker, Deshler, Alley, & Warner, 1983), students with LD were taught a series of writing strategies to master. Once a strategy was mastered, four generalization conditions were implemented. Each condition was used only if classroom data indicated that a student's performance fell below mastery. The four conditions were: review (included practice in easy material), generalization orientation and activation (identification of places to use the strategy and practice in adapting and applying the strategy for these purposes), self-control (included setting goals for using the strategy), and cooperative planning between the resource and regular classroom teacher to promote strategy use. The basic findings of this study were that generalization of strategy use was improved by the inclusion of follow-up procedures, that cooperative planning procedures were not necessary for many of the students, and that the amount and types of generalization conditions needed to obtain generalization varied across students.

Follow-up procedures have also proven to be especially helpful in such diverse areas as giving up smoking (Glasgow & Lichtenstein, 1987), dealing with marital discord (Jacobson, 1989), and losing weight (Brownell & Jeffery, 1987). In these areas, experimenters and practitioners have assumed that relapses will occur and, consequently, have actively included follow-up procedures as part of their therapy. As Kendall (1989) has argued, we need to provide our students with more long-term assistance and help in applying the skills they are taught.

Follow-up procedures that researchers may find especially useful in promoting durable and flexible use of academic strategies include: self-monitoring and recording of strategy use, setting goals for using the strategy, periodic review and practice in using the strategy, peer support in using and adapting the strategy, proactive planning for generalization, homework assignments to use the strategy on new tasks, and problem solving sessions to decide how to deal with set backs and adapt the strategy to new situations. For example, after learning to apply a strategy or several strategies, students might participate in a series of ongoing follow-up support sessions. During these support sessions, students might work together to set and monitor goals for using the strategies, pro-actively identify when and where the strategies should be used, problem solve to identify ways of overcoming setbacks and how to adapt the strategies to new situations, and receive additional review and practice from the teacher or their peers in using the strategies (when necessary).

The Normal Progression of Maintenance and Generalization

At the present time, we know very little about the breadth, depth, and course of development of maintenance and generalization in children (cf. Harris, Graham, & Pressley, 1992; Harris & Pressley, 1991). This re-presents a formidable obstacle for strategy researchers (especially those working with low-achieving students), because it means that we have little more than intuition to guide us in setting reasonable criteria and evalu-ating outcomes in our research. For instance, it is difficult to evaluate how successful a child with a learning disability has been in maintaining and generalizing an academic strategy, if we know little or nothing about how successful regularly achieving students are in adapting and main-taining the use of this or other strategies.

More descriptive developmental studies of academic strategy main-tenance and generalization among students who are progressing normally, and those who are having problems learning, would greatly inform theory and the types of instructional recommendations that we make to teachers. Several ways in which attention to development has already enriched our understanding of strategy instruction include the findings that less explicit instruction is needed to promote durable strategy application with older versus younger children (cf. O'Sullivan & Pressley, 1984), that younger children require more prompting than older children to obtain gener-alization (Bjorklund, 1990); that metacognitive knowledge relevant to strategy use develops with experience and age (cf. Garner & Alexander, 1989; Harris, Graham, & Freeman, 1988), and that short-term memory capacity is an important determinant of whether or not children benefit from certain types of strategy instruction (cf. Pressley, Goodchild, Fleet, Zajchowski, & Evans, 1989). Additional attention to developmental vari-ation in maintenance and generalization and developmental constraints on instructional benefits should also be useful because it would help to develop assessment methodology, assist in determining developmentally and culturally appropriate definitions of competence, and provide insight about the acquisition of competent behavior (Harris, 1985).

In examining the course of development of maintenance and gener-alization in normally achieving and low-achieving students, it is important to study variability in the patterns of development. How do different children of the same age maintain and generalize academic strategies? What strategies does an individual child have available for use when working on similar tasks (e.g., planning a paper) in different contexts?

Other questions in this area that need to be addressed include the following: How is the development of maintenance and generalization related to other aspects of cognitive development? What roles do developmental differences in children's knowledge base play in the development of durable and generalized strategy use? How do developmental differences in children's self awareness (e.g., awareness of the outcome of their actions) contribute to the development of maintenance and generalization? Are there age-related differences in the amount of mental effort required to maintain and generalize academic strategies? How does children's intentionality to maintain and generalize academic strategies change with age?

How Should Strategy Instruction Be Evaluated?

In evaluating the effects of strategy instruction, the researcher must decide what factors are of interest and how they can best be measured. In addition, the researcher's basic approach to studying the problem must be determined; this can range from the use of quantitiative to qualitative methodologies.

Measures

Cognitive strategy instruction approaches typically include some combination of behavioral (e.g., modeling), cognitive (e.g., cognitive or metacognitive strategies), and affective components (e.g., development of adaptive attributions or tolerance for frustration and errors). Moreover, the cognitive components of instruction may create cognitive changes as well as nonspecific behavioral and affective changes, and so on (Harris, 1985). As a result, an evaluation that concentrates on only one of these processes of change and associated outcomes (e.g., modeling and behavioral outcomes) may very likely produce a truncated picture of strategy effects. Evaluation of strategy instruction, therefore, must be multifaceted.

The specific measures chosen for a research study should depend on the composition of the strategy and the accompanying instructional regime as well as the specific hypotheses addressed by the study. For example, if students are taught to set goals for what their written compositions will accomplish, there are a number of cognitive, behavioral, and affective processes that should be measured. Behavioral indices should be included to determine if goals are achieved and if goal acquisition is related to improvement in quality of written products. Because goals motivate the establishment of a plan of action for their attainment, changes in students' approach to the task should also be examined. It would be equally important to determine if students who set goals expend more effort (write longer) and form more accurate perceptions of their writing competence (self-efficacy), since goal setting has a motivational function and provides information that can facilitate self-evaluation (Graham, MacArthur, Schwartz, & Voth, 1992).

Researchers also need to collect evidence on the use of the inculcated strategy. There are at least three benefits to collecting this information. First, documentation showing that students use the strategy effectively provides evidence that the instructional program was successful. Second, such documentation provides evidence on whether the strategy mediates change in students' behavior. Third, by examining how students use the strategy, considerable insight into what students internalize as a result of instruction, and how they effectively modify or subvert a strategy over time can be obtained (Graham & Harris, 1992). Likewise, if students are taught or encouraged to use specific procedures to regulate the use of the inculcated strategy (e.g., goal setting, self-verbalizations, and so forth), the application of these processes should be documented as well.

Finally, possible interactions between the characteristics of students and the outcomes of strategy instruction need to be examined. There is very little data about which student characteristics predict who will benefit from strategy instruction; such data would be especially valuable.

Research Design

While it is beyond the scope of this paper to present a thorough discussion of issues involving research methodology in strategy instruction (see Pressley et al., 1990 for a more complete discussion), we would like to offer several observations. First, there is room for improvement in experimental studies examining the effects of cognitive strategy instruction. This can be illustrated by considering a methodological review conducted by Lysynchuk, Pressley, Ailly, Smith, and Cake (1989). They examined 37 studies of reading comprehension strategy instruction. The most striking design problems in these studies included: (a) failure to randomly assign students or groups to treatment and control conditions (36% of the studies); (b) not using the appropriate unit of analysis (83%); (c) exposing treatment and control students to different training material (30%); (d) failure to assess strategy maintenance (76%) and generalization (92%); and (e) not checking to determine if participants completed the treatment as directed (63%) or actually used the strategy (73%). We have observed similar problems in strategy instructional studies done with students with LD.

Lysynchuk and her colleagues' (1990) investigation makes it clear that researchers have not been successful in guaranteeing all aspects of validity when using traditional experimental methodology to evaluate strategy effects. While the strengths of true experimental designs are well known, some strategy interventions (for example, strategy curriculums designed for a whole school or multiple-year interventions) will probably never be evaluated using such procedures (Pressley et al., 1990). Studies employing true experimental designs can also be criticized in terms of the types of information they have generated. They do not generally provide a rich description of strategy instructional effects for individual students, nor do they usually provide much insight into the daily workings of strategy instructional programs. As a result, other approaches to evaluation, such as applied behavior analysis, the case study approach, quasi-experimental designs, and qualitative research methodology, have an important role to play in evaluating the effects of strategy instruction.

Some examples of how alternative methodologies can be used to more fully investigate cognitive strategy instruction include the following: Detailed descriptions obtained through qualitative research methods on what students with LD learn and teachers do during cognitive strategy instruction are needed. The strategies students with LD use spontaneously under naturalistic conditions need to be more fully described. Correlational data can be used to pinpoint strategies that are worthy of instructional consideration for students with LD. For example, a strategy used by students who are successful at a task is a likely candidate for instruction with other students when those using it on their own outperform those not using it. Students and teachers should be interviewed to obtain their reactions and recommendations regarding strategy instruction.

Cognitive Strategy Instruction in the Schools

If strategy instruction is to fulfill its potential, it must "go to school." Despite its educational potential, cognitive strategy instruction does not appear to be especially common in either special or regular classrooms. Nonetheless, enough is now known so that it is possible to prepare multicomponent strategy instructional packages, as was done by researchers at the University of Kansas (Deshler & Schumaker, 1986). As such packages are developed and implemented, researchers need to study this process. This will provide invaluable information on how the implementation process can be further refined and improved.

An important issue in implementation concerns the role of strategy instruction in the school curricula. Strategy instruction could supplant the existing curricula, supplement it, or be integrated as part of it. We have argued elsewhere (Graham & Harris, 1989a, 1992) that strategy instruction should be a fully integrated part of the school program. In the area of writing, for instance, strategies for planning, revising, and regulating the writing process can be taught within the context of the process approach to writing instruction (e.g., Harris & Graham, in press-b).

Finally, as teachers strive to implement new forms of instruction in their classroom, it is important to ask what is acceptable and what is not. Teachers are not likely to teach strategies or use instructional regimes that they do not view as reasonable, appropriate, or fair. Likewise, students probably will not use strategies they do not view as being effective, efficient, useful, and reasonably easy to use. While there is some reason to believe that teachers view strategy instruction as an acceptable treatment (Harris, Preller, & Graham, 1990), researchers should make it a common practice to gather information on consumer satisfaction.

A Final Comment

Cognitive strategy instruction is an evolving area that offers many practical as well as methodological challenges for researchers. It is also an exciting area for researchers because its great educational promise has yet to be fulfilled. Enough is currently known about cognitive strategy instruction, however, to be optimistic that its potential will be achieved. Research and development conducted during the 1990s will play a major role in determining if cognitive strategy instruction actually does go to school.

References

Bjorklund, D. (1990). *Children's strategies: Contemporary views of cognitive development.* Hillsdale, NJ: Erlbaum.

Brown, A.L. & Campione, J.C. (1990). Interactive learning environments and the teaching of science and mathematics. In M. Gardner, J. Greens, F. Reif, A. Schoenfeld, A. di Sessa, & E. Stage (Eds.), *Toward a scientific practice of science education* (pp. 111–139). Hillsdale, NJ: Erlbaum.

Brown, A.L., Campione, J.C., & Day, J.D. (1981). Learning to learn: On training students to learn from tests. *Educational Researcher, 10*, 14–21.

Brownell, K. & Jeffery, R. (1987). Improving long-term weight loss: Pushing the limits of treatment. *Behavior Therapy, 18*, 353–374.

Case, L., Harris, K.R., & Graham, S. (1992). Improving the mathematical problem solving skills of students with learning disabilities: Self-instructional strategy development. *Journal of Special Education, 26*, 1–19.

Deshler, D.D. & Schumaker, J.B. (1986). Learning strategies: An instructional alternative for low-achieving adolescents. *Exceptional Children, 52*, 583–590.

Englert, C.S., Raphael, T.E., Anderson, L.M., Anthony, H.M., Stevens, D.D., & Fear, K. (1991). Making writing strategies and self-talk visible: Cognitive strategy instruction in writing in regular and special education classrooms. *American Educational Research Journal, 28*, 337–373.

Garner, R. & Alexander, P.A. (1989). Metacognition: Answered and unanswered questions. *Educational Psychologist, 24*, 143–158.

Glasgow, R. & Lichtenstein, E. (1987). Long-term effects of behavioral smoking cessation interventions. *Behavior Therapy, 18*, 297–332.

Goldman, S. (1989). Strategy instruction in mathematics. *Learning Disability Quarterly, 12*, 43–55.

Graham, S. & Harris, K.R. (1989a). Cognitive training: Implications for written language. In J. Hughes & R. Hall (Eds.), *Cognitive behavioral psychology in the schools: A comprehensive handbook* (pp. 247–279). New York: Guilford.

Graham, S. & Harris, K.R. (1989b). A components analysis of cognitive strategy instruction: Effects on learning disabled students' compositions and self-efficacy. *Journal of Educational Psychology, 81*, 353–361.

Graham, S. & Harris, K.R. (1992). Teaching writing strategies to students with learning disorders: Issues and recommendations. In L. Meltzer (Ed.), *Strategy and assessment and instruction for students with learning disabilities* (pp. 271–292). Austin, TX: PRO-ED.

Graham, S., Harris, K.R., MacArthur, C., & Schwartz, S. (1991). Writing and writing instruction with students with learning disabilities: A review of a program of research. *Learning Disability Quarterly, 14*, 89–114.

Graham, S., MacArthur, C., Schwartz, S., & Voth, T. (1992). Improving the compositions of students with learning disabilities using a strategy involving product and process goal setting. *Exceptional Children, 58*, 322–334.

Harris, K.R. (1982). Cognitive-behavior modification: Application with exceptional students. *Focus on Exceptional Children, 15*, 1–16.

Harris, K.R. (1985). Conceptual, methodological, and clinical issues in cognitive-behavioral assessment. *Journal of Abnormal Child Psychology, 13*, 373–390.

Harris, K.R. (1990). Developing self-regulated learners: The role of private speech and self-instructions. *Educational Psychologist, 25*, 35–50.

Harris, K.R. & Graham, S. (1992a). *Helping young writers master the craft: Strategy instruction and self-regulation in the writing process.* Cambridge: Brookline Books.

Harris, K.R. & Graham, S. (1992b). Self-regulated strategy development: A part of the writing process. In M. Pressley, K.R. Harris, & J. Guthrie (Eds.), *Promoting academic competence and literacy: Cognitive research and instructional innovation* (pp. 277–309). New York: Academic Press.

Harris, K.R., Graham, S., & Freeman, S. (1988). Effects of strategy training on metamemory among learning disabled students. *Exceptional Children, 54*, 332–338.

Harris, K.R., Graham, S., & Pressley, M. (1992). Cognitive behavioral approaches in reading and written language: Developing self-regulated learners. In N.N. Singh & I.L. Beale (Eds.), *Learning disabilities: Nature, theory, and treatment* (pp. 415–451). New York: Springer-Verlag.

Harris, K.R., Preller, D., & Graham, S. (1990). Acceptability of cognitive-behavioral and behavioral interventions among teachers. *Cognitive Therapy and Research, 14*, 573–587.

Harris, K.R. & Pressley, M. (1991). The nature of cognitive strategy instruction: Interactive strategy construction. *Exceptional Children, 57*, 392–404.

Hughes, J. & Hall, R. (1989). *Cognitive behavioral psychology in the schools: A comprehensive handbook.* New York: Guilford.

Jacobson, N.C. (1989). The maintenance of treatment gains following social learning-based marital therapy. *Behavior Therapy, 20*, 325–336.

Kendall, P. (1989). The generalization and maintenance of behavior change: Comments, considerations, and the "no-cure" criticism. *Behavior Therapy, 20*, 357–364.

Kendall, P. (1991). *Child and adolescent therapy: Cognitive-behavioral procedures.* New York: Guilford.

Lysynchuk, L., Pressley, M., Ailly, H., Smith, M., & Cake, H. (1989). A methodological analysis of experimental studies of comprehension strategy instruction. *Reading Research Quarterly, 24,* 458–470.

Meichenbaum, D. (1977). *Cognitive behavior modification: An integrative approach.* NY: Plenum Press.

O'Sullivan, J. & Pressley, M. (1984). Completeness of instruction and strategy transfer. *Journal of Experimental Child Psychology, 38,* 275–288.

Palincsar, A.S. (1986). The role of dialogue in providing scaffolded instruction. *Educational Psychologist, 21* (1 & 2), 73–98.

Pressley, M., Goodchild, F., Fleet, J., Zajchowski, R., & Evans, E. (1989). The challenges of classroom strategy instruction. *Elementary School Journal, 89,* 301–342.

Pressley, M., Harris, K., & Marks, M. (1992). But good strategy instructors are constructivists!! *Educational Psychology Review, 4,* 3–31.

Pressley, M., Johnson, C., Symons, S., McGoldrick, J., & Kurita, J. (1989). Strategies that improve memory and reading comprehension of what is read. *Elementary School Journal, 90,* 3–32.

Pressley, M., Snyder, B., & Cariglia-Bull, T. (1987). How can good strategy use be taught to children: Evaluation of six alternative approaches. In S. Cormier & J. Hagman (Eds.), *Transfer of learning: Contemporary research and application.* Orlando, FL: Academic Press.

Pressley, M., Symons, S., Snyder, B., & Carigulia-Bull, T. (1989). Strategy instruction research comes of age. *Learning Disability Quarterly, 12,* 16–30.

Pressley, M., Woloshyn, V., Lysynchuk, L., Martin, V., Wood, E., & Willoughby, T. (1990). A primer of research on cognitive strategy instruction: The important issues and how to address them. *Educational Psychology Review, 2,* 1–57.

Sawyer, R., Graham, S., & Harris, K.R. (1992). Direct teaching, strategy instruction, and strategy instruction with explicit self-regulation: Effects on learning disabled students' composition skills and self-efficacy. *Journal of Educational Psychology, 84,* 340–352.

Schumaker, J., Deshler, D., Alley, G., & Warner, M. (1983). Toward the development of an intervention model for learning disabled adolescents: The University of Kansas Institute. *Exceptional Education Quarterly, 4,* 45–74.

Stokes, T. & Osnes, P. (1989). An operant pursuit of generalization. *Behavior Therapy, 18,* 353–374.

Vygotsky, L. (1978). *The development of higher psychological processes.* Cambridge, MA: Harvard University Press.

Wong, B.Y.L., Harris, K.R., & Graham, S. (1991). Cognitive-behavioral procedures: Academic applications with students with learning disabilities. In P.C. Kendall (Ed.), *Child and adolescent therapy: Cognitive-behavioral procedures* (pp. 245–275). New York: Guilford.

Part IV

Methodological Issues:
Case Study, Qualitative,
and Longitudinal

9
Using Single-Subject Research Methodology to Study Learning Disabilities

John Wills Lloyd, Melody Tankersley, and Elizabeth Talbott

Single-subject research requires repeated, trustworthy measurement of dependent variables and repeated manipulation of one or more independent variables to establish lawful relationships between the dependent and independent variables and to discredit alternative explanations for that relationship. Single-subject researchers intensively study individuals' actions under two or more experimentally controlled conditions; usually behavior, or the product of behavior, is the dependent variable, and presence or absence of an experimentally controlled condition is the independent variable. To judge whether a relationship between the independent and dependent variables exists, the investigator inspects the data visually. These characteristics are shared by the various designs typically discussed in texts on single-subject research methodology (e.g., Johnston & Pennypacker, 1993; Kazdin, 1982; Tawney & Gast, 1984).

In the field of learning disabilities, researchers have employed single-subject designs primarily as a means of testing variations in classroom environments, particularly instructional interventions. The interventions include procedures, techniques, or programs for improving performance in reading (e.g., Rose, 1985), mathematics (e.g., Thackwray, Meyers, Schlesser, & Cohen, 1985), written expression (e.g., Harris & Graham, 1985), social skills (e.g., Strain & Kerr, 1981), and task-related behaviors such as attention (e.g., Lloyd, Bateman, Landrum, & Hallahan, 1989).[1]

In this chapter, we discuss methodological issues surrounding single-subject research in work with individuals with learning disabilities. Although a discussion of method invites us to pontificate about research issues in the field, we will avoid a lengthy discussion here. Furthermore, limitations on length preclude discussion of some other topics that we consider germane to understanding single-subject research applications

---

[1] Readers interested in research about academic interventions with children with learning disabilities may benefit from examining any of many reviews of this literature (e.g., Haring, Lovitt, Easton, & Hansen, 1978; Lahey, 1976; Lloyd, 1988; Rose, Koorland, & Epstein, 1982; Singh, Deitz, & Singh, 1992).

in learning disabilities; we shall not address, for example, procedural reliability (e.g., Billingsley, White, & Munson, 1980) or statistical methods for integrating single-subject research studies (e.g., Scruggs, Mastropieri, & Casto, 1987; White, Rusch, Kazdin, & Hartmann, 1989). Instead, we present a rationale for using single-subject methods in studying learning disabilities, a recitation of developments in design, and a discussion of the issue of the generality of results from single-subject research.

Relevance to Learning Disabilities

Certain features of single-subject methods make them particularly appropriate for research in learning disabilities. One feature is their focus on individual analysis, a focus that corresponds to the heterogeneity among students with learning disabilities. A second feature is that both teachers and researchers can use single-subject designs, a practice that can help to close the gap between teachers and researchers (Barlow, Hayes, & Nelson, 1984; Lovitt, 1975, 1977). However, single-subject research methodology is not universally applicable. Thus, before turning to these topics, we delimit the range of research questions for which single-subject methods are appropriate.

Questions

Single-subject procedures are appropriate for addressing some research questions but inappropriate for others. Table 9.1 provides specific examples and not-examples of the types of questions for which single-subject methods are appropriate. In general, the suitability of single-subject methods derives from the basic features of the approach. Questions must be experimental, must not require between-subjects analysis of the data, and must have dependent variables that can be administered repeatedly and that are sensitive to rapid changes.

As indicated previously, the primary application of single-subject methodology in learning disabilities is the study of independent variables' effects on specific academic and social behavior. Table 9.1 reflects this emphasis. However, the method should not be seen as being restricted to applications with individual students in which only the overt behavior of one or a few pupils may be studied. These methods could readily be applied to other questions as well. For example, a policy of requiring that a specific number and quality of interventions be implemented in a regular classroom setting prior to referral for child study or special education evaluation (perhaps modeled after the recommendations of Graden, Casey, & Christenson, 1985) could be evaluated using single-subject design. In such a study, researchers could collect data frequently on relevant variables such as (a) accuracy of responding on curriculum-based

TABLE 9.1. Appropriateness of types of research questions for single-subject analysis.

Type of question	Example	Amenable to single-subject analysis?	Reason for judgment
Developmental	Whether pupils acquire reading skills in a specific order regardless of curriculum.	No	No manipulable independent variable; requires comparison between subjects
Correlational	Whether we can predict individuals' IQ scores based on SES, level of education, and number of televisions in home.	No	No manipulable independent variable; requires comparison between subjects
Evaluation	Whether teaching procedure P increases the accuracy of children's answers on tasks of type T and also has effects on measures of Q, R, and S.	Yes	Comparison can be made within subjects; manipulable independent variable
Comparative	Whether Ritalin increases attention to task more than does behavior modification.	Yes	Comparison can be made within subjects; manipulable independent variable
Parametric	Whether the accuracy of answers to arithmetic problems varies under three different dosages (mg/kg) of Ritalin.	Yes	Comparison can be made within subjects; manipulable independent variable
Actuarial	Whether boys with LD in mathematics are more likely to graduate from high school than boys with LD in language arts.	No	No manipulable independent variable; requires comparison between subjects
Interactions between types of people and types of instruction (ATIs)	Whether pupils with light-colored eyes benefit more from reading text printed on colored paper than do pupils with dark-colored eyes.	No	Requires comparison between subjects
Interactions among independent variables	Whether the effects of differential reinforcement on rate of problem completion vary when the pupil is working in the resource versus the mainstream classroom.	Yes	Comparison can be made within subjects; manipulable independent variable

assessments and (b) disciplinary referrals and, after establishing baseline levels of performance, researchers could implement the policy across school buildings in the fashion of a multiple-baseline design. Thus, single-subject research permits the intensive study of individuals or groups of individuals treated as one unit (e.g., a class, a school building, a local educational agency).

Using single-subject designs circumvents many of the problems of between-groups research, including (a) the need for large numbers of subjects, (b) the possibility of obscuring individual responses in the grouping of data with statistics, and (c) the ethical problem of never providing treatment to members of a control group (Poling & Grossett, 1986). Because the study of individuals is particularly pertinent in the field of learning disabilities, single-subject designs are especially appropriate for the field. Among its various features, research using this method takes into account the diversity of the students having learning disabilities and variations in the settings where these students are found.

Heterogeneity in the Population

The population of individuals with learning disabilities is regularly acknowledged to be quite diverse (e.g., Gallagher, 1986; Kavale & Forness, 1987). Although it is not explicitly stated in the 1976 federal definition of learning disabilities, definitions offered as improvements on the federal definition (e.g., Hammill, Leigh, McNutt, & Larsen, 1981; Kavanaugh & Truss, 1988)[2] expressly acknowledge this heterogeneity.

One of the results of the diverse character of the group has been an emphasis on defining research populations carefully (Lovitt & Jenkins, 1979). Another result is a growing emphasis on identifying homogeneous subtypes within the heterogenous population (e.g., Feagans, Short, & Meltzer, 1991; McKinney, 1984). In addition, examinations of current policy options (e.g., Bryan, Bay, Lopez-Reyna, & Donohue, 1991) review the literature in the area with an emphasis on how heterogeneity in the population demands diverse program options.

Common sense underscores the population's heterogeneity. Individuals with learning disabilities may display specific academic deficits in reading, writing, or arithmetic; have difficulty in processing information including problems with cognition, memory, metacognition, or attention; or encounter adversity in behavioral, social, or emotional areas. Probably no single individual with a learning disability displays all of these difficulties, yet many individuals with learning disabilities display more than one of them.

---

[2] Although the two definitions cited here differ in important ways (see Kavanaugh & Truss, 1988, pp. 549–551 for a discussion), both explicitly include the phrase "Learning disabilities is a generic term that refers to a heterogeneous group of disorders." It is this aspect of the definitions that we emphasize here.

In traditional between-groups research methods such heterogeneity or (within-group variability) increases error variance. Increased error variance makes it difficult to obtain statistically significant differences between groups. To combat such variability, researchers have adopted diverse strategies including covariation and studying pupils with specific characteristics (i.e., subtypes). Single-subject research methods obviate the need for using such techniques. As Repp and Lloyd described it: A major advantage of single-subject designs is that the differences between individuals (between-subjects variability) do not cloud the evaluation of whether different levels of independent variables have different effects. Between-subjects variability is a major reason for group designs requiring the statistical evaluation of average differences. But, in single-subject designs, between-subject variability is controlled by having the same subject in each condition, there simply is no comparison *between* subjects (1980, p. 78).

Applied research in learning disabilities faces the task of finding interventions to remedy the heterogeneous deficits of individuals with learning disabilities. Because of the heterogeneity among individuals with those deficits, and because professionals have not yet agreed on ways to reduce that heterogeneity, research that investigates interventions demands an idiographic approach. Single-subject research is an idiographic approach that allows us to study interventions for individuals. In addition, single-subject designs are inherently flexible, a characteristic which makes them appropriate for use in the diverse clinical situations in which we encounter individuals with learning disabilities.

Clinical Research

Although schools are typically the clinical settings in which we find these diverse individuals, they are not the only places where we encounter people with learning disabilities. We may also find them in the work place, in hospital settings, or in prisons. Just as single-subject designs are not constrained by the individual characteristics of participating students, they are not limited by the type of setting in which a study is to be conducted, the nature of the procedures to be investigated, and so forth.

Dependent measures in single-subject research may be quite similar to those used in other research, but one of the advantages of single-subject methods is that these measures may be taken from the setting (e.g., the materials that the pupils are customarily using in their classwork). For example, researchers may measure the proportion of correct answers on arithmetic practice pages, the number of words read correctly per minute, the number of words written during composition lessons, the percentage of letters that are correctly formed, and so forth. In addition, single-subject researchers may also assess pupils' performance on more sophisticated measures (e.g., proportion of meaning units included in students' retelling of passages they have read, or the proportion of sentences that meet certain requirements). In any case, these measures are clinically relevant. And although designs can become quite complex, we still examine one independent variable at a time, or one teaching procedure at a time.

Developments in Design

Probably most readers are familiar with the four elementary designs used in single-subject research. These designs include the (a) reversal, ABA, or ABAB designs or variants; (b) multiple-baseline designs across subjects, settings, or responses; (c) multi-element or alternating treatments designs; and (d) changing criterion designs. Each of these has been thoroughly described in various texts (Kazdin, 1982; Kratochwill, 1978; Kratochwill & Levin, 1992; Tawney & Gast, 1984) and are the prototypical procedures for manipulating the independent variable.[3] They share the characteristics noted in the first lines of this chapter: (a) repeated measurement of the dependent variable, (b) repeated manipulation of the independent variable, and (c) analysis of effects within subjects.

However, the elementary designs are neither exclusive prescriptions nor an exhaustive catalog of methods for appropriate research practice. Adherence to them may provide protection against threats to internal validity, but it may restrict the conclusions one can draw about matters relevant to learning disabilities, too. It is often fruitful to go beyond the simple, prototypical designs. Therefore, in this section, we provide some suggestions about applying specific design variations to address some of the aspects of learning disabilities interventions we consider important.

Comparisons

As Lovitt (1975) noted, single-subject designs are especially useful when examining one independent variable, a feature that coincides well with the practice of analyzing one teaching method at a time. Of particular interest and value to those who investigate learning disabilities, we think, are studies in which interventions are compared. In essence, this is always the case with single-subject research: The individual's performance under one condition (often labeled *A*) is compared to his or her performance under another condition (*B*). However, we fear that the *A*, or baseline condition, too rarely provides a strong basis for comparison and is too often poorly defined.

---

[3] We note that some designs with other appellations have been recommended (e.g., Gast & Wolery, 1988; Sindelar, Rosenburg, & Wilson, 1985). We consider these designs variants on the prototypical designs mentioned here.

Baselines that are inadequately described or weak do not permit useful conclusions. The researcher may argue that intervention *B* produced better student performance than baseline *A*, but that tells us little if baseline *A* was chaos or the absence of reasonable instruction. We probably want to know whether *B* produces better student performance than some other, well-known intervention; thus, it is this other, well-known intervention that we should put into effect as *A* or baseline. Who wants to know, for example, that using manipulatives in arithmetic instruction is better than doing nothing? When we can say that our horse beat Seattle Slew and not just the old grey mare, we are making a far more powerful statement about the qualities of our horse.

Birnbrauer, Peterson, and Solnick (1974) identified this concept as one of using active baselines, and recommended that researchers in mental retardation adopt it. Clearly, theirs is a recommendation that we strongly endorse. Studies in which researchers compare active conditions will tell us a good deal more about the qualities of those conditions, an outcome that should help the field of learning disabilities interventions advance much more rapidly.

Joint or Interactive Effects

As indicated in Table 9.1, one type of comparison that single-subject methodology does not permit is a comparison of different subjects under different conditions; that is, studies of aptitude-by-treatment interactions are not possible with this method. However, interactions between independent variables can be examined with single-subject designs. In the case in which two independent variables may have joint or combined interactive effects, these comparisons include (a) What is the effect of condition *A*? (b) What is the effect of condition *B*? and (c) What is the effect of conditions *A* and *B* in combination?

Although all single-subject designs are based on comparisons between two conditions, the design generally considered most appropriate for direct comparisons is the multielement. Whereas, in reversal and multiple-baseline designs, conditions remain in effect for at least three and usually many more measurement occasions, in multielement designs the experimenter creates two or more measurement occasions that are generally comparable (e.g., occur on the same day) and associates a separate condition with each occasion.

However, problems of interference can occur when we compare the effects of two treatments on an individual's behavior. Having each subject experience each level of the independent variable while making direct comparisons of treatments may result in transfer of effects from one treatment to another. This is the threat to internal validity that Campbell and Stanley (1963) identified as "multiple-treatment interference."

Only a few researchers to date have conducted direct investigations of multiple-treatment interference. Shapiro, Kazdin, and McGonigle (1982) and Johnson and Bailey (1977) reported that the sequence in which one presents treatment influences whether interference occurs; McGonigle, Rojahn, Dixon, and Strain (1987) demonstrated that the duration of time between treatment sessions will influence interference. McGonigle et al. clearly see multiple-treatment interference as a problem, especially in applied research, where several active treatments can influence each other.

Hains and Baer (1989), on the other hand, argue that researchers should take advantage of interference in multielement designs by directly assessing its effects. They argue that in applied settings, interference is common, so that direct studies of the phenomenon will give us a more accurate and realistic appraisal of how it works. "So far researchers have investigated the relative effectiveness of two or more treatments in alteration, but they have rarely examined whether the treatments interact, and they have not investigated the generality of the treatments' effectiveness by varying their potentially crucial contextual parameters" (Hains & Baer, 1989, p. 67).

Indeed, by avoiding a direct study of treatment interference, we have avoided contributing to our knowledge of how interventions interact in applied settings. In the field of learning disabilities, for example, teachers may use a skills-training approach to teach arithmetic operations and provide opportunities for students to apply these skills in diverse situations. If we investigate the effectiveness of either of those interventions independently, we will likely obtain different results than if we investigate the effectiveness of the two in concert. The latter scenario is the more frequent one in classrooms: Teachers typically combine interventions in working with students with learning disabilities.

Single-subject analyses that make active comparisons of interventions and assess interactions between independent variables will benefit the study of learning disabilities by providing more precise and detailed information about those interventions. We think that they will also enhance the external validity of the research. But, we believe that the external validity of single-subject research results have been inappropriately questioned.

Generality of Findings

Although the technologies resulting from single-subject research have been used repeatedly, some professionals have questioned the generality of results that have been obtained with so few subjects and in highly specific situations. Indeed, clinicians and teachers of individuals with learning disabilities should have little use for findings that prove to be overly specific or that are not durable. But critics fail to acknowledge that a central goal of single-subject research is to identify relationships that are generalizable beyond the immediate research conditions (Baer, Wolf,

& Risley, 1968; Kazdin, 1982). We believe that both the *external* and the *internal* validity of single-subject research are genuinely compelling.

Issues of generality are particularly critical in applied research with individuals with learning disabilities: We need to know if an intervention will work in settings other than that in which it was tested and with individuals other than those who participated in specific studies. We address this challenge in single-subject research by: (a) applying treatment in settings of concern using measures common to those settings, (b) replicating studies systematically to assess the range of conditions under which treatment is effective, (c) using designs that directly assess transfer of learned behavior, and (d) making circumspect arguments about the generality of results.

Applicability

Because many single-subject studies address research questions about improving people's performance in settings where such performance is of concern, they are immediately applicable for the individuals participating in a study. Because single-subject research can be conducted in specific settings of concern and can incorporate measures that are common to those settings, results are readily generalizable to those situations. The results are of applied importance. Furthermore, single-subject research provides information about the performance of individuals rather than average group performance, easing the task of generalizing to other individuals with similar characteristics (Kazdin, 1982).

The applied importance of single-subject results is demonstrated also in the way in which researchers assess the effects of the intervention. Single-subject researchers typically inspect their data visually to determine whether changes in behavior are the consequence of changes in experimental conditions; they look for (a) discontinuities in the levels of the behavior at the time of phase changes, (b) changes in the trend or slope from one phase to another, (c) differences between the means (or medians) for adjacent phases, and (d) few or no overlaps between lowest data points in one phase and the highest data points in the adjacent phase. Although there is some disagreement about the extent to which visual inspection is robust,[4] advocates of interocular analysis (e.g., Baer, 1978) argue persuasively that it should be a conservative activity. That is, single-subject researchers should rely on the dramatic changes in behavior to establish the effects of independent variables.

This reliance on dramatic changes in behavior increases the probability that the most effective interventions are incorporated in studies. Interven-

---

[4] See DeProspero and Cohen (1979), Jones, Weinrott, and Vaught (1978), and Ottenbacher (1990) for more detailed discussion of issues surrounding visual analysis.

tions that produce dramatic results may be, in turn, more generalizable than interventions that produce statistically significant—yet relatively weaker—results (Kazdin, 1982). Therefore, the stringent criteria used to evaluate the effects of the intervention lead to an increase in the overall generality of results.

Replication

Replication of intervention effects—an essential feature of single-subject research methods—is another way in which single-subject research ensures generality. As the effects of an intervention are replicated within a study, either across phases (as in reversal designs) or across settings, subjects, or behaviors (as in multiple baseline designs), the trustworthiness of the intervention is examined. But, at the same time, preliminary evidence about the generality of that effect is obtained; the researchers can begin to assert that the results are not limited by when, where, or with whom the independent variable is applied.

Further evidence about the generality of an effect is produced when the results of one study can be directly or systematically replicated through initiating another, or several studies, that investigate the same intervention. In this manner, replication can examine the extent to which results obtained in the first study extend, or generalize, to subsequent studies. By conducting what Sidman (1960) called "systematic replications," we are assured of having research that develops the case for generality in an orderly fashion.

Thus, replication provides information regarding the external validity of a study—the extent to which changes in the dependent measure can be reproduced under conditions other than those in which they were originally demonstrated (Johnston & Pennypacker, 1993). The generality of the results is determined when the intervention influences the behaviors of new subjects or of the same subjects in different settings or at different times (Kazdin, 1982). Replication, whether initiated within a design or through other studies, detects the extent to which changes in the dependent variable can be attributed to the effects of the independent variable. In this way, replication permits single-subject researchers to make strong statements about the internal validity of a study as well as the generality of its results.

Replicating a finding does not mean that one obtains the same results repeatedly. Sometimes one obtains only partial replication. Variations in results from study to study do not represent failures, however. Differences in results are probably attributable to variations in treatments under study or to methods used in studying treatments, and they provide valuable information about the phenomenon under study. When one does not obtain consensus across studies of a teaching procedure, for example, one may have found a boundary of the effectiveness of that procedure. Under such circumstances, one has the opportunity to explore that boundary further or to vary other features of the independent variable to resolve other boundaries.

Transfer

Although the inherent features of replication and applicability of single-subject research may increase the likelihood of the generality of results, these features do not *insure* generalization. We must plan for and assess generalization of effects, especially when studying interventions with students who have learning disabilities. Students with learning disabilities may not spontaneously generalize behaviors learned under one set of conditions to other conditions (Hallahan, Kauffman, & Lloyd, 1985). Therefore, professionals in special education advocate that we include transfer of effects in our interventions, rather than hoping that transfer will emerge serendipitously (e.g., Hayes, Rincover, & Solnick, 1980; Thorpe, Chiang, & Darch, 1981).

Researchers using single-subject research methods have begun to do so. "Increasingly, efforts have shifted from investigations that merely demonstrate change to investigations that explore the generalization of changes across situations and settings" (Kazdin, 1982, p. 288). Two single-subject designs that are appropriate for assessing transfer are based on the use of probes, or the systematic withdrawal of treatment.

Probe Designs

Probe designs permit investigations of changes in behaviors when no contingencies are in effect for the behavior. This focus leads to statements regarding the generality of behaviors across responses and situations (Kazdin, 1982). For example, researchers may investigate the effects of a training program designed to increase social skills by assessing the number and duration of initiations made during an organized rehearsal. Setting generalization probes, in which students' social initiations were assessed, could be conducted when students are on the playground. In this manner, the effects of training can be assessed beyond the training situation.

Withdrawal Designs

Withdrawal designs (Rusch & Kazdin, 1981) are also useful for evaluating the generalization of intervention results. Interventions that end abruptly (e.g., contingencies that are suddenly withdrawn as in the reversal phase of an ABA design) may not produce durable effects. Withdrawal designs (i.e., sequential withdrawal, partial withdrawal, and combined sequential and partial withdrawal) are used to help sustain behavior under nonintervention conditions. Using a sequential withdrawal design, for example, different aspects of a multicomponent reading intervention could be eliminated one at a time to assess the maintenance of the effects of the reading program on dependent variables of reading speed, accuracy, and comprehension.

General Comments

In addressing issues of generalization, we profit from replication, the applied nature of interventions, and the flexibility to program for transfer of applied interventions in single-subject research. Although we recognize the need to program for generalization, we believe that single-subject research lends itself well to the discovery of generalizable relationships.

To program for generalization of intervention results for students with learning disabilities, researchers must first consider aspects of the characteristics of these students and of the environment that may influence the generality of results. As previously mentioned, the characteristics of students with learning disabilities are diverse. Such heterogeneity among students with learning disabilities must be considered when programming for the generality of results, underscoring the need to identify pupil characteristics when reporting results of single-subject studies.

Further, students with learning disabilities are often seen in diverse educational settings—regular classrooms, resource classrooms, self-contained classrooms—and may use disparate educational materials or programs. The features of these types of environments, materials, and programs must also be considered when programming for the generality of intervention effects. The applied nature of single-subject research intimates that research is often conducted in the setting of concern, with as few disruptions or changes to programs and materials within that setting as possible. Therefore, it may also be advantageous to identify salient aspects of the intervention setting when reporting results of single-subject research.

Summary

Single-subject designs are appropriate for answering research questions about the behavior of individuals under different experimental conditions. They are particularly appropriate for investigations with students with learning disabilities, because of (a) the heterogeneity in those students' abilities, (b) the flexibility of the designs, and (c) the applicability of the designs to clinical settings. We use single-subject designs to look intensely at individuals and to scrutinize our interventions. For this reason, we endorse the use of active baselines, so that we can find the most effective interventions for individuals and not merely those that work better than no intervention. In fact, we can use single-subject designs to test the effectiveness of combinations of interventions, a practice that would help us to understand the complex relationships that occur daily in classrooms and other environments important in the field of learning disabilities. Finally, we can use single-subject designs to identify relationships that are generalizable beyond the conditions under which they are studied.

References

Baer, D.M. (1978). Perhaps it would be better not to know everything. *Journal of Applied Behavior Analysis, 10*, 167–172.

Baer, D.M., Wolf, M.M., & Risley, T.R. (1968). Some current dimensions of applied behavior analysis. *Journal of Applied Behavior Analysis, 1*, 91–97.

Barlow, D.H., Hayes, S.C., & Nelson, R.O. (1984). *The scientist practitioner: Research and accountability in clinical and educational settings*. New York: Pergamon Press.

Billingsley, F., White, O.R., & Munson, R. (1980). Procedural reliability: A rationale and an example. *Behavioral Assessment, 2*, 229–241.

Birnbrauer, J.S., Peterson, C.R., & Solnick, J.V. (1974). Design and interpretation of studies of single subjects. *American Journal of Mental Deficiency, 79*, 191–203.

Bryan, T., Bay, M., Lopez-Reyna, N., & Donohue, M. (1991). Characteristics of students with learning disabilities: The extant database and its implications for educational programs. In J.W. Lloyd, N.N. Singh, & A.C. Repp (Eds.), *The regular education initiative: Alternative perspectives on concepts, issues, and models* (pp. 113–131). Sycamore, IL: Sycamore.

Campbell, D.T. & Stanley, J.C. (1963). *Experimental and quasi-experimental designs for research*. Boston: Houghton.

DeProspero, A. & Cohen, S. (1979). Inconsistent visual analyses of intrasubject data. *Journal of Applied Behavior Analysis, 1*, 573–579.

Feagans, L.V., Short, E.J., & Meltzer, L.J. (Eds.). (1991). *Subtypes of learning disabilities: Theoretical perspectives and research*. Hillsdale, NJ: Erlbaum.

Gallagher, J.J. (1986). Learning disabilities and special education: A critique. *Journal of Learning Disabilities, 19*, 595–601.

Gast, D.L. & Wolery, M. (1988). Parallel treatments design: A nested single subject design for comparing instructional procedures. *Education and Treatment of Children, 11*, 270–285.

Graden, J.L., Casey, A., & Christenson, S.L. (1985). Implementing a preferral intervention system: Part I: The model. *Exceptional Children, 51*, 487–496.

Hains, A.H. & Baer, D.M. (1989). Interaction effects on multielement designs: Inevitable, desirable, and ignorable. *Journal of Applied Behavior Analysis, 22*, 57–69.

Hallahan, D.P., Kauffman, J.M., & Lloyd, J.W. (1985). *Introduction to learning disabilities* (2nd ed.). Englewood Cliffs, NJ: Prentice Hall.

Hammill, D.D., Leigh, J.E., McNutt, G., & Larsen, S.C. (1981). A new definition of learning disabilities. *Learning Disability Quarterly, 4*, 336–342.

Haring, N.G., Lovitt, T.C., Easton, M.D., & Hansen, C.L. (1978). *The fourth R: Research in the classroom*. Columbus, OH: Charles E. Merrill.

Harris, K.R. & Graham, S. (1985). Improving learning disabled students' composition skills: A self-control strategy training approach. *Learning Disability Quarterly, 8*, 27–36.

Hayes, S.C., Rincover, A., & Solnick, J.V. (1980). The technical drift of applied behavior analysis. *Journal of Applied Behavior Analysis, 13*, 275–285.

Johnson, M.S. & Bailey, J.S. (1977). The modification of leisure behavior in a half way house for retarded women. *Journal of Applied Behavior Analysis, 10*, 273–282.

Johnston, J.M. & Pennypacker, H.S. (1993). *Strategies and tactics of human behavioral research* (2nd ed.). Hillsdale, NJ: Erlbaum.

Jones, R.R., Weinrott, M.R., & Vaught, R.S. (1978). Effects of serial dependency on the agreement between visual and statistical inferences. *Journal of Applied Behavior Analysis, 11*, 277–284.

Kavale, K.A. & Forness, S.R. (1987). The far side of heterogeneity: A critical analysis of empirical subtyping research in learning disabilities. *Journal of Learning Disabilities, 20*, 374–382.

Kavanaugh, J.F. & Truss, T.J., Jr. (Eds.). (1988). *Learning disabilities: Proceedings of the national conference.* Parkton, MD: York Press.

Kazdin, A.E. (1982). *Single-case research designs: Methods for clinical and applied settings.* New York: Oxford University Press.

Kratochwill, T.R. (Ed.). (1978). *Single-subject research: Strategies for evaluating change.* New York: Academic Press.

Kratochwill, T.R. & Levin, J.R. (Eds.). (1992). *Single-case research design and analysis: New directions for psychology and education.* Hillsdale, NJ: Erlbaum.

Lahey, B.B. (1976). Behavior modification with learning disabilities and related problems. In M. Hersen, R. Eisler, & P. Miller (Eds.), *Progress in behavior modification* (Vol. 3, pp. 173–205). New York: Academic Press.

Lloyd, J.W. (1988). Direct academic interventions in learning disabilities. In M.C. Wang, M.C. Reynolds, & H.J. Walberg (Eds.), *The Handbook of special education: Research and practice* (pp. 345–366). London: Pergamon Press.

Lloyd, J.W., Bateman, D.F., Landrum, T.J., & Hallahan, D.P. (1989). Self-recording of attention versus productivity. *Journal of Applied Behavior Analysis, 22*, 315–323.

Lovitt, T.C. (1975). Applied behavior analysis and learning disabilities: Part 1: Characteristics of ABA, general recommendations, and methodological limitations. *Journal of Learning Disabilities, 8*, 432–443.

Lovitt, T.C. (1977). *In spite of my resistance I've learned from children.* Columbus, OH: Charles E. Merrill.

Lovitt, T.C. & Jenkins, J.R. (1979). Learning disabilities research: Defining populations. *Learning Disability Quarterly, 2*, 46–50.

McGonigle, J.J., Rojahn, J., Dixon, J., & Strain, P.S. (1987). Multiple treatment interference in the alternating treatments design as a function of the intercomponent interval length. *Journal of Applied Behavior Analysis, 7*, 649–653.

McKinney, J.D. (1984). The search for subtypes of specific learning disability. *Journal of Learning Disabilities, 17*, 43–50.

Ottenbacher, K.J. (1990). When is a picture worth a thousand *p* values? A comparison of visual and quantitative methods to analyze single subject data. *Journal of Special Education, 23*, 436–449.

Poling, A. & Grossett, D. (1986). Basic research designs in applied behavior analysis. In A. Poling & R.W. Fuqua (Eds.), *Research methods in applied behavior analysis: Issues and advances* (pp. 7–28). New York: Plenum Press.

Repp, A.C. & Lloyd, J. (1980). Evaluating educational changes with single-subject designs. In J. Gottlieb (Ed.), *Educating mentally retarded persons in the mainstream* (pp. 73–105). Baltimore: University Park Press.

Rose, T.L. (1985). The effects of two prepractice procedures on oral reading. *Journal of Learning Disabilities, 17,* 544–548.

Rose, T.L., Koorland, M.A., & Epstein, M.E. (1982). A review of applied behavior analysis interventions with learning disabled children. *Education and Treatment of Children, 5,* 41–58.

Rusch, F.R. & Kazdin, A.E. (1981). Toward a methodology of withdrawal designs for the assessment of response maintenance. *Journal of Applied Behavior Analysis, 14,* 131–140.

Scruggs, T.E., Mastropieri, M.A., & Casto, G. (1987). The quantitative synthesis of single-subject research: Methodology and validation. *Remedial and Special Education, 8*(2), 43–48.

Shapiro, E.S., Kazdin, A.E., & McGonigle, J.J. (1982). Multiple-treatment interference in the simultaneous- or alternating-treatments design. *Behavioral Assessment, 4,* 105–115.

Sidman, M. (1960). *Tactics of scientific research: Evaluating experimental data in psychology.* New York: Basic Books.

Sindelar, P.R., Rosenburg, M.S., & Wilson, R.J. (1985). An adapted alternating treatments design for instructional research. *Education and Treatment of Children, 8,* 67–76.

Singh, N.N., Deitz, D.E.D., & Singh, J. (1992). Behavioral approaches. In N.N. Singh & I.L. Beale (Eds.), *Learning disabilities: Nature, theory, and treatment* (pp. 375–414). New York: Springer-Verlag.

Strain, P.S. & Kerr, M.M. (1981). Modifying children's social withdrawal: Issues in assessment and clinical intervention. In M. Hersen, R.M. Eisler, & P.M. Miller (Eds.), *Progress in behavior modification* (Vol. 11, pp. 203–248). Beverly Hills, CA: Sage.

Tawney, J.W. & Gast, D.L. (1984). *Single subject research in special education.* Columbus, OH: Charles E. Merrill.

Thackwray, D., Meyers, A., Schlesser, R., & Cohen, R. (1985). Achieving generalization with general versus specific self-instructions: Effects on academically deficient children. *Cognitive Therapy and Research, 9,* 291–308.

Thorpe, H.W., Chiang, B., & Darch, C.B. (1981). Programming generalization when mainstreaming exceptional children. *Journal of Special Education Technology, 4,* 15–23.

White, D.M., Rusch, F.R., Kazdin, A.E., & Hartmann, D.P. (1989). Applications of meta analysis in individual-subject research. *Behavioral Assessment, 11,* 281–296.

10
Qualitative Research and Learning Disabilities

CANDACE S. BOS AND VIRGINIA RICHARDSON

More than any other methodology presented in this book, qualitative research has the smallest base of research in learning disabilities yet is gaining growing acceptance as a means of studying the complex questions and issues that arise when understanding learning disabilities from a contextualist perspective. A number of researchers in special education have called for the greater use of qualitative methodologies in special education (e.g., Jacob, 1990; Miller, 1990; Murray, Anderson, Bersani, & Mesaros, 1986; Stainback & Stainback, 1984), but only a handful of researchers in learning disabilities have responded. Therefore, the purpose of this chapter must be necessarily different than the other chapters on methodology. Whereas other chapters have a strong base of research in learning disabilities upon which to draw for determining methodological issues, this chapter is more basic in its approach to qualitative research and naturalistic inquiry. It has been divided into four sections. The first section discusses the parameters of qualitative research and naturalistic inquiry: the purposes, underlying assumptions, characteristics and types. The second section focuses on designing a qualitative study while the third section deals with conducting ethnographies. The fourth section comments on the future directions for research and suggests how qualitative and quantitative methodologies can complement each other when used in the pursuit of a better understanding of learning disabilities. Throughout the chapter, examples from the field of learning disabilities are used to illustrate different aspects of this methodology. It is the intent of this chapter to stimulate interest and provide information valuable to researchers and educators attempting to better understand learning disabilities in educational settings.

What is Qualitative Research?

Smith (1987), in her seminal article signifying to the educational research community that manuscripts based on qualitative research are welcome in the *American Education Research Journal*, notes that qualitative research defies simple description. Researchers conducting qualitative research seek to understand qualities or entities in a particular context. As Dabbs (1982) suggests, "Quality is the essential character or nature of something; quantity is the amount. Quality is the what; quantity is the how much. Qualitative refers to the meaning ... while quantitative assumes the meaning and refers to a measure of it" (p. 13). This focus on meaning is highlighted by Spradley (1980) when he portrays the central aim of ethnography as describing and understanding a culture or another way of life from a native point of view. He suggests that ethnography means *learning from people* rather than *studying people.*

Spradley's analogy of the ethnographer as an explorer and the social science researcher as the petroleum engineer illustrates the different foci of qualitative and quantitative research. Spradley (1980) suggests,

The ethnographer has much in common with the explorer trying to map a wilderness area. The explorer begins with a general problem, to identify the major features of the terrain. Then the explorer begins gathering information, going first in one direction, then perhaps retracing that route, then starting out in a new direction. . . . The explorer would take frequent compass readings, check the angle of the sun, take notes about prominent landmarks, and use feedback from each observation to modify earlier information. . . . Like an ethnographer, the explorer is seeking to describe a wilderness area rather than trying to "find" something.

Most social science research has more in common with the petroleum engineer. . . . The engineer has a specific goal in mind: to find oil or gas buried far below the surface. Before the engineer even begins an investigation, a careful study will be made of the maps which show geological features of the area. Then, knowing ahead of time the kinds of features that suggest oil or gas beneath the surface, the engineer will go out to "find" something quite specific. A great deal of social science research begins with a similar clear idea of something to find; investigators usually know what they are looking for (p. 26).

Qualitative research starts with general questions and requires constant feedback to give the study direction. Planning a study ahead of time is done in only the most general sense since the constant feedback from the information that is being gathered and analyzed helps to steer the study. In fact, Spradley (1980) has suggested that failing to follow this cyclical pattern of data collection and analysis is problematic in that after collecting fieldnotes week after week the researchers become overwhelmed with a mass of unorganized data. They have difficulty knowing when they have enough information. When new questions arise from the data, they cannot ask these questions because it is difficult or impossible to return to the field.

The Purposes of Qualitative Research

The main purpose of qualitative research is to develop an understanding of the qualities of phenomena within their particular contexts. As Wolcott

(1985) suggests, this research must extend beyond description, albeit good or even "exquisite description" (p. 189). The written products of qualitative research describe the *sense or meaning* that the researcher(s) has made of what has been investigated. It leads, then, to the development of theory.

For many qualitative educational researchers, an additional or perhaps overarching purpose is the identification of problems and processes that would help to improve education. This purpose, however, is the subject of some debate. For those who are primarily anthropologists writing about one form of qualitative research, ethnography, such work is viewed with some concern. Wolcott (1985) stated: Most so-called school ethnography, however, is really quick description (not to be confused with "thick description"), the purpose of this is to reveal weaknesses, point out needs, or otherwise pave the way for change and reform. At best, it is ad hoc, pragmatic, and utilitarian ethnography. It reveals far more of the educator commitment to what is *possible* (an important aspect of educator world view, it might be noted), than to the ethnographer's painstaking efforts to document—and even to "respect," in the sense of deferring judgment—what already is (p. 200).

For Wolcott (as well as Chilcott, 1987), ethnographic studies help us understand; they do not suggest ways of improving the social and cultural conditions.

In a recent article on standards for qualitative research, however, Howe and Eisenhart (1990) suggest that challenges to ethnographic methodologies are leading to new conceptions. They attribute this to "logic in use" (p. 4), and provide an example of a dissertation study (Naff, 1987), self-described as an ethnography, that led to the reform of several teacher education programs. Howe and Eisenhart suggest that "there must be some feature(s) of educational research that justify the term *educational* and therefore make it of interest and value to educators" (p. 6). They leave open the possibility that improvement of education could be an aim of educational ethnography.

Certainly, many of the qualitative studies of learning disabilities described in this chapter were designed for purposes of developing understandings that would lead to educational improvement (e.g., Bos & Lloyd, 1989; Miller, Leinhardt, & Zigmond, 1988; Richardson, Casanova, Placier, & Guilfoyle, 1989; Smith, 1982). As Miles and Huberman (1990) suggest: "Deep down, we are meliorists first and researchers second" (p. 352).

Underlying Assumptions

A number of interrelated assumptions underlie qualitative research methodology. First, and oftentimes considered most fundamental, is a phenomenological perspective. "The phenomenologist views human behavior, what people say and do, as a product of how people define their world. The task of the phenomenologist and for us, the qualitative methodologist, is to capture this process of interpretation" (Taylor & Bogdan, 1984, pp. 8–9). Whereas the scientific inquirer views the world as a series of real entities and consistent processes leading to a single reality, the naturalistic inquirer focuses on multiple realities that, like the layers of an onion, nest within or complement one another (Guba & Lincoln, 1981). These layers are interrelated to form a pattern of "truth." It is these patterns that must be searched out in naturalistic inquiry.

A second assumption focuses on the relationship between the inquirer and the inquiry. By design, the inquirer is oftentimes integrally involved in the study. For example, in *Learning Denied* (1991), an artistic ethnography of a child and his parents who interacted with the special education placement process, Denny Taylor, the inquirer, was also the child's tutor. The key is not to ignore the relationship between the inquirer and the inquiry, but to determine the perceptions of the data collector and the effect of those perceptions on the developing information (Guba & Lincoln, 1981).

A third assumption deals with central role of culture. Spradley (1980) defines ethnography as "the work of describing a culture" (p. 3). Inferences about and subsequent understanding of a culture are made from observing cultural behavior, observing cultural artifacts, listening to what people say, and from the tacit knowledge that is inferred by the inquirer. At first, each cultural inference is only a hypothesis. These hypotheses must be tested over and over until the ethnographer becomes relatively certain that the inference is a shared understanding of the particular cultural system (Spradley, 1979).

A fourth assumption focuses on the perspective taken toward generalization or transferability. Rather than searching for generalizations that are relatively unchanged across contexts, the naturalistic inquirer assumes the interactive, complex role that the context plays in understanding phenomena (Donmoyer, 1990). The inquirer opts for "thick descriptions" (Geertz, 1973) of the contexts as the basis for determining whether sufficient basis for transfer exists.

Types of Qualitative Research

Mary Lee Smith (1987) describes four types of empirical qualitative research. These types vary in terms of the degree to which primarily quantitative standards, such as validity and reliability, are applied and used; in terms of conceptions of the nature of knowledge and reality; and in terms of whether or not the data are *emic*, that is, the categories and theories are abstracted from the data and therefore express the meaning of those involved in the context, or *etic*, in which the researcher's language and theory are imposed on the data. Smith does not suggest that these are pure types in the sense that a particular study will always fit neatly into one or another category. However, elements of a study will fit one of the four types in terms of the intentions of the research and methodologies that are used.

1. Interpretive Approach

This type of research, borrowed from anthropology and qualitative sociology, is the one most often written about in educational research (e.g., Bogdan & Biklen, 1982; Chilcott, 1987; Erickson, 1986; Wolcott, 1985). The researcher attempts to understand the meanings that participants in a setting make of events and of their actions. It is primarily emic, suggests that reality is created within the mind, and cannot be determined "objectively." Thus, the goal is to "understand particular actions and meanings in particular contexts" (Smith, 1987, p. 176).

One conclusion of research in this tradition in the area of learning disabilities is that the designation of learning disabilities is socially constructed. For example, on the basis of a set of 25 case studies of handicapped students (Bogdan & Barnes, 1979), Bogdan and Kugelmass (1984) concluded that there are no disabled students in an absolute sense. "Mental retardation, emotional disturbance, learning disability and even blindness and other specific disability categories are ways of thinking about others, attitudes we take towards them, ways of structuring relationships, and accepted processes and frames of mind" (p. 184).

They suggest, therefore, that "Alleged differences, be they physical, behavioural or psychological, have particular meanings in particular settings. Not knowing how to read has a different meaning from one school to another. Its meaning in one class may differ from the meaning in another" (p. 188).

2. Artistic Approaches

The artistic approach is most often reflected in the written product of a piece of qualitative research rather than in the methods of data collection and analysis. It is perhaps the least "scholarly" of renditions, in the sense of tradition, because it seeks to present an artistic, narrative account of what the researcher learned in the setting. A strong proponent of the artistic approach is Elliot Eisner (1981), who suggests that the meaning of the studied case for the researcher is expressed through literary modes such as metaphors. An example of a piece of writing in the artistic mode is Eisner's (1986) description of a videotape of then Secretary of Education, William Bennett, teaching the Federalist Paper No. 10 to a group of students in a Washington, DC high school. Eisner led off his piece in the following way, "In this corner, at 175 pounds we have William, The Cat, Bennett! Reporters surround the ring. Microphones create a small mountain on the desk before him—all the networks, it seems are hooked in. . . . It is the Secretary of Education himself—our educational leader—preparing for this first high school bout with Baneker High's best and brightest" (p. 325).

3. Systematic Approaches

Systematic methodologists seek to discover *and* to verify. Researchers in this tradition believe that there is a reality that is separate from our perceptions, and that it is possible to discover it in a reasonably objective manner. Great attention is paid to standards borrowed from quantitative research such as reliability, validity and objectivity (e.g., Kirk & Miller, 1986). Miles & Huberman (1984) represent this approach in their book on qualitative analysis, and, in another publication, describe their research as violating both quantitative and anthropological methodologies as: "looseness in experimental design where controls are called for, and rigorous models of analysis where, in the social anthropology community at least, softer and less codified modes are more typical" (1990, p. 347).

An example of a systematic qualitative study in the area of learning disabilities is described in Bos and Lloyd (1989) and Chalfant, Bos, and Pysh (1990). The first part of the study examined the social and academic task demands in classrooms with mainstreamed elementary students with learning disabilities, and the students' responses to them. The informants were 18 students, identified as learning disabled, in five schools. Each classroom had 1 to 2 students with learning disabilities as well as 2 to 4 average-achieving students. In addition, each of the teachers was interviewed extensively.

Because of the size and scope of the study, a number of observers were involved in collecting the data. Issues of reliability in classroom observation, interviewing, and coding of data were attended to with care. Observers received extensive training with videotapes, two researchers observed tasks in each classroom, and reliability measures were developed through the examination of sets of interviews and observations that had been coded by at least two different observers.

4. Theory-driven Approaches

Smith's (1987) fourth category describes research that is generated to help explain or clarify social theories that have been accepted by the theorists prior to beginning the research. The meanings that the participants make of the actions in their settings constitute the preliminary data, rather than the conclusions, of such a study. The researcher goes on to explain the deep structure of these meanings within the theoretical framework in which the researcher is operating. Since these meanings are seldom seen or understood by the participants, the research is etic, or explained within the researcher's own categories. Conflict, critical, and structural-functional theories are three examples of current theories that drive such research.

While there are few examples of theory-driven research in the learning disabilities area, several studies are quite critical (e.g., Bogdan & Barnes, 1979; Richardson et al., 1989). Sigmon (1987, 1990) presents an example of a theory-driven, nonempirical study in the learning disabilities area. He describes his methodology as "radical socioeducational analysis" (RSA). "RSA emphasizes historical development within the social context, the difficulty (or perhaps impossibility) of value-free social science, and Karl Marx's (1818–1883) notion of the dialectic within the realm of social class conflict theory" (1987, p. 8). RSA is described as qualitative, interpretive, and historical. It seeks to uncover the roots and underlying assumptions of education. Sigmon's (1987) research is quite different from others described in this chapter because it does not rely on observation and interview techniques. Instead, it examines historical documents and literature and places these within a critical theory framework. With this analysis, he concludes "The alarming increase of the so-called mildly handicapped student population, regardless of the label, may be the most serious ethical and practical dilemma facing American education today. The primary problem is that special education, through LD schooling tracks, has been perverted into a means of child control" (p. 97).

Designing a Study

Whereas the last section was meant to be informative and provide for a basic understanding of the parameters, purposes, and assumptions associated with qualitative research and naturalistic inquiry, this and the next section are meant to be more instructive. This section deals with issues related to designing a qualitative study, and specifically addresses the developmental nature of the research design and constant comparative analysis as the most common design strategy employed in qualitative research with learning disabilities.

Developmental Nature of the Research Design

Naturalistic inquiry involves open-ended inquiry. This does not mean that the inquirer approaches the research from a haphazard perspective, but that the design requires constant feedback to give the study direction. Hence, the design contrasts designs in scientific inquiry which are oftentimes thoroughly explicated and piloted before the study begins. Spradley (1979, 1980) has referred to naturalistic designs as being cyclical in nature in that the ongoing analysis of the data guides the direction and further questions of the research. In fact, his books, *Participant Observation*

TABLE 10.1. Developmental research sequence method for participant observation and ethnographic interviewing.

Steps	Participant observation	Ethnographic interviewing
One	Locating a social situation	Locating an informant
Two	Doing participant observation	Interviewing an informant
Three	Making an ethnographic record	Making an ethnographic record
Four	Making descriptive observations	Asking descriptive questions
Five	Making a domain analysis	Analyzing ethnographic interviews
Six	Making focused observations	Making a domain analysis
Seven	Making a taxonomic analysis	Asking structural questions
Eight	Making selected observations	Making a taxonomic analysis
Nine	Making a componential analysis	Asking contrast questions
Ten	Discovering cultural themes	Making a componential analysis
Eleven	Taking a cultural inventory	Discovering cultural themes
Twelve	Writing an ethnography	Writing an ethnography

(1980) and *The Ethnographic Interview* (1979), are based on a developmental research sequence method that forms the framework for the discussions presented in this and the next section. This developmental research sequence (see Table 10.1) has been depicted for participant observation and ethnographic interviewing, the two most frequently used procedures in ethnographic research. The cyclical nature of the design is evident from the steps in which data are collected, analyzed, additional questions and hypotheses posed, and then data are again collected and analyzed.

The type of questions addressed in naturalistic inquiry also lend themselves to a developmental process in which questions are initially posited, then reformulated, expanded, or narrowed based on what is gleaned during the course of the study. In Erickson's chapter on qualitative methods in the *Handbook of Research on Teaching* (1986), he suggests that fieldwork is best at answering the following questions in educational research:

1. What is happening, specifically, in social action that takes place in this particular setting?
2. What do these actions mean to the actors involved in them, at the moment the actions took place?
3. How are the happenings organized in patterns of social organization and learned cultural principles for the conduct of everyday life—how, in other words, are people in the immediate setting consistently presented to each other as environments for one another's meaningful actions?
4. How is what is happening in this setting as a whole (i.e., the classroom) related to happenings at other system levels outside and inside the setting (e.g., the school building, a child's family, the school system, federal government mandates regarding mainstreaming)?

5. How do the ways everyday life in this setting is organized compare with other ways of organizing social life in a wide range of settings in other places and at other times? (p. 121; see Erickson, Florio, & Buschman, 1980, of which these remarks are a paraphrase).

Clearly, such broad questions as these will be revisited and refined as the study progresses, and the particulars from the data are grouped and patterns emerge.

Design Strategies

Because the research design is developmental in nature, it is important to consider the procedural strategies used by the inquirer when conducting the study. While design flexibility is important for the exploratory, discovery nature of qualitative research, the study cannot be conducted haphazardly and be expected to produce findings worthy of consideration (Lincoln & Guba, 1985). The design strategy employed in much of the qualitative research on learning disabilities has been *constant comparative analysis* (Glaser & Strauss, 1967). This design strategy focuses on the development and refinement of theory based on a number of cases. The cases are collected and then categories, patterns, and themes are analyzed to build a pattern of relationships that evolve into a theory (Stainback & Stainback, 1988). Such a theory is faithful to the everyday realities of the substantive area under study since it has been carefully induced from diverse field data (Glaser & Strauss, 1967).

This strategy was employed by Richardson and her colleagues (Richardson et al., 1989) as they explored what happens to at-risk children, including some with identified learning disabilities, in the context of two particular schools. They note:

We had no hypotheses to test, just a number of initial lenses through which we viewed schooling and at-risk children, and a set of guiding questions.

The assumptions that existed at the onset of the study were:

- The concept at-risk may be viewed as a combination of personal and background characteristics of a child and the social and academic context of the school. It is therefore necessary to look at the interaction between the school and the at-risk students as well as the child's background factors: socio-economic environment, ethnicity, language, family mobility, etc.
- The particular organization of the school and classroom, the norms of its teachers, the academic expectations held for its students and the academic tasks encountered by the students may affect the students' at-risk status.
- The labeling of children within a school setting as deprived, learning disabled, mentally retarded or at-risk could be more damaging to a child than the characteristics of the child that lead to the designation.

. . . our guiding questions were as follows: (i) Who are the students designated as at-risk? (ii) What is the organization of the schools and classrooms in which the students are operating? (iii) What are the beliefs held by the teachers and other adults in the school setting about the term at-risk? (iv) What happens to the at-risk students in their classrooms and schools? (v) What perceptions do the at-risk students express about school? and (vi) What do the parents of the at-risk students believe about their children and about school? (pp. 9–10)

In their study, Richardson and her colleagues proceeded to collect data for a set of nested case studies focusing at the district, school, classroom, and student levels. In the analysis of their data they followed the guidelines for constant comparative analysis suggested by Bogdan and Biklen (1982) in that they looked for recurrent events that became categories; worked with the data and emerging categories to discover basic patterns, relationships, and themes; and continually compared specific incidents in the data, refined the categories, relationships, and themes, and integrated them into a coherent theory of at-risk populations.

While constant comparative analysis is used when a specific hypothesis is not developed early in the study, an *analytic induction design* strategy (Katz, 1983) can be used when the researcher wants to quickly develop a specific hypothesis or has a specific hypothesis in mind and wants to use additional cases to confirm and modify the hypothesis. Regardless of the design strategy, it is important to focus at multiple levels as indicated by the use of nested case studies in the previously described research. Erickson (1986) suggests that "in fieldwork one never considers a single system level in isolation from other levels" (p. 143).

Conducting a Study

In conducting qualitative research, the process and procedures vary based on the aim of the study. For example, Bos and Lloyd (1989) constructed and orchestrated a series of teacher, student, and principal interviews, classroom observations, school climate interviews, and document analysis to construct a snapshot of and context for the functioning of several students with learning disabilities in their regular education classrooms. In contrast, Taylor (1991) used similar types of techniques—interviews, informal conversations, participant observations, and document analysis— but collected the data as the events unfolded over several years as she followed her case study.

This section discusses general guidelines and procedures for conducting qualitative research or naturalistic inquiry. This discussion is necessarily limited. A number of methodological books have been written, and a list is provided in the Appendix. Critical to naturalistic inquiry is the role of the researcher and the informant. Therefore, the discussion of methodology begins with these considerations. The next section on data collection and analysis highlights two of the most frequently used techniques: participant observation and interviewing. The final two sections deal with the triangulation of data and the written reports associated with qualitative research.

The Role of the Researcher

Naturalist inquiry presupposes that the researcher will enter the context being studied. In that context the researcher becomes not only a keen observer and listener, but oftentimes a participant in the culture. While the aim of scientific inquiry is to view the phenomena from an outsider's perspective, naturalistic inquiry focuses on the insider's viewpoint (Stainback & Stainback, 1988). In the same light, naturalistic inquiry assumes that research is necessarily value-bound—in other words, influenced by the values of the researcher in the selection of the issues for study, the manner in which the questions are framed, the design of the study, and the analysis and interpretation of the data (Lincoln & Guba, 1985).

Consequently, it becomes the job of the researcher to understand those values and to report them as part of the study. Michael Agar, in his book *The Professional Stranger*, characterizes the role of the researcher:

Ethnography is really quite an arrogant enterprise. In a short period of time, an ethnographer moves in among a group of strangers to study and describe their beliefs, document their social life, write about their subsistence strategies, and generally explore the territory right down to their recipes for the evening meal. . . . To some extent, the area covered depends on the ethnographer. On entering the community, an ethnographer carries more baggage than a tape recorder and a toothbrush, having grown up in a particular culture, acquiring many of its sometimes implicit assumptions about the nature of reality. . . . These aspects of "who you are" deserve some careful thought. They raise problems for ethnographers, and for all social scientists. Even at this early stage, they show that ethnography is much more complicated than collecting data, and that "objectivity" is perhaps best seen as a label to hide problems in the social sciences. The problem is not whether the ethnographer is biased; the problem is what kinds of biases exist—how do they enter into ethnographic work and how can their operation be documented. By bringing as many of them to consciousness as possible, an ethnographer can try to deal with them as part of methodology and can acknowledge them when drawing conclusions during analysis. In this sense, ethnography truly is a personal discipline as well as a professional one (1980, pp. 41–42).

The discussion of the role of the researcher is evident in the naturalistic inquiry conducted by Mary Lee Smith (1982) into the process by which educators decide whether particular children referred to them have learning disabilities. In describing the methodology and methods, she comments:

Because in naturalistic inquiry the researcher is the instrument, I will describe something about the instrument employed here. I am not learning disabled nor do I have a child who is or has been considered such. I am not an expert in the field of learning disabilities. . . . I am a research methodologist and secondarily a psychologist. My approach to this problem was an intellectual one. My motivation to do the study had less to do with its substance than its method. I did it because I wanted to do a case study, and this problem afforded the opportunity. . . .

It would be difficult to tag me with a political label, the only exception to this being my frequently stated observation that planned, centralized government has worked poorly. No doubt this belief affected and was reinforced by this project. If the data had shown otherwise, I would have believed the data (pp. 235–236).

Not only does the role of the researcher need to be explained and taken into account for data analysis and reporting purposes, but also in terms of presenting the study to the participants when access to a setting is being requested. The aim of the research should be communicated as clearly as possible to the participants, and participants should have the right to remain anonymous. Agar (1980), at the end of a discussion regarding the ethics associated with presenting the research and researcher to the participants, concludes, "Your goal is to begin your work honestly by presenting yourself and your task in some way that will make sense to group members" (p. 61).

The Role of the Informant

Critical to naturalistic inquiry are the informants who serve to provide the researcher with an avenue into the culture or community. Spradley (1979) suggests that informants are first and foremost native speakers in that they speak the language of the community and can serve as a model for the ethnographer to imitate. This modeling is clearly critical when the ethnographer is studying another culture with a language other than his/her own. However, this modeling is also critical as the ethnographer studies learning disabilities and the placement process. For example, Richardson and her colleagues (1989) found the interviews with the learning disabilities specialists and psychologists invaluable in understanding the professional language associated with placement procedures for special education.

The informants also serve as a valuable source of information. Spradley (1979) suggests that they become the teacher for the ethnographer. One barrier to a productive relationship is when this role of informant or teacher is confused with the scientific inquiry roles of subject and respondent. In considering informants, Spradley (1979) recommends that the informant be thoroughly enculturated and currently involved in the cultural setting under study.

Data Collection and Analysis

Naturalistic designs are oftentimes cyclical in nature in that ongoing data collection and analysis guides the direction of the research. For example, in collecting field notes, it is generally recommended that they are collected during an observation or interview. After the observation, the researcher is encouraged to immediately review the notes, elaborating on the notes to further explain what has been observed or discussed. This reflective process immediately after data collection oftentimes serves as the beginning of the analysis, for the researcher has the opportunity to study the information for patterns and themes. This section demonstrates this cyclical pattern using participant observation and ethnographic interviewing, the two fundamental techniques for data collection used in naturalistic inquiry.

Participant Observations

The purpose of participant observation is to describe in detail all aspects of the setting including physical description, the activities that took place, the people who participated, and the meaning(s) of the activities and setting as perceived by those people being observed (Stainback & Stainback, 1988). Although the participant observer's goals are oftentimes to blend into the situation, they inherently engage in activities different from the participant including collecting and organizing the observations around a framework of social science theory, keeping detailed notes of what occurs, occasionally detaching oneself from the situation to reflect on it, and monitoring observations and notes for personal bias (Dobbert, 1982). Spradley (1980) suggests five levels of participant observation:

Nonparticipation—only observes, no involvement in the activities,
Passive participation—a spectator present at the scene but does not participate or interact to any great extent,
Moderate participation—maintains a balance between being a participant and an observer,
Active participation—begins with observation but moves to doing what the participants are doing to more fully learn the cultural rules, and
Complete participation—studies a situation in which the observer is ordinarily a participant.

While one might imply from these levels that complete participation is ideal, it is considered the most difficult role to assume due to the difficulty in maintaining a questioning stance and reflective awareness necessary to understand and describe the tacit knowledge in the situation (Spradley, 1980; Stainback & Stainback, 1988).

Observations usually move from more general descriptive observations to more focused and selected observations. During the initial stages of the study, the participant observer's goal is to understand the nature and context of the situation being observed. For example, Bos and Lloyd (1989) were interested in observing students with reading/learning disabilities as they participated in literacy tasks in mainstreamed classrooms.

At first, rather than limiting themselves to observations of only literacy tasks, they began their observations by observing for the entire day so as to get a picture of the variety of activities in which the students participated. Spradley (1980) suggests that such observation might be called "grand tours," for the purpose is to record the major features of the classroom. He suggests the use of nine major dimensions: (a) space—physical place, (b) actors—people involved; (c) activities—the acts in which the participants engage; (d) objects—the things that are present; (e) acts—single actions of people; (f) events—sets of related activities; (g) time—the sequencing of events; (h) goals—the tasks that people are trying to accomplish, and (i) feelings—the emotions felt and expressed.

These types of descriptive observations lend themselves to data analysis that focuses on general domains or categories of study. Bos and Lloyd (1989) found that their general observations could be organized into several major domains when addressing the functioning of the students with learning disabilities in their mainstreamed classrooms. Adapting the framework of Miller et al. (1988), they considered two major domains: teacher/context accommodation and student assimilation. Within each domain they further delineated social/participatory aspects and cognitive/academic aspects.

TABLE 10.2. Typical semantic relationships.

Relationship	Form	Example
Strict inclusion	X is a kind of Y	Repeating directions is a kind of teacher accommodation.
Spatial	X is a place in Y X is a part of Y	The reading corner is a place in the classroom.
Cause-effect	X is a result of Y	Not receiving directions for a task is the result of being in the resource room when the directions are given.
Rationale	X is a reason for doing Y	Students asking clarification questions is a reason for elaborating on the directions.
Location for action	X is a place for doing Y	The classroom is a place for making plans for out-of-school activities with friends.
Function	X is used for Y	Assertive discipline is used as a system for monitoring student behavior.
Means-end	X is a way to do Y	Copying from a friend is a way to complete the task.
Sequence	X is a step in Y	Reading the directions is a step in completing work sheets.
Attribution	X is a characteristic of Y	Concern and caring are characteristics of the teacher.

Adapted from Spradley, J.P. (1980). *Participant observation.* New York: Holt, Rinehart & Winston.

Spradley (1980) suggests that a domain is made up of three basic elements: cover term, included terms, and a single semantic relationship. For example, from the observations collected by Bos and Lloyd (1989), one cover term was teacher accommodation for academic tasks. Using the semantic relationship of "is a kind of" they found a number of included terms (e.g., repeating directions, demonstrating the task, further describing the task, guiding the students as they work on the task). Table 10.2 presents a list of what Spradley (1979; 1980) considers universal semantic relationships with examples from the Bos and Lloyd (1989) study.

Two trends are evident in many studies that use participant observations as one of the major sources for obtaining data. First, the observations become more focused and selected as they continue across time. Again in the Bos and Lloyd study, the observations moved from a grand tour of the social situation to focus specifically on literacy tasks in which the students with learning disabilities participated. Second, the observer oftentimes assumes a more participatory role as the observations continue. While observers during the first days of the Bos and Lloyd study might be categorized as nonparticipants (only observers), the observers became passive participants (spectators present at the scene but not participating or interacting to any great extent).

Ethnographic Interviewing

Another major tool for the naturalistic inquirer is the interview. The goal of interviewing is to have the participants or informants talk about things of interest to them and yet to cover topics of importance to the inquirer in such a way that the participants use their own concepts and language (Spradley & Spradley, 1988). Consequently, these interviews usually range from semistructured (i.e., a set of topics or general questions to be covered) to informal or casual conversations and discussions. "The fundamental principle of qualitative interviewing is to provide a framework within which respondents can express their own understandings in their own terms" (Patton, 1980, p. 205).

One assumption of ethnographic interviewing is the interactive nature of the question-answer relationship. The manner in which a question is framed by the inquirer reflects his/her culture and necessarily influences the manner in which the informant answers the questions. Therefore, in ethnographic interviewing, both questions and answers must be discovered from the informant (Spradley, 1979). One way to learn about the questions of a culture is to listen and observe conversations to discover the types of questions that are asked. For example, both Smith (1982) and Taylor (1991) discuss the types of questions that are asked at placement meetings by the various participants. It is also helpful for the interviewer to directly inquire about questions used by participants. In a recent study of special education teacher planning (Duffy, 1991), informants viewed videotapes of their teaching a unit in science or social studies. At different points in the tape, the teachers were asked to discuss if and what questions they were asking themselves about planning.

Spradley (1979) suggests that using *descriptive questions* is yet another way in which to provide opportunity for the informant to shape the discussion and lessen the influence of the questions asked by the inquirer. Descriptive questions aim to elicit a large set of utterances using the informant's language. In the same way that Spradley suggests the use of grand tour observations to get a "big picture" of the cultural situation, he suggests grand tour questions as a means of getting rich, global descriptions of places, situations, or sequences of events or activities. These types of questions are well represented in the interviews that Richardson et al. (1989) used with the students, teachers, principals, and parents in their study of at-risk students. For example, the students were asked to tell about their teacher, school day, classroom, classmates, things they did in school, and things they used in school. Other types of descriptive questions include *example questions*, in which the interviewer asks the informant to provide an example of a specific event or situation, and *experience questions*, in which the interviewer asks the informant to provide an experience related to a specific event or situation.

One important aspect of ethnographic interviews is to ask questions that capture the *native language* of the informant. Spradley (1979) provides several strategies for assisting the interviewer in this endeavor, including using key questions such as "How would you refer to———?" "If you were talking to (another person in the situation), how would you say———?" and "What are some sentences I would hear that include (the key word or phrase)?"

In the same way that general observations lend themselves to data analysis that focuses on general domains or categories of study, descriptive questions lend themselves to the same kinds of domain and category analyses which allow the researcher to search for patterns within the data. For example, Schiller (1990) interviewed special education teachers prior to and after they participated in a staff development program designed to increase their understanding and application of discipline-based art education (DBAE). After transcribing and coding the data using 15 categories (e.g., memories of art in elementary school, reasons for using art in special education, knowledge of DBAE, self-perception as an artist), common domains were identified across the seven participating teachers using the semantic relationships of X is a kind of Y, X is a characteristic of Y, X is the reason for Y, and X is a statement about Y. For example, the following domain analysis was generated: No sink, lack of administrative support, lack of time, difficulty obtaining materials, personal inadequacy as an artist, and lack of funds (included terms) is a kind of (semantic relationship) barrier (cover term). To further delineate the relationships among the included terms, Schiller used taxonomic analysis (Miles & Huberman, 1984; Spradley, 1979). In this case, types of barriers were divided according to internal and external barriers, with personal inadequacy as an artist being viewed as an internal barrier and the others being grouped under external barriers. Schiller compared the taxonomic analyses for barriers from the pre-study and post-study interviews to demonstrate change in teacher attitudes. She found internal barriers regularly represented in the pre-study analysis by such statements as: "I can't draw," "I'm a new teacher," "I need help from an art specialist," and "I'm not an artist." However, on the post-study analysis internal barriers were no longer evident, with no references made to a negative perception of oneself as an artist.

While descriptive questions provide a rich core of data, *structured and contrast questions* provide the researcher with the opportunity to fine-tune, clarify, and verify analysis categories. Asking structural and contrast questions allows the researcher to test hypothesized categories and domains and to discover additional included terms. Spradley (1979) suggests nine principles be used in asking structural and contrast questions. These include:

1. *Concurrent Principle*: Ask structural and contrast questions concurrently with descriptive questions. They complement descriptive questions.
2. *Explanation Principle*: Let the informant know you are asking a structural or contrast question for they are not typical in ordinary conversation. For example, the interviewer might say, "We've been talking about how (student) interacts during reading group. How does (student) compare to the other students in the group?" (contrast question)
3. *Repetition Principle*: Repeat structural and contrast questions to be sure that all examples or comparisons have been made. For example, the interviewer might say, "You have told me how (student) compares to the other students in terms of oral reading, how does he compare in terms of understanding what he/she reads?"
4. *Contextual Principle*: Provide the informant with contextual information, particularly when a structural or contrast question is first being introduced. For example, the interviewer might say, "You work with (student) and four other students four times a week in a small reading group. Think for a minute about this group. How would you compare (student's) performance in that group with the other students?"
5. *Cultural Framework Principle*: Provide a cultural framework for structural and contrast questions. Informants oftentimes discuss a topic or domain in relation to their own personal experiences. If the goal is to obtain an exhaustive list of all the included terms in a domain, then it will be important to have the informant go beyond his/her personal

experiences. For example, in trying to obtain an exhaustive list for the cover term "difficult to teach" children, the interviewer might say, "You have described 'difficult to teach' children based on the ones that you have had in your classroom. Could you describe any additional characteristics of 'difficult to teach' children regardless of whether or not you have had students with these characteristics in your classroom?"

6. *Relational Principle*: Provide opportunities for the informant to describe how one idea, category, or domain is related to another. For example, when trying to clarify the informant's definition of learning disabilities, the interviewer might inquire, "How does the term 'learning disabilities' relate to the term 'learning problems'?"

7. *Use Principle*: Ask how something is used rather than asking what it means. Spradley (1979) suggests, "If we ask for meaning, we will only discover the explicit meanings, the ones that people can talk about. If we ask for use, we will tap that great reservoir of tacit meanings which exists in every culture" (p. 156).

8. *Similarity Principle*: Ask how one term is similar to a related term. This will assist in clarifying and discovering the boundaries associated with the term. For example, the inquirer could ask: "How is the term 'learning disabilities' similar to the term 'learning problems'?"

9. *Contrast Principle*: Ask how one term is different from a related term. The meaning of a term is based as much on what is does not mean as what it does mean. For example, the inquirer could ask: "How is the term 'learning disabilities' different from the term 'reading disabilities'?"

One trend is evident in studies that use ethnographic interviews as one of the major sources for obtaining data. The interviews move from simply descriptive discussions and questions to interspersing structural and contrast questions as the inquirer attempts to clarify and verify the information. Chalfant, Bos, and Pysh (1990) used teacher interview pre- and post-study to ascertain regular classroom teachers' beliefs and attitudes about students with learning disabilities. The initial use of descriptive questions followed by the interspersing of structural and contrast questions is evident in these interviews, particularly in the follow-up questions asked during the interviews.

Triangulation

Triangulation is a process by which multiple methods or sources of data that focus on the same phenomenon are collected. This process provides for different perspectives on the same activities and context, and is thought to guard against researcher bias. It is also felt that triangulation may increase both validity, since it provides the researcher with deeper and more extensive understandings of the context and its participants, as well as generalizability. As Sevigny (1981) points out: "The triangulated approach asks whether plausible interpretations are allowed from differing participant perspectives, while allowing for cross-validation measurement" (p. 73). Triangulation can be accomplished through the collection of multiple sources of data and through the use of *team research*, or two or more field workers collecting data in the same setting (Taylor & Bogdan, 1984). Many researchers also advocate the involvement of the informants in a review of analyses and findings of the study (e.g., Schon, 1991; Spradley, 1979). As can be deduced from the language used in the description of triangulation (reliability, validity, generalizability), this process is particularly stressed in the systematic approaches to qualitative research.

Miller, Leinhardt, and Zigmond (1988) provide examples of triangulation in their case study of a high school that had an unusually low dropout rate given the student population. The researchers followed a small number of adolescents with and without learning disabilities to understand the features of the school that might influence them to graduate or drop out. They used four forms of triangulation to overcome bias: multiple observers; multiple data sources, which they used to explore emerging trends; two independently conducted data analyses; and a search for disconfirming evidence.

The Written Product

There are few guidelines to use in writing an article or book from a qualitative study, other than the fact that it is best to maintain a distinction between the study itself and the written product. Unlike experimental studies, in which there is something of a formula for the organization of an article and the data analyses are conducted with the written product in mind, we have no formulae in qualitative research and seldom is all data collected in a qualitative study used in one book or article. Faced with mounds of data, many analyses at different conceptual levels, and lots of ideas floating in the head, what is the researcher to do?

It is important to understand the various purposes for writing a qualitative study. The first relates to writing to learn. Writing helps the researcher discover and express ideas that have been germinating throughout the study. For this reason, writing should begin soon after the study commences, and the first draft of any piece of formal writing from the study should be just that: a first draft used to help the researcher develop and articulate burning issues.

The second purpose is to develop a record of the following: methodologies; context of the study; processes of gaining entry, interviewing, observing (with dates); methods for storing data; descriptions of different levels of data used for analysis; and the results of the analyses. This, basically, becomes a final report of the project. It will be extremely long, with considerable data. Again, many pieces of it may be developed during the course of the study. If it is anticipated that several formal written products will be developed from the study, it would be useful to archive the final report in a system such as ERIC. In writing articles, the author is then able to refer readers to the final report for the details of process and results.

The third purpose is to communicate what has been learned to the national or international community of scholars with whom the researcher associates. This requires a very different mindset and set of processes than the preceding two purposes. The writing-to-learn document emphasizes those elements that the researcher is grappling with and ignores aspects that the researcher has already conceptually solved. The final report document is generally not publishable, primarily because it is descriptive, all-inclusive, and long. For the publishable article or book, the researcher must turn his/her attention to the reader. What are the issues in the field that are of interest to the reader and that can be addressed by the study?

One place to look to answer this question, of course, is in the literature. The literature search is conducted throughout the course of the study, and provides information on many different aspects of the study. For this purpose, the literature can help provide clues toward theory development, gaps in the community's understandings, and areas of interest that are being pursued. This literature analysis, in interaction with the material in the final report, provides the story line of an article or book. The writing of a publishable qualitative article requires just that: a good story line. It is possible, then, to select from the final report those elements of the data and analyses that support the story line.

The form that the written product takes may vary. Van Maanen (1988) writes about three types in ethnographies: realistic tales, confessional tales, and impressionist tales. These vary in terms of the presence of the author, the degree of description of mishaps in fieldwork, the feelings while conducting research, the number of "voices" represented, and the ways in which the sequence of events are portrayed. The choice of form would depend to a certain degree on the research approach taken. The written product of a systematic study could, for example, resemble a realistic tale. The events would be described as quite separate from the researcher's feelings and cognitions. Numbers and tables could be employed to indicate themes and conclusions. An artistic approach would resemble an impressionist tale and would be quite novelistic in character.

However, regardless of the form taken, the author must consider audience both in terms of the story that is being presented, and in the traditions of form within the community. Many journals have recently been responsive to different forms of presentation for studies. However, prior to writing an article, the author had best carefully review the published articles in a given journal to determine its traditions and whether it might be possible to "break the mold."

Future Directions for Research

Clearly, the field of learning disabilities is ripe for qualitative research. We are in the midst of asking difficult questions regarding policy and practices for students with learning disabilities, including issues of definition, identification, and service delivery. Qualitative research can provide us with differing perspectives on these issues and inform our practice. In much the same way that Salomon (1991) used qualitative and quantitative research to study both sides of the coin with regard to the hypothesis that interaction with a computer would improve writing ability, several recent studies (Allington & McGill-Franzen, 1989; Gersten, Darch, & George, 1991; Meyers, Gelzheiser, Yelich, & Gallagher, 1990) have integrated qualitative and quantitative methodologies to better understand the mainstreamed environment and the participants within that environment. Such flexible use of methodologies holds promise for the field of education in general, and specifically for the field of learning disabilities.

References

Agar, M.H. (1980). *The professional stranger: An informal introduction to ethnography*. Orlando, FL: Academic Press.

Allington, R.L. & McGill-Franzen, A. (1989). School response to reading failure: Instruction for Chapter 1 and special education students in grades two, four, and eight. *Elementary School Journal, 89*, 529–542.

Bogdan, R. & Barnes, E. (1979). A qualitative-sociological study of mainstreaming. National Institute of Education Proposal (mimeographed). Syracuse, NY: Syracuse University, Center for Human Policy.

Bogdan, R. & Biklen, D. (1982). *Qualitative research for education: An introduction to theory and methods*. Boston: Allyn & Bacon.

Bogdan, R. & Kugelmass, J. (1984). Case studies of mainstreaming: A symbolic interactionist approach to special schooling. In L. Barton & S. Tomlinson (Eds.), *Special education and social interests* (pp. 173–191). London: Croom Helm.

Bos, C.S. & Lloyd, C. (1989). *Teacher and student perceptions of literacy tasks: Looking for congruence*. Paper presented at the annual meeting of the National Reading Conference, Austin, TX.

Chalfant, J.C., Bos, C.S., & Pysh, M.V. (1990). *Interim final report of the TEAM project*. Report submitted to the U.S. Department of Education, Office of Special Education and Rehabilitation Services. Tucson: University of Arizona, College of Education.

Chilcott, J. (1987). Where are you coming from and where are you going? The reporting of ethnographic research. *American Educational Research Journal, 24*, 199–218.

Dabbs, J.M., Jr. (1982). The rescue from relativism: Two failed attempts and an alternative strategy. *Educational Researcher, 14*(10), 13–20.

Dobbert, M. (1982). *Ethnographic research*. New York: Praeger.

Donmoyer, R. (1990). Generalizability and the single-case study. In E.W. Eisner & A. Peshkin (Eds.), *Qualitative inquiry in education: The continuing debate* (pp. 175–200). New York: Teachers College Press.

Duffy, M.L. (1991). *Special education teacher planning: A qualitative study.* Unpublished doctoral dissertation, Unversity of Arizona.

Eisner, E. (1981). On the differences between scientific and artistic approaches to qualitative research. *Educational Researcher, 10*, 5–9.

Eisner, E. (1986). A secretary in the classroom. *Teaching and Teacher Education, 2*, 325–328.

Erickson, F. (1986). Qualitative methods in research on teaching. In M. Wittrock (Ed.), *Handbook of research on teaching* (3rd ed., pp. 119–161). New York: Macmillan.

Erickson, F., Florio, S., & Buschman, J. (1980). *Fieldwork in educational research* (Occasional Paper No. 36). East Lansing, MI: Michigan State University, Institute for Research on Teaching.

Geertz, C. (1973). Thick description: Toward an interpretative theory of cultures. In C. Geertz (Ed.), *The interpretation of cultures* (pp. 174–198). New York: Basic Books.

Gersten, R., Darch, C., & George, N. (1991). Apprenticeship and intensive training of consulting teachers: A naturalistic study. *Exceptional Children, 57*, 226–236.

Glaser, B. & Strauss, A. (1967). *Theoretical sensitivity: Advances in the methodology of grounded theory*. Mill Valley, CA: Sociology Press.

Guba, E.G. & Lincoln, Y.S. (1981). *Effective evaluation: Improving the usefulness of evaluation results through responsive and naturalistic approaches*. San Francisco: Jossey-Bass.

Howe, K. & Eisenhart, M. (1990). Standards for qualitative (and quantitative) research: A prolegomenon. *Educational Researcher, 19*(4), 2–9.

Jacob, E. (1990). Alternative approaches for studying naturally occurring human behavior and thought in special education research. *Journal of Special Education, 24*, 195–211.

Katz, J. (1983). A theory of qualitative methodology: The social science system of analytic fieldwork. In R.M. Emerson (Ed.), *Contemporary field research* (pp. 127–148). Boston: Little, Brown.

Kirk, J. & Miller, M.M. (1986). *Reliability and validity in qualitative research.* Newbury Park, CA: Sage.

Lincoln, Y.S. & Guba, E.G. (1985). *Naturalistic inquiry*. Newbury Park, CA: Sage.

Meyers, J., Gelzheiser, L., Yelich, G., & Gallagher, M. (1990). Classroom, remedial, and resource teachers' views of pullout programs. *Elementary School Journal, 90*, 533–545.

Miles, M. & Huberman, A.M. (1984). *Qualitative data analysis: A sourcebook of new methods*. Newbury Park, CA: Sage.

Miles, M. & Huberman, A.M. (1984). Drawing valid meaning from qualitative data: Toward a shared craft. *Educational Researcher, 16*, 20–30.

Miles, M. & Huberman, A.M. (1990). Animadversions and reflections on the uses of qualitative inquiry. In E. Eisner & A. Peshkin (Eds.), *Qualitative in-*

quiry in education: The continuing debate (pp. 339–357). New York: Teachers College Press.

Miller, M. (1990). Ethnographic interviews for information about classrooms: An invitation. *Teacher Education and Special Education, 13*, 233–234.

Miller, S.E., Leinhardt, G., & Zigmond, N. (1988). Influencing engagement through accommodation: An ethnographic study of at-risk students. *American Educational Research Journal, 25*, 465–487.

Murray, C., Anderson, J., Bersani, H., & Mesaros, R. (1986). Qualitative research methods in special education: Ethnography, microethnography, and ethology. *Journal of Special Education Technology, 7*(3), 15–31.

Naff, B. (1987). *The impact of prescriptive planning models on preservice English teachers' thought and on the classroom environments they create: An ethnographic study.* Unpublished Ed.D. dissertation, Virginia Polytechnic Institute and State University.

Patton, M. (1980). *Qualitative evaluation methods.* Newbury Park, CA: Sage.

Richardson, V., Casanova, U., Placier, P., & Guilfoyle, K. (1989). *School children at-risk.* Philadelphia: Falmer Press.

Salomon, G. (1991). Transcending the qualitative-quantitative debate: The analytic and systemic approaches to educational research. *Educational Researcher, 20*(6), 10–18.

Schiller, M.A. (1990). *An interpretive study of teacher change during staff development with teachers of special education.* Unpublished doctoral dissertation, University of Arizona.

Schon, D. (1991). Concluding comments. In D. Schon (Ed.), *The reflective turn: Case studies in and on educational practice* (pp. 343–359). New York: Teachers College Press.

Sevigny, M. (1981). Triangulated inquiry—a methodology for the analysis of classroom interaction. In J. Green & C. Wallat (Eds.), *Ethnography and language in educational settings* (pp. 65–86). Norwood, NJ: Ablex.

Sigmon, S.B. (1987). *Radical analysis of special education: Focus on historical development and learning disabilities.* Philadelphia: Falmer Press.

Sigmon, S.B. (1990). Toward a radical methodology for rational discourse on special education. In S. Sigmon (Ed.), *Critical voices on special education* (pp. 71–82). Albany, NY: State University of New York Press.

Smith, M.L. (1982). *How educators decide who is learning disabled.* Springfield, IL: Charles C. Thomas.

Smith, M.L. (1987). Publishing qualitative research. *American Education Research Journal, 24*, 173–183.

Spradley, J.P. (1979). *The ethnographic interview.* New York: Holt, Rinehart & Winston.

Spradley, J.P. (1980). *Participant observation.* New York: Holt, Rinehart & Winston.

Stainback, S.S. & Stainback, W. (1984). Broadening the research perspective in special education. *Exceptional Children, 50*, 400–408.

Stainback, S.S. & Stainback, W. (1988). *Understanding and conducting qualitative research.* Reston, VA: Council for Exceptional Children.

Taylor, D. (1991). *Learning denied.* Portsmouth, NH: Heinemann.

Taylor, S. & Bogdan, R. (1984). *Introduction to qualitative research methods* (2nd ed.). New York: Wiley.

Van Maanen, J. (1988). *Tales of the field: On writing ethnography*. Chicago: University of Chicago Press.

Wolcott, H. (1985). On ethnographic intent. *Educational Administration Quarterly*, *21*, 187–203.

Appendix

Suggested Resource Books for Conducting Qualitative Research and Naturalistic Inquiry

Agar, M.H. (1980). *The professional stranger: An informal introduction to ethnography*. Orlando, FL: Academic Press.

Bogdan, R.C. & Biklen, S. (1982). *Qualitative research for education: An introduction to theory and methods*. Boston: Allyn & Bacon.

Eisner, E.W. & Peshkin, A. (Eds.). (1990). *Qualitative inquiry in education: The continuing debate*. New York: Teachers College Press.

Glaser, B. & Strauss, A. (1967). *Theoretical sensitivity: Advances in the methodology of grounded theory*. Mill Valley, CA: Sociology Press.

Guba, E.G. & Lincoln, Y.S. (1981). *Effective evaluation: Improving the usefulness of evaluation results through responsive and naturalistic approaches*. San Francisco: Jossey-Bass.

Kirk, J. & Miller, M.M. (1986). *Reliability and validity in qualitative research*. Newbury Park, CA: Sage.

Lincoln, Y.S. & Guba, E.G. (1985). *Naturalistic inquiry*. Newbury Park, CA: Sage.

Marshall, C. & Rossman, G.B. (1989). *Designing qualitative research*. Newbury Park, CA: Sage.

Miles, M. & Huberman, A.M. (1984). *Qualitative data analysis: A sourcebook of new methods*. Newbury Park, CA: Sage.

Spradley, J.P. (1979). *The ethnographic interview*. New York: Holt, Rinehart & Winston.

Spradley, J.P. (1980). *Participant observation*. New York: Holt, Rinehart & Winston.

Stainback, S. & Stainback, W. (1988). *Understanding and conducting qualitative research*. Reston, VA: Council for Exceptional Children.

Taylor, S. & Bogdan, R. (1984). *Introduction to qualitative research methods* (2nd ed.). New York: Wiley.

Yin, R.K. (1989). *Case study research: Design and methods* (rev. ed.). Newbury Park, CA: Sage.

11
Methodological Issues in Longitudinal Research on Learning Disabilities

JAMES D. McKINNEY

The purposes of this chapter are to discuss (a) the definition of longitudinal research and the types of research questions addressed by longitudinal designs, and (b) the practical and methodological issues involved in designing and conducting longitudinal studies and in performing longitudinal data analyses. In addition, the limitations of longitudinal research will be discussed. Therefore, this chapter does not review that research on learning disabilities that has used longitudinal designs, but rather illustrates the purpose and methods of longitudinal research with selected studies of individuals with learning disabilities and presents both the strengths and limitations of a longitudinal approach.

Although longitudinal research has a long and prominent history in the fields of epidemiology and human development, it is nevertheless an underused design in the child development literature relative to the overall number of scientific studies that are conducted (Gallagher, Ramey, Haskins, & Finkelstein, 1976). It is particularly rare in the field of learning disabilities (Kavale, 1988; Keogh, 1988; McKinney, 1989). While it is the case that the field of learning disabilities is relatively new (compared to the history of theory and research on mental retardation) and that research on learning disabilities has been more issue-driven than theory-driven (Kavale, 1988; Keogh, 1988; McKinney, 1988), these factors alone are not sufficient to account for the paucity of longitudinal research on learning disabilities. Nor is it the case that longitudinal research has not been done.

Recent reviews of longitudinal research on learning disabilities cite numerous studies, albeit fewer than those in many other disciplines (Horn, O'Donnel, & Vitulano, 1983; Kavale, 1988; Nichols & Chen, 1981). However, these reviews also reveal that the bulk of longitudinal evidence is based on follow-up studies that are mostly retrospective rather than prospective in focus and seriously flawed methodologically (see Kavale, 1988). Although there are notable examples of strong prospective studies to the contrary, most of these still focus on outcomes as the major findings of interest, and/or the correlative relationships between antecedent variables and outcomes.

Therefore, apart from methodological problems that limit current knowledge about outcomes and risk factors, it appears that a major failing is simply not taking full advantage of the descriptive and explanatory power of the longitudinal method itself. Accordingly, we still lack basic knowledge about the natural history of learning disability.

Specifically, we know little about how the various risk factors that have been associated with the disorder interact over time to produce learning disabilities, or how the manifestations of the disorder evolve and change over time as a function of biologic and environmental factors. Also, we have little direct knowledge that can be applied to prevent or ameliorate the educational consequences of learning disabilities by altering the course of faulty development. Such are the broader purposes of longitudinal research.

This is not to say that significant progress has not been made in the field of learning disabilities over the past decade, nor to say that longitudinal research can address all of the relevant and important questions concerning the nature of learning disabilities. However, it remains an underused but powerful tool in understanding the development of individuals with learning disabilities and its full impact on practice has yet to be realized.

Definition, Purpose, and Design of Longitudinal Research

The Definition of Longitudinal Research

As noted by Baltes and Nesselroade (1979) and Menard (1991), longitudinal research is defined by both the design and the data analysis strategies that are used. Longitudinal designs are used to describe patterns of change in individuals (or other units of measurement) over time and to establish the direction (positive/negative, increasing/decreasing) and magnitude of relationships among conditions, events, treatments, and later oucomes measured as dependent variables. Thus, longitudinal research is characterized by the following:

1. Observations are made on each unit (individual) at each of two or more distinct periods of time;
2. The same individuals (units) are assessed successively from one period to the next; and
3. The analysis involves the evaluation of within-subjects variance between or among periods.

Cohort, Period, and Age Effects

In conceptualizing and describing a longitudinal research design, the terms *cohort*, *period*, and *age* need to be understood and carefully operationalized to draw proper conclusions about the nature of change over time. In classic developmental studies, the term *cohort* usually refers to the time of birth. *Age* refers to the point since birth when an observation is taken, and *period* refers to the length of time between observations. The term *event cohort* is used to denote cohorts that are selected based on some event that occurs after birth, for example, time of identification as learning disabled, but is not necessarily correlated with age.

In the classical single-cohort design, cohort, period, and age are linearly dependent, and each varies as a function of the other two. Thus, the data collection schedule for each individual must ensure that the time of each observation has a constant lag from the date or age of entry into the study. For example, if age varies as yearly intervals (e.g., 6, 7, and 8 years) and children enter at different times during their sixth year, then a child who is observed first at 76 months (6 years, 4 months) is observed the second time at or about 88 months (7 years, 4 months) to have a measure of age that is not confounded by variation in cohorts or periods. The term "panel" refers to the time span for taking all the observations for all the individuals in a given cohort (also called a wave of data collection).

This design feature allows the investigator to draw causal inferences about the relationship between age-dependent trends (i.e., development) on various dependent variables and the independent variables (e.g., group membership, treatment) that are manipulated in the design. Although this relationship is intuitively simple, it presents significant problems in the interpretation of the data when cohorts and periods interact to produce inexplicable age effects.

The Purposes of Longitudinal Research

To justify longitudinal research in comparison with other design options, one must distinguish between research questions that are uniquely appropriate for longitudinal research and those that are better or more efficiently addressed by other designs. In general, the purposes of longitudinal research are similar to other types of research, that is, to describe the phenomenon of interest, to predict other variables, to evaluate the efficacy of intervention/treatments, and to explain directional (presumably causal) relationships. Beyond these similarities, longitudinal designs alone have the following common features:

1. They assess the magnitude and direction of change over time;

2. They are sensitive to intraindividual variation relative to time as opposed to individual variation relative to sample means; and
3. They establish true temporal order for inferring cause and effect relationships.

Description of Change over Time

Longitudinal research is necessary to address questions pertaining to the patterns or rates of developmental change displayed by different individuals. At present, little is known about the different developmental paths children with learning disabilities take to a given outcome. Fundamental assumptions related to the concepts of developmental delays and specific ability deficits are largely untested from a longitudinal perspective.

For example, Piaget's concept of stage invariance suggests that developmental delay could occur if a child failed to make the transition from preoperational to concrete operational thought or to progress through a given stage at an age-appropriate rate. Speece and McKinney (1986) compared longitudinally 6- and 7-year-old children with learning disabilities with average-achievers on a series of conservation tasks, and found that children with learning disabilities were delayed in attaining the stage of concrete operations. However, they acquired specific concepts (e.g., number, quantity, weight) at the same rate as average achievers once they experienced the transition.

A major weakness of longitudinal follow-up studies is that they have tended to focus on average outcomes for heterogeneous groups (Kavale, 1988) and to ignore individual differences in academic progress over time—the essential reason for doing longitudinal research. While evidence from cross-sectional and prospective follow-up studies tend to support the Matthew effect (Stanovich, 1986) with respect to a decreasing trend in achievement for children with learning disabilities, longitudinal evidence on individual patterns of academic progress is needed to explain individual variation in outcome as a function of antecedent child characteristics, and environmental and educational experiences.

For example, three studies from the Carolina Longitudinal Learning Disabilities Project (McKinney & Feagans, 1984) indicated that some subtypes of children with learning disabilities showed relatively stable but below-average patterns of academic progress over a 3-year period, while other subtypes showed decreasing patterns relative to average-achievers (Feagans & Appelbaum, 1986; McKinney, Short, & Feagans, 1985; McKinney & Speece, 1986). Thus the Matthew effect was not evident for all children in the longitudinal sample. More recently, Osborne, Schulte, and McKinney (1991) related longitudinal trends in classroom behavior, achievement, and grade retention to changes in special education placement (e.g., mainstream vs. special education) as an alternative way to view antecedents and outcomes longitudinally.

Prediction of Developmental Outcomes

In general, the research question addressed in these studies pertains to the relative contributions of different variables to the prediction of later events, child characteristics, or group membership. For example, Nichols and Chen (1981) identified a large sample of children with learning disabilities and their controls at age 7 from a total cohort of 30,000 subjects in the Collaborative Perinatal Project. They related approximately 62 variables assessed during the first year of life with later group membership. Discriminant analysis showed strong relationships for a number of socioeconomic status (SES) and demographic factors; however, medical indexes of perinatal risk which predicted developmental growth at the end of the first year did not predict group membership.

An example of a longitudinal cross-time predictive study is McKinney's (in press) follow-up study of children in the Carolina Longitudinal Project sample who were identified as learning disabled when they were 6 and 7 years of age and assessed repeatedly over 5 years. The regression model included measures of child IQ, mother's educational level, grade retention, and classroom behavior measured over 3 years prior to the follow-up assessment. While mother's educational level and teacher perceptions of child ability (with IQ) predicted achievement scores consistently over time for average-achievers, attentional behavior and a history of academic failure predicted consistently for children with learning disabilities.

In another example, Yeats, McPhee, Campbell, and Ramey (1983) used path analysis to compare the relative and cumulative contributions of maternal IQ and home environment to the prediction of child IQ in a high-risk sample of children from low-income families. They found that while the variables combined to show a monotonic increase in prediction between 24 and 48 months of age, there was a shift in their relative contribution such that the correlation between maternal IQ and child IQ decreased while the correlation between child IQ and home environment increased and replaced maternal IQ as a significant predictor beyond 36 months. Research questions of this nature are theoretically interesting because they elucidate the interactions that occur between intrinsic and environmental influences (Sameroff & Chandler, 1975) that vary with age to increase or reduce risk for poorer outcomes (Keogh, in press; Werner, 1986; Werner & Smith, 1982).

Prediction of Sequential Change across Periods

McKinney and Speece (1983) used IQ and two measures of classroom behavior (rating scales and observations) to predict the residual gains of children with learning disabilities from Period 1 of the longitudinal study to Period 2, and from Period 1 to Period 3. IQ was a better predictor of achievement measured concurrently at each period than was classroom behavior. However, classroom behavior was the sole predictor when academic progress was measured as change across periods. This study illustrates the utility of longitudinal research in identifying potentially modifiable variables that are educationally relevant due to their association with changes in outcomes as opposed to variables that merely covary with achievement at a given point in time.

Evaluation of Intervention

One of the basic purposes of longitudinal research on intervention is to test the hypothesis that treatment alters individuals' patterns of change with respect to the magnitude and direction of response trends over time. Accordingly, it is particularly suited to studies that seek to prevent or ameliorate poor developmental outcomes. In most examples of this kind of research, the intervention was designed to accelerate normal development in children who were at risk for developmental delay and school failure due to environmental disadvantage.

The Carolina Abecedarian Project (Ramey & Campbell, 1991, Ramey, Yeates, & Short, 1984) illustrates the interaction between treatment groups and longitudinal trends in the dependent variables. In this study, children who were at high risk for school failure were randomly assigned to an experimental group that received an intense preschool educational treatment in a day-care setting, or to a control group that, like the experimental group, received pediatric care and family support services—but not the intensive preschool curriculum that was based on age-appropriate cognitive, linguistic, motor, and social intervention.

Although the results of the Abecedarian Project showed that children who received intensive intervention gained the advantage early and outperformed the control children at each observational period on measures of intelligence (Ramey & Campbell, 1991), the most important findings from a theoretical and practical perspective concerned the interaction between treatment groups and pattern of change over time. Although both groups had comparable average ability in infancy, children in the control group showed a steeply decreasing pattern of performance between 9 and 24 months, and showed no recovery until 36 months. While the control children did recover and showed a slightly increasing trend between 36 and 60 months, their performance was still below that of the experimental group from 60 months through 96 months (8 years). Thus, the intervention did appear to alter the early onset of developmental delay and promote more stable rates of growth throughout the preschool period. These findings illustrate the strength of longitudinal research in identifying critical periods of development that provide a window of opportunity for prevention as well as specifying the means for accelerating growth. Additional examples of longitudinal studies of early intervention programs can be found in Lazar, Darlington, Murray, Royce, and Snipper (1982).

Cumulative Impact of Treatment

In addition to the implications of longitudinal research for the age-appropriate timing of intervention for specific periods of development, longitudinal designs also have the capacity for assessing the cumulative impact of sequential treatments aimed at the further enhancement of growth and/or the maintenance of beneficial effects. For example, some studies of early intervention found that treatment effects tended to "fade out" early in the elementary period or that they are obviated by control group gains from school experience (see Lazar et al., 1982).

Anticipating this problem, the investigators in the Abecedarian Project randomly subdivided the experimental and control groups at school entry into secondary treatment groups that received a follow-up treatment that was delivered by home/school resource teachers (Ramey & Campbell, 1991). The completely randomized design varied the intensity of intervention such that one group had 8 years of intervention (preschool and follow-through), one had 5 years (preschool only), one had 3 years (school-age only), and one had no special intervention.

Longitudinal analysis of IQ scores for the four groups indicated that children who received continuous preschool intervention maintained their superiority over preschool control children regardless of follow-through intervention (Ramey & Campbell, 1991). However, clear linear trends were obtained for academic achievement which were ordered by intensity of intervention from greatest (preschool plus follow-through) to least (control). The practical value of these effects was further demonstrated by data on grade retention and referral for special education. While preschool plus follow-through children were less likely to be retained by the eighth grade than children who had only preschool (16% vs. 29%), both were less likely to be retained than follow-through only (38%) and control children without special intervention (50%).

Impact of Intervention on Children with Biologic Risk

Another longitudinal study on early intervention is worthy of mention because of its findings with respect to the interaction between environmental factors and biologic risk, as well as its overall scope and well-conceptualized design. The Infant Health and Development Project (IHDP, 1990) is a national eight-site randomized experimental study to test the efficacy of early educational intervention and pediatric follow-up care in preventing adverse developmental and health problems associated with low birth-weight. The sample consisted of 985 infants who were randomly assigned to a comprehensive intervention program that incorporated three features (preschool day-care curriculum, home support, and pediatric care) or to pediatric care with no intervention. The children were stratified by site and birth-weight (less than 2,000 grams and 2,001 to 2,500 grams).

Educational treatment began when they were discharged from the neonatal nursery, and outcomes were measured at 36 months with cognitive, behavioral, and health status measures. The project is still underway. However, initial findings at 36 months indicated that the intervention groups scored higher than the control group on IQ tests, had fewer behavior problems as reported by parents, and showed no differences on health status. Thus, it appeared that educational treatment was instrumental in offsetting this form of biologic risk.

In sum, these examples demonstrate the superiority of long-term longitudinal research with respect to explanatory power and practical application. Also, the utility and validity of research in this vein for program planning and the implementation of educational policy are evident.

Serendipity and Intentional Outcomes

In addition to the stated purposes of longitudinal research, it should be noted that it also has the capability of detecting unanticipated findings of interest. This capability often enhances the importance of longitudinal studies from a policy-analytic perspective, which must consider the likely intended and unintended consequences of investing resources in various alternative solutions to some significant social problem. For example, one unanticipated benefit that was observed as the result of the Abecedarian Project was that center-based day-care intervention with on-site health services allowed a significant number of mothers in poverty to improve their education and economic condition. In the same vein, one implication drawn from the Kauai longitudinal study was that the evidence concerning factors related to successful outcomes for children who were at risk had greater implications for preventative intervention than the evidence concerning factors related to poor outcomes (Werner & Smith, 1982).

Causal Relationships/Model Testing

The final purpose of longitudinal research is to draw causal inferences from the relationship between independent variables and change assessed by dependent variables. According to Baltes and Nesselroade (1979) and Menard (1991), three criteria must be met to infer cause and effect:

1. The independent and dependent variables in question must covary such that differences between groups (experimental and control) are a function of group membership or such that a correlation exists (nonzero) between the two variables or sets of variables;

2. The relationship must not be spurious, that is, it cannot be attributable to rival explanations due to the effects of uncontrolled variables, or it must be evident by the existence of a partial correlation (non-zero) between the independent and dependent variables with other variables held constant; and
3. The presumed cause must precede or occur simultaneously with the supposed effect, that is, the change in cause occurred no later than the associated change in the effect.

As Menard (1991) notes, some argue that additional criteria might be imposed, such as an inference concerning the mechanism that links cause with effect, that is, theoretically inferred intervening variables related to the manipulation (e.g., task instructions designed to heighten test-taking anxiety or treatments that presumably compensate for disability). Others argue that the term "cause" is not used properly and that it is not necessary to draw inferences about the strength of a relationship in the behavioral sciences. The reader may wish to refer to Menard (1991) on pages 17–20 and page 75 (Note 2) for a more elaborate discussion of this issue.

In any event, the major point is that all three criteria apply to causal inference from all experimental designs. However, the third criterion is addressed uniquely by longitudinal designs when the investigator's question pertains to the magnitude *and* direction of individuals' changes over time. Perhaps it should be noted that single *n* operant learning designs can also address this question because they use repeated measures to assess change in the pattern of learning curves that reflect both magnitude and rate, and they also meet the third criterion by the sequential manipulation of events. At the same time, the explanatory power of longitudinal designs is particularly evident when the investigator is interested in the temporal order of events that explain outcomes.

For example, Menard and Elliott (1990) tested two competitive theories about peer group influence on delinquent behavior. One theory implied that involvement with delinquent friends produces delinquent behavior (social learning theory), while the other suggested that delinquent behavior leads to involvement with delinquent friends (control theory). They applied causal modeling and found support for social learning theory in that the association with delinquent friends more often preceded an individual's delinquent behavior. However, they noted that this finding was "typical" of the relationship. Accordingly, Menard (1991) concluded that temporal order is necessary but not sufficient to establish true causality (one contrary case violates "absolute" truth). However, temporal order in longitudinal studies does provide sufficient evidence to accept one theory as more plausible than another when tested in this fashion as opposed to simply rejecting the null hypothesis of no group differences and then inferring the truth of the theory when plausible alternatives were not tested.

Types of Longitudinal Designs

In this section, alternative designs will be discussed for assessing change over time and change as a function of treatment and/or experimental manipulation. Types of alternative designs are displayed in Figures 11.1 and 11.2.

Classical Birth Cohort Design

With classical longitudinal designs, the investigator begins with a large birth cohort and takes repeated measures on the same individuals over an extended period of time. This design is illustrated by Werner and Smith's (1982) study, which began with all live births ($n = 1,963$) on the island of Kauai between 1954 and 1957 who were followed prospectively for 25 years.

The purposes of classical designs are to describe developmental change, determine the antecedents of later outcome, and assess the interaction between indexes of developmental status and changes in events and prior developmental status. The design does not evaluate treatments systematically except as they occur as natural events, for example, low birth-weight and other perinatal risk factors are free to vary and are related correlatively to later outcome. The principal strength of this design follows from its scope and detailed portrait of individuals' developmental course. However, it is limited by its initial assumptions and methodology. Also, long-term studies are particularly subject to the perils of missing data and subject (as well as investigator) attrition. As a result, scientists have sought to develop more flexible and less costly longitudinal designs, although this frequently occurs at the expense of the elegance and simplicity of the classical design.

Population Designs

Total Population Designs

The purpose of these designs is to capture periodic change in representative samples of a total population. In these designs, temporal changes can be assessed both cross-sectionally across periods and longitudinally within a given cohort across periods if (a) sufficient numbers of subjects who represent the population across periods are retained, and (b) the number of periods is sufficient for meaningful comparison.

For example, the United States census data permits cross-sectional comparisons on changes in sociodemographic characteristics by state, region, and locality over successive 10-year periods. Although all the cases are not the same from one year to the next due to population entry via birth and immigration and exit via death and out-migration, sufficient numbers of individuals are available for life span developmental analysis

TOTAL POPULATION DESIGN

Panels X Age

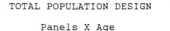

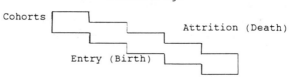

REPEATED CROSS SECTIONAL LONGITUDINAL PANEL DESIGN

Age within Panels

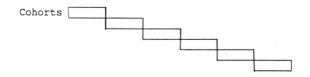

REVOLVING PANEL DESIGN

Overlapping Age within Panels

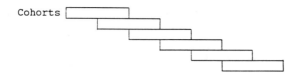

LONGITUDINAL PANEL/MULTIPLE COHORT DESIGN

Panels X Age

Cohorts	Age 6				Age 10
	Age 7				Age 11
	Age 8				Age 12
	Age 9				Age 13
	Age 10				Age 14

FIGURE 11.1. Alternative longitudinal panel designs.

(Menard, 1991). Unfortunately, this is not the case with the child-count data collected by the Office of Special Education and Rehabilitative Services (DOE) on the number of children served in special education each year because no attempt is made to identify the same children who are served from year to year, or to identify those who change category or type of service received. Accordingly, this data, collected at great expense nationally, is useless for most epidemiological purposes.

Figure 11.1 illustrates common alternative longitudinal designs which can be compared to the total population design. In describing these designs the term "panel" refers to the entire wave of data collection across periods for each cohort.

Repeated Cross-Sectional Designs

Repeated cross-sectional designs are often used for survey research. In this design, independent separate samples that are representative of the population of interest are drawn at each period of observation. The basic purpose is to gather common data on a specific age group over time (e.g., self-reported delinquent behavior of adolescents with learning disabilities). Although the subjects are comparable from period to period, the amount of overlap varies from period to period, which may or may not permit an analysis of longitudinal trends across periods. The major advantage of this design is that it does provide for the replication of cross-sectional age trends over periods. However, it is not appropriate for studying developmental trends within cohorts and is not capable of testing temporal order effects. For these reasons Baltes and Nesselroade (1979) argue that it is not a true longitudinal design. Basically, it merely provides a description of changes in opinions or behavior within a defined population of individuals by repeatedly sampling the population over time (e.g., a weekly index of voter preference for candidates during a campaign).

Revolving Panel Designs

These longitudinal designs use multiple independent cohorts but feature planned overlapping panels of measurement (see Figure 11.1). With revolving panel designs data may be collected either retrospectively or prospectively within or across periods such that there is a common subset of individuals that overlap. These designs are applicable for both long-term and short-term studies. Revolving panel designs are useful when the investigator wishes to assess short-term (days, weeks, months) changes in a discrete dependent variable as in a learning experiment where rate of acquisition, generalization, and transfer effects are of interest. By retaining some subjects but not others in each successive panel, the investigator can also test for cohort, age-related task difficulty, and practice effects in explaining patterns of change. For example, repeated assessment on cognitive tasks often facilitates incidental learning, which biases inferences about ability. On the other hand, repeated assessment might be the purpose of the study (e.g., the effect of different lengths of practice on strategy acquisition and use).

Developmental issues that might be addressed by this design include short-term studies of age-dependent transitions from one level of cognitive development to another (preoperational to concrete operational thought), or in isolating the factors and events that immediately precede age-specific manifestations of behavior (e.g., teenage pregnancy, school dropout). Educational applications might concern questions about the developmental readiness of children or the most effective sequences of instruction to enhance long-term memory or promote generalization.

Longitudinal Panel Design

This design samples multiple cohorts at successive ages at the beginning of the study. Unlike repeated cross-sectional designs, data are collected on the same individuals (units) at each period and the same cohorts are retained throughout the study. The major advantage of this design is protection against lost data on populations that are known to have high attrition rates due to uncontrollable factors such as high migration and death rates. Examples might include studies of health and educational services for children in families of migrant workers, the special education needs of children with medically complex conditions, and research on culturally, legally, or personally sensitive topics such as teenage substance abuse and illegal behavior (Elliott, Huizinga, & Menard, 1989).

Virtually all longitudinally relevant questions concerning age, period, and cohort effects, the descriptions of developmental change, and analysis of temporal order can be addressed with the longitudinal panel design. Assuming that individuals in each of the age cohorts are representative of the population of interest and vary in comparable ways other than age, the longitudinal panel design is powerful and protects against attrition by allowing the substitution of comparable data from adjunct cohorts for missing individuals, observations on individuals, and entire panels if necessary.

On the other hand, it requires tight control over cohort membership and periods of observation to have good estimation of age effects for cases that may be substituted. Also, the design requires extensive data collection within multiple panels, which may make it prohibitively expensive compared to alternative designs.

Single- and Multiple-Cohort Treatment/Experimental Designs

Single- and multiple-cohort designs are often used to manipulate subject characteristics (e.g., birth-weight, presence or absence of learning disability) and/or environmental determinants (e.g., SES, home environment) and/or treatment conditions. In such designs, the manipulated variables become between-subject factors in a classical factorial design, and individuals are assessed repeatedly over periods. Figure 11.2 shows a single-cohort randomized (R) treatment design, compared to the classical single-cohort longitudinal design and the multiple-cohort design. The classical design involves no between-Ss analysis, and the latter designs involve partitioning the cohorts, treatment groups, and Cohort × Treatment effects as between-Ss factors, and the age effects as a within-Ss factor with the resulting interactions with cohorts and treatment groups.

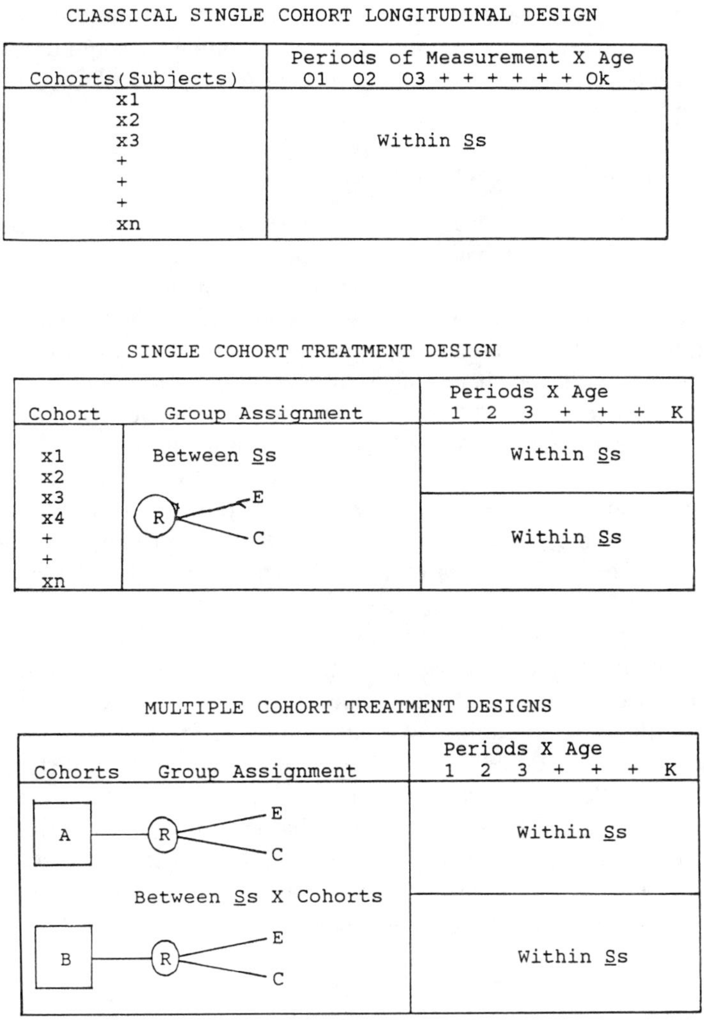

CLASSICAL SINGLE COHORT LONGITUDINAL DESIGN

Cohorts(Subjects)	Periods of Measurement X Age O1 O2 O3 + + + + + + Ok
x1 x2 x3 + + + xn	Within $\underline{S}$s

SINGLE COHORT TREATMENT DESIGN

MULTIPLE COHORT TREATMENT DESIGNS

FIGURE 11.2. Longitudinal treatment/experimental designs.

Thus, the single-cohort design assures the comparability of cohorts with respect to treatment groups and evaluates patterns of change in response to treatment, that is, the extent to which linear, quadratic, and cubic trends in change over periods can be attributed to treatment. Multiple-cohort designs evaluate either the extent to which patterns of change can be attributed to cohorts or treatments, or their interaction. Although these designs address all of the longitudinal research questions addressed by the classical single-cohort design, they can provide a more direct inference of causal relationships among manipulated antecedent factors and resulting changes over time. A good example of a multiple-cohort randomized treatment design is the Carolina Abecedarian Project (Ramey & Campbell, in press).

Cross-Sectional Repeated Measures Designs

In this design, separate age or event cohorts are drawn at the same point in time and then the individuals in each cohort are followed longitudinally with repeated measures. This design provides a between-groups cross-sectional analysis of age differences summed over repeated measures in the same fashion as the classical cross-sectional design without repeated measures. In addition, it permits within-cohorts longitudinal analyses of change; however, while the comparison of change between cohorts can be used to assess replication for different groups, it is not longitudinal because the cohorts differ historically. When age or grade level is varied as cross-sectional cohorts, the prior experience of the cohorts (e.g., second vs. fourth graders) is uncontrolled. Thus, this design is basically a compromise in that it has features of both cross-sectional and longitudinal designs.

This design is useful for studying the sequential acquisition of skills longitudinally within a narrow age range (e.g., 3 to 5 years) compared to the sequence within an adjacent range (5 to 7 years). Also, it is useful in evaluating the durability of treatment effects for children who are identified cross-sectionally at different grade levels (e.g., first, second, and third) and followed with repeated measures over the entire school year. In this regard, it should be noted that the design must include three or more repeated measures to be considered "longitudinal." Only two measures would make it a simple pre-posttest cross-sectional design which assesses change, but not trends in change.

Prospective Case-Control Designs

A major problem with long-term prospective longitudinal studies that attempt to address epidemiological questions about the prevalence, developmental course, and early indicators of risk for various childhood disorders, is that the majority of children in a randomly constituted population sample are not likely to develop the disorder the investigator wants to predict and further study (Bell, 1986; McKinney, 1986; Scott, Shaw, & Urbano, in press). This is the case even with high-incidence conditions such as learning disability, which has a latency of 7–8 years for identification and an estimated prevalence of 2.5–3.5% in samples that are independent of school-referral bias. Thus, an initial randomized population sample of 1,000 children drawn at birth would likely generate a longitudinal research sample of 25 to 30 children with learning disabilities after 7 years of study, not counting attrition.

Unless the study is broadly aimed at predicting school failure per se or a spectrum of related disorders, the cost in relation to the knowledge gained must be justified adequately based on substantial significance for theory, practice, and policy. The prospective case-control approach provides a more economical and robust test of the relationship between early risk factors and later outcomes by using purposive sampling based on the hypothesized link between specific, well-defined antecedents and outcomes, rather than using population samples.

In prospective case-control studies of risk, children who do and do not present the antecedent risk factor(s) are sampled from a representative population and followed until they reach an age where the outcomes typically occur. For example, Carran, Scott, Shaw, and Beydoin (1989) used a historical design to identify three birth cohorts of Very Low Birth-weight (VLBW = less than 1,500 grams), Low Birth-weight (LBW 1,501 to 2,500 g), and Normal Birth-weight (NBW = greater than 2,500 g) from hospital records of live births in 1974–1975 and 1978–1979). Children were then tracked in the local public schools using a surveillance system that tied school records to birth and early childhood records to assess the relative risk of being classified as educationally handicapped due to low birth-weight.

Retrospective case-control studies draw samples defined by outcome, and then search for risk factors retrospectively from available data. The Nichols and Chen (1981) analysis of data from the Collaborative Perinatal Project is an example of this approach. Although it is a "not quite" longitudinal design since data were not collected until outcomes were measured, the analysis was prospective in focus and the control group was sampled from the same birth cohort. This is not the case in most clinical follow-up studies that characterize long-term research on children with learning disabilities. Clinical follow-up studies often have no control group, or one is selected that coincides with the time of outcome rather than the time the target sample was collected. While case-control studies can suffer from attrition and cohort effects that are inexplicable, they are much superior to follow-up studies that are based on samples of convenience and a hypothetical control group.

Longitudinal Data Analysis

As noted early in this chapter, longitudinal research is defined by both the design and the analysis. Since the purpose of this chapter is to discuss methodological issues, I will not dwell on various types of statistical analyses. Menard's recent (1991) book on longitudinal research is an excellent reference that provides many examples of studies that used various strategies. Also, he provides a nice classification scheme for describing alternative techniques for different types of dependent variables that are analyzed as a function of independent variables that are either quantitative/continuous, mixed continuous and categorical, or qualitative/ categorical. This scheme can be used to classify analysis strategies in relation to research questions.

Suffice it to say that most parametric univariate and multivariate analysis strategies that are used with other designs are appropriate for longitudinal designs with the exception that they involve the analysis of repeated measures. Since the conceptualization and measurement of change are complex and often problematic in longitudinal analysis, it is only this aspect of the analysis that requires considerable additional expertise and experience on the part of the investigator.

The significance of problems with repeated measures analysis were called to attention in the classic article by Cronbach and Furby (1970) entitled "How should we measure change—or should we?" Since then, the problems in conceptualizing and measuring change have been the subject of serious methodological study and debate in and of themselves. Significant strides have been made in the development of statistical techniques that correct or obviate for violations of assumptions about the homogeneity of covariances among repeated measurements (McCall & Appelbaum, 1973) with ANOVA, the unreliability of raw change scores (Chronback & Furby, 1970), and multicollinearity (Overall & Klett, 1972) with regression analysis.

In addition to parametric analyses, Menard (1991) provides an overview and additional references on problems in nonparametric analyses for categorical data. Also, he describes a number of techniques that are not commonly used in special education concerning the analysis of trends, transitions from one state or period to the next, and model testing. Among these are time-series analysis, latent variable structural equations models or path analysis, regression with dummy variables, log-linear analysis, logit/probit analysis, and hazard/survival/event history analysis. Examples of studies with children with learning disabilities that use probit and latent variable structural equations are McKinney and Speece (1983) and Sawyer (1992).

Problems in Longitudinal Data Analysis

Most of the problems that are presented in longitudinal research concerning data quality and internal validity are the same as those that affect cross-sectional research. There are no fundamental differences in the procedures used to enhance precision and reliability of measurement. However, since longitudinal studies collect data repeatedly on the same subjects and also differ in scope and breadth from most cross-sectional studies, common problems tend to be exacerbated. Also, some problems that can be attributed to repeated assessment are particular to longitudinal research.

Subject Attrition

Attrition is the bane of most longitudinal studies and is particularly damaging to long-term studies that use total-population and single-cohort designs. Attrition rates in larger national studies have varied from lows of 5% to highs of 75–80% (Menard, 1991). The Kauai longitudinal study retained 88% of the subjects over 18 years (Werner & Smith, 1982), whereas the Carolina Longitudinal Learning Disabilities Project retained only 68% over 5 years. Sources of attrition also vary across studies, but include failure to obtain permission in successive years, family mobility, illness and mortality. Also, the nature of the research questions and particular outcomes may result in attrition. For example, it may be difficult to retain individuals who use illicit drugs or engage in criminal acts.

In reporting longitudinal research, it is important to perform analyses to determine whether attrition was systematic or random, and to assess the effect on relevant variables. For example, differences in sociodemographic characteristics between those subjects who were lost and those who remain should be assessed and reported. Similarly, differences in initial levels of response on dependent variables and the strength or structure of correlations among proposed predictor variables can be assessed with conventional statistics.

Generally, studies of attrition show a high negative association between attrition rate and investigators' efforts to maintain frequent and systematic contact with subjects. Strategies for doing so have been described in some detail by Burgess (1989) and Ellickson, Bianca, and Schoeff (1988). Large-scale projects with adequate funding often employ staff whose major responsibilities are to maintain contact with subjects, schedule data collection sessions, and follow-up on missed contacts and observations. Finally, it is helpful if data collection and follow-up are combined with services and other incentives, such as free consultation for parents, social services assistance or transportation for after-school meetings and project activities. However, incentives can also create other problems because they increase research costs and can present ethical issues concerning the use of incentives in exchange for participation.

Missing Data

The problem of missing data is related to the problem of subject attrition. The failure to collect a single observation on a given occasion may be minor if the observation can be collected within the overall period or be estimated statistically. On the other hand, large numbers of missing observations on a given subject may lead to the exclusion of the subject and thereby contribute to overall attrition. Additionally, missing data reduce the power of the analysis by reducing the number of degrees of freedom for the analysis by the number of subjects lost. If the number of missing observations is many and randomly dispersed across subjects or variables, this would result in substantial variation in the power of tests on one variable compared to another. In the case of MANOVA analysis, an entire set of variables could be lost if missing data were distributed randomly across many subjects.

Accordingly, this problem is more serious in longitudinal analyses than cross-sectional analyses because, while standard between-subjects ANOVA in cross-sectional results is robust against nonorthogonality (Appelbaum & Cramer, 1974), this is not the case with repeated measures analysis, which depends on complete data for every subject on each variable in the within-subject analysis.

In general, the remedies for missing data are the same as those for subject attrition, except that the periodic schedule for data collection must include time for follow-up contacts and extra days for data collection. Otherwise, the expense, time, and effort devoted to prior data collection on lost subjects may be wasted.

Sample Size

Longitudinal studies are frequently criticized because they end up with smaller than desirable samples. Thus, standard multivariate techniques such as MANOVA, multiple regression, and factor analysis are often not feasible because of limited subject-to-variable ratio. Most often, the problem is due to either attrition, poor planning, or both. The former is often unavoidable, but can be prevented with adequate effort and resources; however, the latter reflects a failure to appreciate the problems involved in longitudinal research, or at least undue optimism.

In planning for adequate sample size, prior knowledge of the sociodemographic characteristics of the community are essential, as well as knowledge about the stability and school feeder patterns of the local schools. (For instance, school systems that serve large military bases are not good candidates for longitudinal research). In planning the study, a good strategy is to calculate the minimum sample size that would provide sufficient power for the analyses that are planned at the anticipated endpoint of the study, along with the anticipated subject/variable ratio for any planned multivariate analyses that would be performed. Given the desired sample size, it is then necessary to assume a base yearly attrition rate that would be tolerable to the investigator given the cost of data collection and the availability of resources needed to protect against avoidable losses. These estimates are of course very dependent on the investigator's experience and knowledge of the research problem and the population of interest. The strategy is then one of over-sampling the population initially to account for anticipated attrition. This process is analogous to the way insurance companies set premiums based on risk of mortality.

Another strategy is to select a design that is more appropriate for research on subjects and topics that are known to produce high attrition rates due to unavoidable but anticipated causes (e.g., risk of mortality). For example, longitudinal panel and revolving panel designs have distinct advantages because different subjects are studied for briefer periods of time, and subjects in succeeding cohorts can be substituted for lost cases. However, these designs can introduce other serious problems such as unanticipated cohort effects, which complicate the generalization of findings and disallow the aggregation of data across cohorts for similar periods of observation.

Problem of Too Many Variables

Multivariate longitudinal data can either provide a rare opportunity to advance knowledge or entrap the investigator in a morass of information. The difference between these two fates rests with the development of efficient data management and data reduction procedures as part of the study design. Presumably, a conceptual framework would have been devised to provide a rationale for the selection of the variables of interest based on theory and practical issues which specify the major domains and constructs to be measured. This framework then provides a way of systematically reducing the number of variables to avoid the next problem. The solution to both problems rests with an a priori conceptual framework and an implementation plan for systematic data reduction.

Problem of Too Many Analyses

This problem is a related consequence of the problem of too many variables: the more variables, the more potential analyses. As the number of analyses increases, the probability of a Type I error increases for the variable set as a whole due to multiple collinearity (most measures cannot be assumed to be independent of one another). Collinearity is a greater threat in longitudinal analyses because the same variables are analyzed over time, and the variables are interrelated. In order to deal with both problems (too many variables and too many analyses), a systematic data reduction strategy should be considered as part of the study design.

Preliminary checks can be made on the distributional qualities of variables as well as their covariance structure. Univariate analysis of the distributions of the sample often identify variables with restricted variances and/or poor reliability that can be eliminated as poor measures. Also, the intercorrelation matrices can be examined to determine whether factor analysis might reduce the larger variable set to a more manageable smaller set that reflects the major constructs of interest.

The solution to this problem is critical to achieving a favorable subject-to-variable ratio for multivariate analyses, which are preferable to uni-variate analyses because of the need to protect against inflated alpha level, which occurs across a series of univariate tests (McCall & Appelbaum, 1973). In some cases, principal components analysis can be used to aggregate distinct but correlated variables (e.g., task-oriented behavior, verbal intelligence, and independent classroom behavior) with factor scores (e.g., academic competence vs. social competence). Change can then be measured for an entire domain of discrete variables assessed by their principal component which reflects the underlying construct developmentally. Alternatively, MANOVA can be performed on a smaller subset of discrete variables that are the best measures of distinct constructs as determined by prior factor analysis.

Standardization and Changes in Measurement

Consistency of measurement is particularly problematic for long-term longitudinal research (Bell, 1986). One common problem in developmental research is that the age-appropriate items in tests are not the same across successive periods of growth. A classical example can be found in studies that attempt to assess change in ability level and achievement. A study evaluating intraindividual trends in intellectual growth might begin with Bailey scales during infancy, shift to the Stanford-Binet at 24 months, give a Wechsler Preschool and Primary Scale of Intelligence (WPPSI) at 60 months, and then give the Wechsler Intelligence Scale for Children-Revised (WISC-R) through 96 months. In such cases, it may be difficult to parse out test effects from growth trends because available measures do not permit counterbalancing (which might actually be worse). Also, the nature of the construct is changing (e.g., from perceptual motor to verbal) as weell as the covariance structure of the test items from one point in time to the next (see Ramey & Campbell, in press).

In such cases, standard scores based on the test norms may not be helpful because they are relative to different population samples that vary in composition and representativeness. One solution is to use principal components analysis to identify the factor that represents the greatest amount of common variance among the items which can be assumed to the best estimates of the contruct (e.g., general intelligence) for the research sample as a whole. A given individual's factor score could vary over time relative to the sample mean at each period of observation, thereby allowing the investigator to assess increasing or decreasing trends over time for individuals or subgroups of individuals in the sample (see McCall et al., 1973). Finally, it is important to note that in special education we are often attempting to measure behavior and performance at the extremes of the normal distribution, wherein lies the maximum error of measurement. Accordingly, some thought should be given to the selection of variables.

Repeated Measures Effects

Another common problem in longitudinal research is age-related basal and/or ceiling effects which come about when (a) measures are not sufficiently sensitive to age-related variation in difficulty level, and (b) the repeated measures' effects are confounded with practice (also referred to as "panel conditioning"). Of course, how children learn and develop strategies from experience could be the purpose of the study. Nevertheless, rate of learning as the result of experience or intervention can be confounded by repeated assessment on the same tasks.

The basic problem is that as children in the sample learn, the sample becomes more homogeneous with respect to individual differences in performance, which violates the homogeneity of variance assumption such that change in variance is correlated with change in the means (the former decreases while the latter increases). Standard univariate repeated measures ANOVA produces artificially high F values under these conditions; however, repeated measures MANOVA as described by McCall and Appelbaum (1973) corrects for this problem.

In addition to counterbalancing (which is not always possible) and using repeated measures control groups, it is advisable to conduct cross-sectional pilot studies to determine the age range for the proposed tasks when they have not been well-established by previous studies on the same population. When the research question pertains to the transition from one period of development to another, a revolving panel design might be more efficient for studying short-term change because it can be used to assess bias in developmental trends due to repeated measurement (Menard, 1991).

Factors that Impede Longitudinal Research

Longitudinal research is expensive, cumbersome in many ways, and not always responsive to larger changes in the state-of-the-art in science and major funding priorities nationally. A number of factors can be identified that influence both the feasibility and impact of longitudinal research.

Cost of Longitudinal Research

Some have argued that longitudinal research is not cost-effective in relation to the knowledge gained and that it ties up scarce resources over an extended period of time that could be redirected to more pressing research priorities at the moment. On the other hand, the costs of a six-panel longitudinal study are probably the same as those for a similar number of cross-sectional multiple-year studies (Wall & Williams, 1970). The issue in some of these arguments is not so much cost per se as it is waste and disappointing findings.

Many of the earlier longitudinal studies were essentially descriptive in purpose and lacked theoretically based hypotheses. Massive data banks were developed that suffered from many of the problems described above and perhaps benign neglect. Some studies did not have the anticipated impact and left the "so what?" question unanswered. For example, many of the prospective follow-up studies on learning disabilities have focused solely on the correlation between early risk factors and later outcome and were not longitudinal in scope. The significant practical and theoretical impact of longitudinal research for education rests in explaining the pathways from one point in development to a given outcome. Accordingly, like all types of research, the rationale for longitudinal studies must be compelling to justify the cost regardless of its relation to the cost incurred by cross-sectional or any other approach. Viewed this way, the issue is really the justification of the research question.

It is the case that for some research questions, longitudinal designs are the only acceptable options. If the research questions pertain to historical or developmental change over time, a prospective longitudinal design is the only design. Cross-sectional designs cannot separate age, period, and cohort effects, and are almost always left with competing hypotheses that explain the age effects and changes that are inferred. Hypotheses derived from theory about causal relationships are best tested by experimental designs, and experimental designs that are also prospective longitudinal designs are the only designs for testing true temporal causality because they assess antecedent events and conditions directly (Menard, 1991).

Therefore, when these conditions are met with respect to the compelling questions addressed only by longitudinal designs, as well as other conditions pertaining to the scientific and practical merit of the research itself, the cost of longitudinal research can be justified, given the importance and potential benefits of the knowledge gained.

At the same time, the cost of long-term prospective studies will continue to be debated for other reasons. Since special education is still a relatively young and evolving field, there is an inherent conflict between short-term, highly applied research and development aimed at improving current school practices, and long-term programmatic research aimed at producing basic knowledge and theory about faulty development. Thus, we frequently choose to accept the bird in the hand while we yearn for the two in the bush.

Consistency of Funding

The problem of obtaining and maintaining continued funding for longitudinal research is related to the debate about cost and impact, but is more clearly due to the fluctuating nature of research priorities. Research priorities change predictably with the political agendas of the Congress and federal administration. Private support varies with the specific interests and support strategies of individual donors. The states generally assume the role of providing funds for program implementation and leave research to the universities and the federal government.

Although support for research on 3- to 5-year timelines is generally available through most federal grant competitions, it is difficult for an agency to tie up funds for longer periods of time and still have funds to address new initiatives. Also, the politics of science is that there are always more deserving proposals than can be funded, and investigators who seek funding for individual research projects often cry foul play when agencies tie up disproportionately large resources in long-term research and/or shift resources to respond to politically based initiatives, or when the lion's share goes to large research centers in the most prominent research universities.

In any event, an investigator's choice of whether to pursue a longitudinal versus a cross-sectional research strategy is influenced by the availability of sufficient resources and the major priorities of the time. A reasonable compromise of some investigators who wish to do longitudinal studies is to propose repeated measures, cross-sectional, or revolving panel designs to study three to four periods of development, or to study short-term treatment effects. Even so, 5 years of support would usually be necessary to complete the data collection for three yearly panels of observations for most developmental studies.

Changes in the State-of-the-Art of the Field

The twentieth century has been marked by an explosion of knowledge and advances in the technology that serves science in most disciplines. New knowledge in a rapidly growing field such as special education changes the way research problems are conceptualized and the way basic constructs are operationalized. Theories and models are revised or discarded, new and better measures are developed, new statistical and computerized procedures become available. Long-term longitudinal studies are cumbersome in that it is difficult and in some cases impossible to modify variables and data collection methods to accommodate such changes in the field. Any design modification that alters the standardization of data collection, the nature of the sample in new cohorts, or the comparability of measures across periods affects cost, and may compromise data analysis.

Also, changes in the state-of-the-art may lessen the importance of long-term studies that cannot adapt or respond to contemporary knowledge. For these reasons, it is often difficult to use extant longitudinal data bases to address contemporary research questions. For example, the generality of older longitudinal studies on learning disabilities that used school-defined samples can be questioned if the data are not available to classify subjects by contemporary criteria. On the other hand, extant data bases are often extremely valuable for methodological purposes and model testing. Examples of advances produced from extant data bases are those of McCall, Appelbaum, & Hogarty (1973) who provided an innovative way to analyze longitudinal trends and Menard and Elliott's (1990) causal model analysis of drug use and illegal behavior using the National Youth Survey data.

Investigator Attrition

Longitudinal research is difficult to move. While investigators may move to other universities, research samples do not. Research and support staff stability is essential to longitudinal research, but is often overlooked when longitudinal research is proposed. Conducting longitudinal research can be particularly problematic for young investigators who have a set timeline for demonstrating the research productivity required for tenure. On the other hand, young investigators often benefit substantially if they are associated with a collaborative ongoing project.

At the same time, senior investigators are often sought by other universities because they have established the scientific credibility necessary to obtain funds for large programmatic research. In any event, the career choices of investigators may make or break a longitudinal study and will certainly influence the nature and impact of its contributions. Also, career plans and choices frequently influence the decision to pursue longitudinal versus other design options.

Institutional Capability

Universities and other research institutions must often commit resources in the form of support personnel and facilities that exceed the direct and indirect costs covered by grants that only support research activity. For example, it is difficult to provide a controlled environment for conducting longitudinal intervention research on handicapped preschool children unless the university has appropriate facilities, is willing to provide and/or renovate existing facilities, and to commit facilities for that purpose. The same is true of public and private schools that might be asked to support such research.

In the same vein personnel policies might not be amenable to the hiring of permanent support staff who do not fit existing categories or who fall outside the primary mission of the university (e.g., certified early childhood special educators, medical technicians, teacher aides). Similarly, there may be problems recruiting and maintaining doctoral level research associates who have no faculty status, no graduate teaching responsibilities and who are not eligible for tenure.

For all of these reasons, institutional capability is a necessary condition for larger long-term longitudinal projects. Beyond scientific merit, institutional capability is perhaps the most important factor in successful funding. Accordingly, not all universities are suited or competitive for some longitudinal projects.

Conclusion

In sum, I have attempted to make a case for longitudinal research as an under-used but powerful tool for advancing knowledge about the nature and development of learning disabilities. Longitudinal research is elegant and uniquely equipped to answer many of the most fundamental questions that remain concerning the phenomenon of learning disabilities and also holds great promise for the improvement of prevention and intervention practices. It could alter the course of the field. A classical example was the role played by longitudinal research in establishing the efficacy of early childhood intervention and its impact on policy and special education with the implementation of P.L. 99-457. Such are the promises.

At the same time I have also attempted to point out the major problems and limitations of this approach. Longitudinal research should be viewed as but one of many designs that are available to the scientist. The questions in design choice are straightforward: Does the design answer the questions that are asked? Can the research be defended on the grounds of scientific and practical merit? Is it feasible and cost-effective, given what it is intended to accomplish? Longitudinal research is not the panacea for all the ills of the field (and perhaps not the majority), but the fact is that it is the only approach that can address some of our most important and vexing questions.

References

Appelbaum, M.I. & Cramer, E.M. (1974). Some problems in the nonorthogonal analysis of variance. *Psychological Bulletin, 1*, 272–274.

Baltes, P.B. & Nesselroade, J.R. (1979). *Longitudinal research in the study of behavior and human development.* New York: Academic Press.

Bell, R.A. (1986). Age-specific manifestations in changing psychosocial risk. In D.C. Farran & J.D. McKinney (Eds.), *Risk in intellectual and psychosocial development* (pp. 168–182). Orlando, FL: Academic Press.

Burgess, R.D. (1989). Major issues and implications of tracing survey respondents. In D. Kasprzyk, G. Duncan, G. Kalton, & M.P. Singh (Eds.), *Panel surveys.* New York: Wiley.

Carran, D.T., Scott, K.G., Shaw, K., & Beydouin, S. (1989). The relative risk of educational handicaps in two birth cohorts of normal and low birthweight disadvantaged children. *Topics in Early Childhood Special Education, 9*, 14–31.

Cronbach, L.J. & Furby, L. (1970). How should we measure change—or should we? *Psychological Bulletin, 74*, 68–80.

Ellickson, P.L., Bianca, D., & Schoeff, D.C. (1988). Containing attrition in school-based research: An innovative approach. *Evaluation Review, 12*(4), 331–351.

Elliott, D.S., Huizinga, D., & Menard, S. (1989). *Multiple problem youth: Delinquency, substance use, and mental health problems.* New York: Springer-Verlag.

Feagans, L. & Appelbaum, M.I. (1986). Language subtypes and their validation in learning disabled children. *Journal of Educational Psychology, 78*(5), 373–481.

Gallagher, J.J., Ramey, C.T., Haskins, R., & Finkelstein, N.W. (1976). Use of longitudinal research in the study of child development. In T.D. Tjossem (Ed.), *Intervention strategies for high risk infants and young children* (pp. 161–186). Baltimore: University Park Press.

Horn, W.F., O'Donnell, J.P., & Vitulano, L.A. (1983). Long-term follow-up studies of learning disabled persons. *Journal of Learning Disabilities, 16*, 542–555.

Infant Health and Development Program (IHDP). (1990). Enhancing the outcomes of low-birth-weight, premature infants. *Journal of the American Medical Association, 263*(22), 3035–3042.

Kavale, K.A. (1988). The long term consequences of learning disabilities. In M.C. Wang, M.C. Reynolds, & H.J. Walberg (Eds.), *Handbook of special education* (Vol. 2, pp. 303–344). Oxford, England: Pergamon Press.

Keogh, B.K. (1988). Learning disability: Diversity in search of order. In M.C. Wang, M.C. Reynolds, & H.J. Walberg (Eds.), *Handbook of special education* (Vol. 2, pp. 225–252). Oxford, England: Pergamon Press.

Keogh, B.K. (in press). Risk and protective factors in longitudinal studies of risk. *Learning Disabilities Research and Practice.*

Lazar, I., Darlington, R., Murray, H., Royce, J., & Snipper, A. (1982). Lasting effects of early education: A report from the Consortium for Longitudinal Studies. *Monographs of the Society for Research in Child Development, 47*(2-3, Serial No. 195).

McCall, R.B. & Appelbaum, M.I. (1973). Bias in the analysis of repeated measures designs: Some alternative approaches. *Child Development, 44*, 401–415.

McCall, R.B., Appelbaum, M.I., & Hogarty, P.S. (1973). Developmental changes in mental performance. *Monographs of the Society for Research in Child Development, 38*(3, Serial No. 150).

Menard, S. (1991). *Longitudinal research* (Series No. 07-075). Newberry Park, CA: Sage.

Menard, S. & Elliott, D.S. (1990). Longitudinal and cross-sectional data collection and analysis in the study of crime and delinquency. *Justice Quarterly, 1*, 11–85.

McKinney, J.D. (1986). Reflections on the concept of risk for developmental retardation. In D.C. Farran & J.D. McKinney (Eds.), *Risk in intellectual and psychosocial development* (pp. 121–124). Orlando, FL: Academic Press.

McKinney, J.D. (1988). Research on conceptually and empirically derived subtypes of specific learning disabilities. In M.C. Wang, M.C. Reynolds, & H.J. Walberg (Eds.), *Handbook of special education* (Vol. 2, pp. 253–281). Oxford, England: Pergamon Press.

McKinney, J.D. (1989). Longitudinal research in the behavioral characteristics of children with learning disabilities. *Journal of Learning Disabilities*, *22*(3), 141–150.

McKinney, J.D. (in press). Academic and behavioral consequences of learning disabilities: Longitudinal follow-up at eleven years of age. *Learning Disabilities Research and Practice*.

McKinney, J.D. & Feagans, L. (1984). Academic and behavioral characteristics: Longitudinal studies of learning disabled children and average achievers. *Learning Disability Quarterly*, *5*, 45–52.

McKinney, J.D., Short, E.J., & Feagans, L. (1985). Academic consequences of perceptual-linguistic subtypes of learning disabled children. *Learning Disabilities Research*, *1*(1), 6–17.

McKinney, J.D. & Speece, D.L. (1983). Classroom behavior and the academic progress of learning disabled students. *Journal of Applied Developmental Psychology*, *4*, 149–161.

McKinney, J.D. & Speece, D.L. (1986). Academic consequences and longitudinal stability of behavioral subtypes of learning disabled children. *Journal of Educational Psychology*, *78*(5), 365–372.

Nichols, P.J. & Chen, T.C. (1981). *Minimal brain dysfunction: A prospective study*. Hillside, NJ: Erlbaum.

Osborne, S.S., Schulte, A.C., & McKinney, J.D. (1991). A longitudinal study of students with learning disabilities in mainstream and resource programs. *Exceptionality*, *2*, 81–95.

Overall, J.E. & Klett, C.J. (1972). *Applied multivariate analysis*. New York: McGraw-Hill.

Ramey, C.T. & Campbell, F.A. (1991). Poverty, early childhood education and academic competence: The Abecedarian experiment. In A. Huston (Ed.), *Children in poverty: Child Development and Public Policy* (pp. 190–221). New York: Cambridge University Press.

Ramey, C.T., Yeates, K.O., & Short, E.J. (1984). The plasticity of intellectual development: Insights from preventive intervention. *Child Development*, *55*, 1913–1975.

Sameroff, A. & Chandler, M.J. (1975). Reproductive risk and the continuum of caretaking casualty. In F.D. Horowitz, M. Hetherington, S. Scarr-Salapatek, & G. Siegel (Eds.), *Review of child development research* (Vol. 4, pp. 187–244). Chicago: University of Chicago Press.

Sawyer, D.J. (1992). Language abilities, reading acquisition, and developmental dyslexia: A discussion of the hypothetical and observed relationships. *Journal of Learning Disabilities*, *25*(2), 82–95.

Scott, K.G., Shaw, K.H., & Urbano, J.C. (in press). Developmental epidemiology. In S.L. Friedman & H.C. Haywood (Eds.), *Developmental follow-up: Concepts, genres, domains, and methods*. Academic Press.

Speece, D.L. & McKinney, J.D. (1986). Longitudinal development of conservation skills in learning disabled children. *Journal of Learning Disabilities*, *19*(5), 302–307.

Stanovich, K.E. (1986). Matthew effects in reading: Some consequences of individual differences in the acquisition of literacy. *Reading Research Quarterly*, *21*, 360–406.

Wall, W.D. & Willams, H.L. (1970). Longitudinal studies and the social sciences. London: Heinemann.

Werner, E.E. (1986). A longitudinal study of perinatal risk. In D.C. Farran & J.D. McKinney (Eds.), *Risk in intellectual and psychosocial Development* (pp. 3–26). Orlando, FL: Academic Press.

Werner, E.E. & Smith, R.S. (1982). *Vulnerable but invincible: A longitudinal study of resilient children and youth.* New York: McGraw-Hill.

Yeates, K.O., MacPhee, D., Campbell, F.A., & Ramey, C.T. (1983). Maternal IQ and home environment as determinants of early childhood intellectual competence: A developmental analysis. *Developmental Psychology, 19*(5), 731–739.

Part V
Assessment and Instrumentation

12
Academic Assessment and Instrumentation

LYNN S. FUCHS AND DOUGLAS FUCHS

Because learning is one of the major goals of education, we frequently find measures of amount learned, or achievement, used in educational research (Borg & Gall, 1989). When research addresses the problems of individuals with learning disabilities, for whom poor achievement in relation to intellectual potential represents the key identifying variable, we certainly expect to find research focusing on achievement and investigating ways to effect better achievement outcomes. In fact, among primary, data-based studies published over the past 3 to 5 years in three major research journals dedicated to learning disabilities, that is, *Learning Disabilities: Research and Practice* (formerly *Learning Disabilities Research*), *Learning Disability Quarterly*, and the *Journal of Learning Disabilities*, approximately 60% (as an average across the three journals) incorporated academic achievement among the variables investigated (this does not include studies that used academic measures only for demographics). Approximately 25% of the primary, data-based studies investigated strategies to effect better academic growth.

In discussions of how to select measures of academic achievement, writers frequently suggest that researchers consider the following issues: (a) the measure's traditional psychometric reliability and validity, (b) administration time, (c) test difficulty (i.e., avoiding test ceilings indicating the test is too easy for many pupils and test floors indicating the test is too difficult for many pupils), and (d) the relationship of the test to the school district's testing program.

In this chapter, however, we have opted to avoid these typically covered, albeit important, topics. Instead, we have focused our discussion on three critical, but frequently overlooked, considerations in selecting academic achievement measures in research on students with learning disabilities. In this paper, we focus on the following three interrelated topics, which are particularly relevant for intervention research focusing on ways to engineer enhanced achievement outcomes:

- the relationship of the measure to the treatment incorporated within the study;

233

- the distinction between content coverage and content mastery in indexing student learning; and
- the importance of the scoring unit in enhancing sensitivity of the measurement to student growth.

In the discussion that follows, we treat each consideration separately. First, we explain the relevant issue, and then we provide examples from our own research to illustrate and highlight the importance of each issue.

The Relationship of the Measure to the Nature of the Treatment

Explanation of the Issue

In designing a study that assesses the effects of an intervention on student achievement, a key consideration is how different measures correspond to the substance of the treatment. Even within a seemingly focused content area, testing procedures for alternative measures can vary in dramatic and critical ways in terms of the types of behaviors sampled. For example, a test of "reading comprehension" may require students to (a) read a sentence, paragraph, or story silently or orally and write or say answers to multiple-choice, short-answer, or essay questions; (b) orally or silently read sentences or passages that contain blanks and restore those blanks with semantically correct words either orally or in writing; or (c) read paragraphs or stories and write or tell summaries of the content read. Although each type of measure taps some dimension of reading comprehension, it should be clear that the testing requirements differ dramatically, and student performance may vary accordingly.

The first challenge to the researcher is to select, from available achievement tests, those measures that are well aligned with the substance of the intervention and that will be sensitive to, or register, treatment effects if and when they occur. The second—and often competing—challenge, however, is for the researcher to select measures sufficiently broad and robust to (a) avoid criticism of "teaching to the test" through the specific intervention and (b) demonstrate that generalizable skills have been successfully taught through the treatment.

Sometimes, selecting a series of measures requiring increasingly closer approximations to the treatment content can represent a satisfactory solution. By doing so, the researcher can simultaneously increase the power of the study to detect treatment effects using measures that incorporate behaviors closely aligned to the treatment dimensions. Yet, at the same time, the researcher can evaluate the robustness and generalizability of treatment effects using measures that are increasingly distal from the specific dimensions of the treatment.

Example Highlighting the Importance of the Issue

A study by Fuchs, Fuchs, and Hamlett (1989c) illustrates this problem and the proposed potential solution. This study investigated the effects of two teacher feedback systems when monitoring reading growth using student recalls. Participants were 22 special education teachers and 44 students, 78% of whom had been classified as learning disabled according to state regulations that comply with P.L. 94-142. All 44 pupils were assessed twice each week with a reading retell procedure: The pupils had 3 minutes to read silently a different passage during each assessment. Then, they had 4 minutes to write a summary of what they had read. These assessments were administered and scored by computer.

Teachers were assigned randomly to two feedback conditions, both of which were mediated by computer. In one condition (i.e., the quantitative-plus-qualitative-feedback condition), teachers saw the student's retell score in terms of how many "matched" (i.e., content) words the student had written in the retell. Additionally, teachers in this condition were prompted by computer to study samples of the student's retells, in light of the corresponding text the students had read, and to provide the computer information about the extent to which the student had included different story grammar components in the retell. Based on the information the teacher provided, the computer recommended a story retell instructional activity focusing on one of the student's missing components. In the second teacher feedback condition (i.e., the quantitative-feedback-only condition), teachers saw only the student's matched words score, and they made decisions about how to develop the student's instructional program without any advice or additional structure.

Most relevant to the current discussion are the types of measures included in this study. We were, of course, interested in how the two types of teacher feedback would determine the teachers' instructional programming decisions and how the achievement of the students, in turn, would be affected. As might be expected, teachers who received quantitative plus qualitative feedback identified greater numbers of story grammar elements for instruction than teachers who received only the quantitative feedback.

What is more interesting, however, is the pattern of achievement. We employed the reading comprehension subtest of the Stanford Achievement Test (SAT; Gardner, Rudman, Karlsen, & Merwin, 1982) and the Comprehensive Reading Assessment Battery (CRAB), a measure based on the work of Brown and Smiley (1977) and Jenkins, Heliotis, Haynes, and Beck (1986). The SAT requires pupils to read short passages and answer multiple-choice questions about the content they have read. The CRAB relies on four 400-word traditional folktales which serve as stimuli for all tasks; passages are counterbalanced across tasks, pre- and post-testing, and treatment conditions. The CRAB measures student reading proficiency in multiple ways: oral reading fluency, question answering, and written retelling with two types of scoring (total words written and matched words written). Consequently, in this study, we indexed reading achievement in a variety of ways, which could be ordered in terms of their proximity to or alignment with the study intervention.

Across these measures, effects became stronger as the indices became more closely related to the nature of the treatment. For the measure least related to the ongoing student assessment and to the teachers' instructional programming (i.e., the CRAB oral reading fluency measure, which requires students to read aloud), essentially no difference between treatment groups was identified. For the SAT, which requires students to read passages and respond to multiple-choice questions, the effect size was a moderate .37, favoring the students whose teachers received both qualitative and quantitative feedback and who incorporated more story grammar comprehension-related instruction. For the total-words-written score on the CRAB retell task, the effect size was .53; for the measure most directly related to the nature of the study's treatment (i.e., the matched-words score of the CRAB retell measure), the effect size was .67. Both effect sizes again favored students whose teachers received the quantitative and qualitative feedback and who provided more retell-related instruction. In addition, significance levels associated with the effects for the various measures decreased as the measure increasingly resembled the study treatment. Importantly, only the GRAB matched-words retell score, the measure most aligned to the study intervention, actually achieved significance.

Consequently, the pattern of results was similar for three of four outcomes: the SAT, the CRAB total-words score on the retell, and the CRAB matched-words score on the retell. Yet, the size of group differences was related to the degree of similarity of the outcome measure to the treatment embedded in the study: Larger effects were associated with more direct measures, and if any of the more distant measures had been selected as the sole measure of student achievement, the study would have produced only null effects. With the one statistically significant finding, however, the effect sizes for all four measures are more interpretable, interesting, and convincing.

This pattern of findings recurs in the measurement and intervention literatures (e.g., Fuchs, Fuchs, & Hamlett, 1989b; Leinhardt, Zigmond, & Cooley, 1981). The related problem in selecting achievement measures for intervention research with students labeled as learning disabled should be considered carefully in terms of the power of an intervention study to detect treatment effects, on the one hand, and to assess the generalizability and importance of the treatment provided, on the other hand.

The Distinction between Content Coverage and Content Mastery

Explanation of the Issue

A related issue concerns the tension between describing content mastery and studying content coverage. *Content mastery* refers to a high level of accuracy and fluency with a relatively circumscribed set of material, which has been taught in a relatively intense manner. *Content coverage* refers to student proficiency with a broader set of information, which has been presented in classroom instruction, but not necessarily taught as thoroughly.

Some have proposed (for example, see Slavin, 1987) that, although some interventions may improve student mastery of the skills specified within the treatment, they actually may *reduce* the extent to which teachers allocate instructional time to a broader curricular scope. Within such a framework, the hypothesis favors an experimental group on achievement tests that tap content mastery measures of the skills addressed within the intervention. The hypothesis, however, simultaneously predicts that the *control* group will exceed the experimental group on broader measures of achievement, because teachers in the control group have covered more material—as a function of *not* having participated in the treatment.

In designing studies addressing the efficacy of interventions for students with learning disabilities, researchers should be sensitive to this issue. Treatments designed specifically for students with learning disabilities frequently are highly structured, with the content controlled tightly. The hypothesis certainly seems plausible that whereas experimental students may outperform controls on material addressed during the treatment, they also may perform reliably lower than control students on broader measures, because the control teachers have covered more material in their instruction. To address this possibility, researchers may incorporate a series of tests that can be conceptualized as content mastery versus content coverage measures.

Example Highlighting the Importance of the Issue

Research examples highlighing this principle are readily available. We describe a study on Curriculum-based Measurement (CBM) conducted in the area of mathematics operations (Fuchs, Fuchs, & Hamlett, 1989a) to illustrate the point. Participants were 30 special educators, along with 60 students with mild handicaps, 77% of whom had been labeled learning disabled according to state regulations that comply with P.L. 94-142.

Teachers were assigned randomly to three treatments. In the first condition, "dynamic goal CBM," teachers monitored student progress toward mathematics operations goals with a prescribed CBM system that required them to raise individual student goals whenever student performance indicated that students might surpass stated goals. In a second condition, "static goal CBM," teachers monitored student progress with the same CBM system; they were not, however, required by the system to raise goals. The third condition was a control group; these teachers monitored student progress using conventional special education monitoring methods. Teachers implemented treatments for 15 weeks.

Two types of math achievement tests were employed. The Math Computation Test (MCT) served as the *content mastery measure*. The MCT samples problems across grades 1–6 from the mathematics operations objectives of the Tennessee state curriculum. This curriculum encompasses a statewide set of competencies that are expected for promotion across grades and assessed annually in a statewide criterion-referenced testing program. Pupils are provided directions in standard format and have 10 minutes to complete 36 problems (or 78 digits). Performance is scored in terms of number of correct digits written in answers. Digits allow credit for partially correct problems and, as an index of achievement, appear to be more sensitive to student growth than correct problems (see related discussion below).

This measure was deemed useful and appropriate as an index of content mastery for the following reasons. Because it was derived from a statewide curriculum, equally applicable to the experimental and control groups, it should have assessed achievement on curriculum targeted for *all* groups, including experimental and control students (see Slavin, 1987 for related discussion). Moreover, the MCT represents more than a simple index of mastery of each individual's CBM curriculum. It encompassess the entire grade 1–6 mathematics operations curriculum—and, as such, represents a typical framework for a global achievement test. We could have selected a more narrow outcome measure, which would have focused *only* on the curriculum actually taught to each student—as reflected by the content incorporated within each student's CBM. However, such a narrow testing framework, which would have differed for students at different grade levels, would have been unusual as an achievement outcome measure for a treatment study. Consequently, our "content mastery" measure was relatively broad.

The Concepts of Number (CN) subtest of the Stanford Achievement Test (Gardner, Rudman, Karlsen, & Merwin, 1982) was our *measure of content coverage*. On the CN, pupils respond to multiple-choice questions concerning number concepts by marking their selected answers. As an index of content coverage, the CN assessed the extent to which teachers had covered materials beyond the scope of the CBM mathematics operations curriculum.

The MCT was administered in small groups before and after the 15-week intervention; the CN also was administered in small groups, but only after the completion of the study. Multivariate analysis of covariance was employed, using the MCT and CN posttreatment scores as the dependent variables and using the MCT pretreatment scores as the covariate. Results indicated that the dynamic goal CBM treatment group's adjusted achievement level was greater than that of controls on the content mastery measure, the MCT. This reliable difference was associated with an effect size of one-half standard deviation. There were no reliable differences among the treatment groups, however, on the measure of content coverage. Nevertheless, contrary to the hypothesis that predicted higher achievement for the control group on this content coverage measure, the direction of the means favored the CBM groups. The effect size for the dynamic goal CBM group versus the control group was .39; for the static goal CBM group versus the control group, .35.

By incorporating contrasting measures of content mastery and content coverage in this study, we were able to address a potential criticism of our treatment, that is, that the close connection between measurement and instruction may result in better content mastery of the measured domain, but may decrease content coverage of skills related to, but not synonomous with, the measured domain (Slavin, 1987). Our results indicated either that the CBM teachers did cover a curriculum broader than that encompassed in the CBM procedures, or that students who grew in mathematics operations concurrently progressed in or generalized their newly acquired skills to a broader curricular scope. Either way, results did not support the contention that a close connection between measurement and instruction leads to more limited achievement on content coverage measures.

Researchers who work with learning disabled populations of students and with highly structured treatments that focus on well-circumscribed, delimited content should attend to the issue of content coverage versus content mastery in their selection of outcome measures. On the one hand, incorporating diverse measures to address this issue can help researchers address potential critics; on the other hand, incorporating both types of measures can help researchers understand the limitations or generalizability of their treatments.

Importance of the Scoring Unit to Enhance Sensitivity to Growth

Explanation of the Issue

Sensitivity refers to the responsiveness of a measure to change. Borrowing from Deno (1985), we provide the following example. Most bathroom scales are designed to index weight in 1-pound intervals. With these scales, we can detect weight loss or gain whenever weight changes by 1 pound. By contrast, however, if your bathroom scale were notched at 5-pound units (and did not show 1-pound intervals), you would have to lose five pounds before the scale would register any change. This 5-pound scaling would decrease the sensitivity of the measure to change (and probably increase the frustration of the dieter).

In a similar way, in math, if we scale student performance in terms of problems correct, we have to wait until a student learns how to complete every part of a new problem type correctly before the measure will register change. By scaling the measurement in terms of digits correct, however, we can award credit for correct parts of answers, and the measure will indicate student growth more quickly or sensitively.

For spelling, we can enhance sensitivity to student growth in an analogous way by scaling the measurement in terms of letter sequences (or correct pairs of consecutive letters). With letter sequences, we can detect student improvement whenever the student learns morphemic patterns or phonetic spelling rules—even if the student has not yet entirely mastered new words.

Such heightened sensitivity of a measure to change is important because, with increased sensitivity, (a) the effects of trying to enhance achievement (as in trying to lose weight) become apparent more quickly, (b) the experience is more gratifying for both teacher and student, and (c) treatment efficacy can be detected more easily. Consequently, in designing or selecting measures of academic achievement, consideration of the measure's sensitivity to student growth is critical.

Example Highlighting the Issue

We draw on two examples from our research to highlight the importance of this issue of sensitivity of the academic measure to student growth: research on treatment efficacy and research on monitoring student growth over time.

Research on Treatment Efficacy

We rely on a series of two studies examining the efficacy of teachers' use of Curriculum-based Measurement (CBM) in the area of math. These studies provide a corroborating pattern of performance supporting the principle that scaling measurement in terms of finer units of behavior increases the sensitivity of the measurement to change.

In the first study (Fuchs, Fuchs, Hamlett, & Stecker, 1990), 30 special educators were assigned randomly to three groups: (a) computer-managed CBM that provided graphed performance indicators to teachers as feedback, (b) computer-managed CBM that provided graphed performance indicators plus supplementary skills analysis as teacher feedback, and (c) no systematic performance monitoring (i.e., control). Teachers implemented their respective treatments for 15 weeks with a total of 91 students with mild or moderate handicaps, 70 (77%) of whom had been classified as having a learning disability. Students were pre- and posttested with the Math Computation Test-Revised (MCT-R). The MCT-R is a revision of the MCT, described above. It samples math problems across grades 1–6 of the Tennessee statewide mathematics operations curriculum. Pupils are provided directions in standard format and have 10 minutes to complete 50 problems, or 142 digits. Performance is scored in terms of numbers of correct problems and digits written in answers.

In terms of correct problems, students registered a mean change from pre- to posttreatment of 2.35 problems for the CBM with graphed performance indicators group; 3.02 problems for the CBM with graphed performance indicators plus skills analysis group; and .85 problems for the control group. By contrast, mean growth in terms of digits correct for these three groups, respectively, was 9.15, 14.60, and 4.50. Of course the standard deviations for the two metrics were different (average standard deviation for problems correct was 6.86; for digits correct, 18.14); means cannot be interpreted without corresponding information on standard deviations. Nevertheless, even in terms of effect size (which takes into account the size of the standard deviation), digits correct made treatment efficacy more visible than did problems correct. For problems correct, the effect size comparing the CBM with graphed performance indicators group and the control group was .11, and the effect size comparing the CBM with graphed performance indicators plus skills analysis group and the control group was .28. On the other hand, for digits correct, the effect size comparing the CBM with graphed performance indicators group and the control group was .55; the effect size comparing the CBM with graphed performance indicators plus skills analysis group and the control group was .67.

Additionally, it is critical to note that differences were statistically different only for the digits metric; not for the problems score. Consequently, if the MCT-R had been scored only in terms of problems correct, we would have incorrectly concluded lack of efficacy for the CBM treatment; that is, we would have committed a Type II error for lack of power due to a measure relatively insensitive to treatment effects. Clearly, treatment efficacy was revealed only through the use of the finer metric: digits correct, which awards students credit for parts of the problems they calculate correctly. (It is important to note that the relatively small effect sizes for the CBM with graphed performance indicators feedback group can be attributed in part to the fact that, with computerized data collection and scoring, teachers who saw only graphs had no other access to information about how students did on segments of the curriculum. With noncomputerized CBM applications, teachers have routine access to student performance on segments of the curriculum when they score tests.)

A subsequent study (Fuchs, Fuchs, Hamlett, & Stecker, in press) corroborates this pattern of performance. The purpose of this study was to assess the effects of CBM and expert system instructional consultation in the area of mathematics operations. Thirty-three teachers were assigned randomly to three treatment groups: CBM with expert system instructional consultation, CBM with no instructional consultation, and control (i.e., no CBM). Teachers implemented treatments for 20 weeks with 63 students with mild disabilities, all of whom had chronic difficulty in the area of mathematics. Fifty-six of these 63 pupils (89%) had been classified as having a learning disability.

Again, the MCT-R was employed to assess student achievement before and after the study. Student growth, in terms of problems correct, was 6.99 for the CBM plus expert system consultation group, 3.09 for the CBM without consultation group, and 1.82 for the control group (the average standard deviation was 7.37). Analogous figures for the digits correct score were 21.45, 7.63, and 5.96 (average standard deviation = 22.36). Again, however, even taking into account differences in standard deviation for the two metrics, effect sizes were larger for the digits correct score. In terms of the problems score, the effect size comparing the CBM plus expert system consultation group with the control group was .84; the effect size comparing the CBM without consultation group with the control group was .64. By contrast, in terms of the digits correct score, the effect size comparing the CBM plus expert system consultation group with the control group was .94 (a difference of .10); the effect size comparing the CBM without consultation group with the control group was .64 (a difference of .20). Although in this study, results were statistically significant for both metrics (i.e., problems and digits correct), treatment efficacy was more evident with the finer scaling unit, that is, digits correct—the measure more sensitive to growth.

Research on Monitoring Student Growth over Time

In a similar way, when practitioners employ ongoing measurement systems to monitor their students' academic progress, they require data that will be sensitive to student growth. In our work on CBM, we have monitored student progress over time using various measures, and one major criterion we use to judge the adequacy of the different measures is sensitivity to student growth.

For example, over 2 years of research (Fuchs, Fuchs, Hamlett, Walz, & Germann, 1991), we have monitored math, spelling, and reading progress of 1,067 students, 13% of whom had been diagnosed as having a learning disability. Each student was measured in one of the three academic areas over the course of the academic year. In our first year of study, each student was measured weekly; in the second year, each student was measured monthly. In each academic area, we contrasted two different scoring metrics. In math, we compared digits and problems; in spelling, we compared letter sequences and words; in reading, we compared number and percentage correct.

In math, the average weekly amount of growth registered when student performance was scored in terms of digits was .50 during Year 1 and .47 during Year 2. By contrast, when performance was scaled as problems correct, the average amount of growth made per week was .23 during Year 1 and .21 during Year 2. Clearly, when teachers are using the measurement information to judge the success of their instructional programs, it is both more gratifying and more useful to expect graphs to show a 1-digit increase every 2 weeks—rather than waiting for approximately 5 weeks to detect a 1-digit increase. Moreover, for students who hope to see improvement in their performance, a system that more easily registers change is potentially more reinforcing.

In a similar way, the average weekly increase in student performance, when letter sequence was used as the scoring metric, was .49 in Year 1 and .55 in Year 2. By contrast, the average weekly increase in student performance, when number of correct words was used as the scale, was .10 in Year 1 and .12 in Year 2. Here the contrast is even more dramatic than for the digits-problems contrast. With letter sequences, we expect to see students improve by 1 scoring unit every 2 weeks; by contrast, with words, we expect to see pupils change by 1 scoring unit every 10 weeks!

In reading, we employed a maze test. For the maze, we have students read 400-word passages at their instructional grade level, from which every seventh word is deleted and replaced with three choices. Only one choice is semantically correct. The pupil has 2.5 minutes to read the passage and replace blanks with semantically correct choices. Using the number of correct restorations as the score, we expect to see a weekly increase of .39 words. Using percentage of correct restorations, however, we see a weekly increase of only .04. Consequently, the scoring metric of number (rather than percentage) represents a better way of indexing students' academic growth.

When selecting measures of academic growth, consequently, it is important to consider the scoring metric and how the scale employed will reflect, be sensitive to, or register student improvement. As we have demonstrated here through treatment efficacy studies, as well as with ongoing academic monitoring systems, different ways of scoring students' academic performance can (a) for researchers, increase the power of the measurement to detect student growth and actually modify the results of studies, and (b) for teacher practitioners and for students, result in more useful and gratifying measurement systems.

Summary Remarks

Within educational intervention research, where external funding for the development of educational treatments is poor (Fuchs & Fuchs, 1990), we unfortunately labor with small sample sizes that make treatment differences difficult to detect: The statistical power to identify treatment effects, when they truly exist, typically is poor. Consequently, we chronically suffer the undesirable possibility of rejecting treatments that actually do make important differences for student achievement.

Given our small sample sizes (along with the low probability of better external funding to increase sample sizes in the near future), it is incumbent on the research community to utilize other research design features to increase power. Such strategies include decreasing measurement error, insuring treatment fidelity, and—most relevant to the current chapter—selecting outcome measures that increase the probability of detecting treatment differences where they exist.

In this chapter, we have reviewed three key considerations in selecting measures of academic achievement within intervention research that includes students with learning disabilities to increase the probability of detecting treatment effects where they exist. These three considerations are: the relationship of the achievement measure to the treatment incorporated within the study, the distinction between content coverage and content mastery in indexing student learning, and the importance of the scoring unit within achievement measurement to insure sensitivity to student growth.

References

Borg, W.R. & Gall, M.D. (1989). *Educational research: An introduction* (5th ed.). New York: Longman.

Brown, A.L. & Smiley, S.S. (1977). Rating the importance of structural units of prose passages: A problem of metacognitive development. *Child Development*, *48*, 1–8.

Deno, S.L. (1985). Curriculum-based measurement: The emerging alternative. *Exceptional Children, 52*, 219–232.

Fuchs, D. & Fuchs, L.S. (1990). Making educational research more important. *Exceptional Children, 57*, 102–108.

Fuchs, L.S., Fuchs, D., & Hamlett, C.L. (1989a). Effects of alternative goal structures within curriculum-based measurement. *Exceptional Children, 55*, 429–438.

Fuchs, L.S., Fuchs, D., & Hamlett, C.L. (1989b). Effects of instrumental use of curriculum-based measurement to enhance instructional programs. *Remedial and Special Education, 10*(2), 43–52.

Fuchs, L.S., Fuchs, D., & Hamlett, C.L. (1989c). Monitoring reading growth using student recalls: Effects of two teacher feedback systems. *Journal of Educational Research, 83*, 103–111.

Fuchs, L.S., Fuchs, D., Hamlett, C.L., & Stecker, P.M. (1990). The role of skills analysis in curriculum-based measurement. *School Psychology Review, 19*, 6–22.

Fuchs, L.S., Fuchs, D., Hamlett, C.L., & Stecker, P.M. (in press). Effects of curriculum-based measurement and consultation on teacher planning and student achievement in mathematics operations. *American Educational Research Journal*.

Fuchs, L.S., Fuchs, D., Hamlett, C.L., Walz, L., & Germann, G. (1991). *Indexing academic progress with curriculum-based measurement: Standard for judging improvement over time*. Manuscript submitted for publication.

Gardner, E.F., Rudman, H.C., Karlsen, B., & Merwin, J.C. (1982). *Standard achievement test*. San Antonio: Psychological Corp.

Jenkins, J.R., Heliotis, J., Haynes, M., & Beck, K. (1986). Does passive learning account for disabled readers' comprehension deficits in ordinary reading situations? *Learning Disability Quarterly*, *9*, 69–75.

Leinhardt, G., Zigmond, N., & Cooley, W. (1981). Reading instruction and its effects. *American Educational Research Journal*, *18*, 343–362.

Slavin, R.E. (1987). Mastery learning reconsidered. *Review of Educational Research*, *19*, 199–204.

13
The Study of Cognitive Processes in Learning Disabled Students

H. Lee Swanson and Marilyn Ransby

This chapter focuses on various approaches and measures used to study the cognitive processes of students with learning disabilities. This is a particularly difficult task since there are no published studies systematically comparing the predictive validity and reliability of process measures. This may be due, in part, to the fact that process measures are interpreted within highly inferential frameworks that attempt to explain the mental operations that occur between stimulus presentation and a subject's response. As such, a greater emphasis is placed on understanding individual differences, rather than on the psychometric characteristics of the task. Given this limitation, however, the present chapter will outline four approaches, as well as some general measures, that assess the cognitive processes of students with learning disabilities. The approaches are not mutually exclusive, but focus on: (a) global structures and processes, (b) cognitive correlates, (c) domain-specific processing, and (d) stage-sequence processing.

The present chapter draws heavily from the information processing literature, since this is the most influential model in cognitive psychology to date (see Anderson, 1990, for a review). The central assumptions of the information processing model are: (a) A number of operations and processing stages occur between a stimulus and a response, (b) The stimulus presentation initiates a sequence of stages, (c) Each stage operates on the information available to it, (d) These operations transform the information in some manner, and (e) This new information is the input to the succeeding stage. In sum, the information processing approach focuses on how input is transformed, reduced, elaborated, stored, retrieved, and used.

Global Processes and Structures

One popular means of explaining students with learning disabilities' cognitive performance is by drawing upon fundamental constructs that are inherent in most models of information processing (e.g., see Brainerd & Reyna, 1991; Ceci, 1986; Siegel & Ryan, 1989; Swanson, 1991). Three constructs are fundamental: (a) a constraint or *structural* component, akin to the hardware of a computer, which defines the parameters within which information can be processed at a particular stage (e.g., sensory storage, short-term memory, working memory, long-term memory); (b) a *strategy* component, akin to the software of a computer system, which describes the operations of the various stages; and (c) an *executive* component, by which learners' activities (e.g., strategies) are overseen and monitored. These constructs are represented in Figure 13.1.

In terms of definition, sensory memory refers to the initial representation of information that is available for processing for a maximum of 3 to 5 seconds; short-term memory processes information between 3 and 7 seconds and is primarily concerned with storage, via rehearsal processes. Working memory also focuses on the storage of information, as well as the active interpretation of newly presented information. Long-term memory is a permanent storage with unlimited capacity. The executive component monitors and coordinates the functioning of the entire system (see Baddeley, 1986, for a review). Some of this monitoring may be automatic, with little awareness on the individual's part, whereas other types of monitoring require effortful and conscious processing. Let us briefly review the research in each area as it applies to assessing students with learning disabilities' cognitive abilities.

Sensory Memory

As shown in Figure 13.1, basic environmental information (e.g., visual, auditory) is assumed first to enter the appropriate sensory register. A common paradigm used to assess the processing of sensory information is recognition. The subject is asked to determine whether information that was presented briefly (i.e., millisecond) had occurred. The task may be a simple "yes" or "no" answer to individual items, or it may require selecting among a set of items. Common dependent measures are correct detection and response time (Rt's).

Information in this initial store is thought to include a mental representation of the physical stimulus. For example, the mental representation of a visual stimulus usually includes an image or icon. If an array of letters is presented tachistoscopically and the child is then asked to write those letters after a 30-second delay between instructions, the child can reproduce about six or seven letters from the images represented in the sensory register. The mental representations may vary between subjects within and across stimulus presentations. For example, students who are presented a letter of the alphabet may produce a photographic trace that decays quickly, or they may physically scan the letter and transfer the information into an auditory (e.g., echo or sound)-linguistic (meaning)

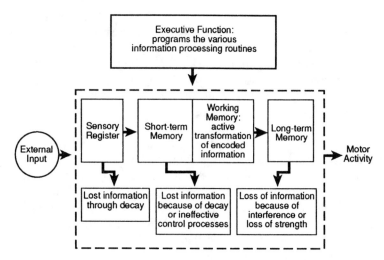

FIGURE 13.1. A simplified model of information processing.

representation. Information that is presented visually may also be recorded into other modalities (e.g., auditory). The transfer of visual information to an auditory-linguistic store is made at the discretion of the person.

In general, research on the sensory register of learning disabilities (LD) children suggests that it is somewhat intact. For example, Elbert (1984) has provided evidence that LD and non–learning disabilities (NLD) students are comparable at the encoding stage of word recognition, but that LD children require more time to conduct a memory search (also see Manis, 1985; Mazer, McIntyre, Murray, Till, & Blackwell, 1983). Additional evidence that LD and NLD children are comparable at the recognition stage of information processing was provided by Lehman and Brady (1982). Using a release from proactive inhibition procedure (see Dempster & Cooney, 1982), Lehman and Brady found that poor and normal readers were comparable in their ability to encode word information (e.g., indicating whether a word was heard or seen and information concerning a word's category). However, children with reading disabilities relied on smaller subword components in the decoding process than did normal readers.

Many accounts of poor recognition of quickly presented information by LD students has been attributed to attention deficits (e.g., see Hallahan & Reeve, 1980, for review), although this conclusion has been questioned (e.g., see Samuels, 1987a, 1987b; Swanson, 1981, 1983a). For example, using a psychological technique free of memory confounds, McIntyre, Murray, Coronin, and Blackwell (1978) reported a lower-than-normal span of attention in students identified with LD. Mazer et al. (1983) attributed the lower span of attention to a slower rate of information pickup from the sensory store. Despite the common assumption of differences between LD and NLD children in attention to visual and auditory stimuli, Bauer (1979a) has argued that the attentional resources of LD children are adequate for performance on a variety of memory tasks. In other words, the residual differences are not great enough to account for the differences in memory performance. For example, LD and NLD children are comparable in their ability to recall orally presented sets of three letters or three words within 4 seconds after presentation (Bauer, 1979a). Similarly, LD and NLD students are comparable in their ability to recognize letters and geometric shapes after a brief visual presentation when recognition is less than 300 milliseconds after stimulus offset (Morrison, Giordani, & Nagy, 1977). In view of these findings, the retrieval of information from sensory storage is an important, although not a major, factor in the cognitive processing deficits exhibited in LD students (also see Jorm, 1983, for a review).

Short-Term Memory

From the sensory register, information is transferred into the limited capacity short-term memory. Information lost in this memory is assumed to decay or disappear, but actual time of decay is longer than time available in the sensory register. Exact rate of decay of information cannot be estimated, because this component is controlled by the subject. The short-term memory retains information in auditory-verbal-linguistic representations. Using the example of a child recalling letters, the child may subvocally rehearse a letter by voicing the letter.

The major measures used to assess short-term memory are a set of recall tasks: distractor task, probe recall, free recall, and serial recall. In distractor tasks the subject is presented with a sequence of items to be recalled, followed by some distractor activity, and then asked to recall. The probe-recall task requires the subject to recall particular elements within a sequence, whereas free recall requires the subject to recall presented words or digits but without any constraints placed on the order in which they are recalled. Serial recall requires the subject to remember items, such as numbers, letters, or words in the same order they were presented. A variation of these tasks is cued recall, in which subjects are given a portion of an item from previously presented stimuli, and the subject is asked to reproduce the remainder of the items. This measure has been employed to determine the extent to which recall may be prompted by appropriate cues, thus highlighting the difference between item accessibility and availability.

Because short-term memory is one of the most actively researched areas related to cognitive processing problems of children with LD, it was necessary to summarize the literature, via a meta-analysis (Swanson, manuscript in preparation; see Glass, 1977, for discussion of calculation procedures). To this end, a standard ERIC and PSYCHINFO search, spanning the years 1975 to 1990, was used to identify experimental studies comparing the performance of LD and NLD students on short-term memory tasks. The search initially identified 70 studies. Studies lacking nondisabled controls, matched IQ scores, and achievement scores were excluded from the analysis. The two groups also had to differ significantly in reading achievement. The LD group had to be performing one or more years below grade level, whereas the NLD group had to be performing at or above grade level. Only 25 studies met this criteria. The studies sampled included approximately 1,700 subjects averaging 10.6 years of age with an average IQ of 102.94. The unit of analysis for comparing these studies was effect size (ES), defined as the mean difference between experimental (LD) and control (NLD) groups divided by the control group standard deviation. A positive ES indicates better performance by the LD group, whereas a negative ES shows a better performance by the NLD group. The studies yielded 88 effect sizes with a mean effect size of -1.18. This indicates that approximately 85% of the LD subjects scored below the NLD subjects on short-term memory measures. Selected findings from this meta-analysis by task, are as follows. For free recall, means effect sizes and representative studies were: $-.87$ for the recall of words (e.g., Bauer, 1979a; Lorsbach, 1982); $-.60$ for the recall of picture stimuli (e.g., Dallego & Moely, 1980; Shephard, Gelzheiser, & Solar, 1985); and $-.77$ for cued recall of words (e.g., Wong, Wong, & Foth, 1977). For serial recall, mean effect sizes and representative studies were: -1.15 for the recall of words (e.g., Richie & Aten, 1976; Torgesen & Houck, 1980, Exp. 7); $-.90$ for the recall of pictures (e.g., Haines & Torgesen, 1979; Torgesen, 1978); -1.16 for the recall of letters (e.g., Hall, Wilson, Humphreys, Tinzmann, & Bowyer, 1983; Siegel & Ryan, 1988); -1.46 for the probe recall of named nonsense shapes (e.g., Swanson, 1978, 1983b); .09 for the probe recall of unnamed nonsense shapes (Swanson, 1978); and -2.41 for the recall of digits (e.g., Torgesen & Houck, 1980, Exp. 1–4 & 6). In general, LD and NLD subjects differ most on tasks that require serial and probe recall. The greatest ability group-differences are observed on tasks that employ digits or verbal material as a stimulus. For example, an oral presentation of strings of digits, increasing in length, and immediate, oral, serial recall are the conditions that show the greatest difference between LD and NLD subjects in their performance on short-term memory tasks (also see Torgesen, Rashotte, Greenstein, & Portes, 1991, for a review).

Given that LD students differ on measures of short-term memory, what cognitive processing deficits underlie such differences? In general, variations in short-term memory performance of LD students have been attributed to control processes (such as rehearsal) and the meaningfulness of the material (see Swanson & Cooney, 1991, for a review). A crucial factor in LD students' performance is their ability to encode units or sequence the items so that they can be recoded into smaller units (Torgesen et al., 1991). Other factors that affect capacity include: (a) information load (Swanson, 1984b), (b) similarity of items (Shankwieler, Liberman, Mark, Fowler, & Fischer, 1979), (c) number of items processed during subsequent activities (Bauer, 1979a; Swanson, 1983a), and (d) passage of time (Worden & Nakamura, 1983). The exact nature of problems with the capacity of short-term memory is somewhat obscure in LD students (see Cooney & Swanson, 1987, for a review). Research has been unclear as to whether the limitation is one of processing capacity, storage capacity, or some interaction between the two (e.g., see Swanson, 1984b).

Control processes in short-term memory reflect choices as to which information to scan as well as choices of what and how to rehearse. Rehearsal refers to the conscious repetition of information, either subvocally or orally, to recall information at a later date. Learning a telephone number or street address illustrates the primary purpose of rehearsal. Additional control processes also involve organization (ordering, classifying, or tagging information to facilitate retrieval) and mediation (comparing new items with items already in memory).

Various organizational strategies of which LD students are deficient may include (see Gelzheiser, Cort, & Shephard, 1987; Pressley, Scruggs, & Mastropieri, 1989; Scruggs & Mastropieri, 1989; Scruggs, Mastropieri, Levin, & Gaffney, 1987; Swanson & Rathgeber, 1986; Swanson et al., 1989; Wong et al., 1977, for example studies of the points below):

1. Chunking: Grouping items so that each one brings to mind a complete series of items (e.g., grouping words into a sentence);
2. Clustering: Organizing items into categories (e.g., animal, furniture);
3. Mnemonics: Idiosyncratic methods for organizing materials); and
4. Coding: Varying the qualitative form of information (e.g., using images rather than verbal labels, substituting pictures for words).

Learning disabled students' mediation of information may be facilitated by:

1. Making use of preexisting associations, thereby eliminating the necessity for new ones;
2. Utilizing instructions, asking the child to mediate information verbally or through imagery, to aid in retrieval and organization; and
3. Cuing at recall by using verbal and imaginary information to facilitate mediation.

There are a number of important studies that have provided a foundation for much of the processing research that occurs to date. For example, concerning research on short-term memory control processes, Torgesen and Goldman (1977) studied lip movements of children during a memorization task. LD children were found to exhibit fewer lip movements than the NLD students. To the extent that these lip movements reflect the quantity of rehearsal, these data support a rehearsal-deficiency hypothesis. Haines and Torgesen (1979) and others (e.g., Dawson, Hallaban, Reeve, & Ball, 1980; Koorland & Wolking, 1982) also reported that incentives could be used to increase the amount of rehearsal and subsequent recall by LD students. Bauer and Embert (1984) have suggested that the difference between LD and NLD students is in the quality of the rehearsal rather than the quantity of rehearsals per se.

Another major source of difficulty that LD students experience during their attempts to memorize material has been highlighted by Gelzheiser, Solar, Shepard, and Wozniak (1983). These authors recorded a brief statement made by an LD student following an attempt to retain a passage containing four paragraphs about diamonds. The student reported that she could identify major themes of the story but could not categorize the various pieces of information under these major items. She was able to abstract the essence of the story but was unable to use this as a framework to organize the retention of the specific passage. Swanson (1983c) found that LD students rarely reported the use of an organizational strategy when they were required to rehearse several items. He reasoned that, because these students were capable of rehearsal, the problem was not a deficiency in rehearsal but was, instead, a failure to perform elaborative processing of each word. Elaborative processing was defined as processing that goes beyond the initial level of analysis to include more sophisticated features of the words and ultimately the comparison of these features with others in the list (also see Swanson, 1989).

Another major source of difficulty related to short-term memory processing has been related to LD students' inefficient use of phonological codes (sound units). Torgesen (1988) conducted studies on a small group of subjects who performed in the retarded range of verbatim recall on sequences of verbal information. His analysis of LD students' performance deficits suggests that they are due to coding errors and represent the phonological features of language. He suggests that LD students' short-term memory problems relate to the acquisition of fluent word identification and word analysis skills. Additional support for the notion of phonological coding errors comes from studies suggesting that good and poor readers differ in the extent to which they recall similar- and dissimilar-sounding names (Shankwieler et al., 1979). An interaction is sometimes found in which poor readers perform better on "rhyming-word and similar letter-sounding tasks" because they have poor access to a phonological code (e.g., Shankweiler et al., 1979; Siegel & Linder, 1984). That is, good readers recall more information for words or letters that have distinct sounds (e.g., *mat* vs. *book*, *A* vs. *F*) than words or letters that sound alike (*mat* vs. *cat*, *b* vs. *d*). In contrast, poor readers are more comparable in their recall of similar and dissimilar words or sounds than skilled readers. This finding suggests that good readers are disrupted when words or sounds are alike because they process information in terms of sound (phonological) units (see, however, Hall et al., 1983). In contrast, poor readers are not efficient in processing information into sound units (phonological codes) and, therefore, their performance is not as disrupted if words or letters sound alike (see Johnson, Rugg, & Scott, 1987).

In summary, LD students' poor short-term memory has been related to problems in rehearsal, organization, elaborative processing, and phonological coding; that is, the previous studies suggest that LD students suffer short-term memory difficulties and these problems manifest themselves by the manner in which information is strategically processed (e.g., rehearsal) and how information is mentally represented (e.g., phonological codes).

Working Memory

Working memory is viewed as a dynamic and active system because it simultaneously focuses on both processing and storage demands, whereas short-term memory primarily focuses on the storage of information and is considered a more passive system (Baddeley, 1986; Daneman & Carpenter, 1980; Swanson, 1992). Thus, short-term memory is partly understood as a component of a limited capacity system from accumulating and holding segments of information in order (e.g., speech or orthographic units) as they arrive during a listening or reading task. Material in short-term memory is retained if it is rehearsed. In contrast, working memory is concerned with the interpretation and integration of information with previously stored information (see Siegel & Ryan, 1989; Swanson et al., 1990 for application to learning disabilities).

How does the construct of working memory help us understand LD students' memory problems better than the concept of short-term store? First, it suggests that verbal rehearsal plays a smaller role in learning and memory (Baddeley, 1986), an important point because some studies do show that performance deficits of LD students are not related to rehearsal per se (e.g., see Swanson, 1983b). For example, previous studies of LD students' short-term memory operations such as rehearsal (Bauer, 1979a) have not explained how constraints in long-term memory contribute to academic performance; specifically, they have not shown how word knowledge, associations, and attentional capacity contribute to some of the problems we see occurring in short-term memory tasks. Furthermore, measures (e.g., digit span) commonly used in assessing differences between LD and NLD students' memory are weakly correlated with academic ability (Daneman & Carpenter, 1980, 1983), suggesting that such short-term tasks may not capture the essence of academic performance, namely, the combination of processing and long-term memory storage functions. Second, the idea of a working memory system is useful because it is viewed as an active memory system directed by a central executive (to be discussed) and the resources stored in long-term memory (Baddeley, 1986).

A recent study (Swanson, Cochran, & Ewers, 1989a) sought to determine the *extent* to which less skilled readers suffer from working memory deficiencies. A sentence span task (Daneman & Carpenter, 1980) was used to measure the combined efficiency of storage and processing operations. The task requires recalling the last word of several sentences as well as answering a comprehension question about a sentence. Materials for the sentence span task were unrelated declarative sentences, 7–10 words in length, arranged into sets of two, three, four, or five sentences. Examples of the sentences for recalling the last word in a series of three sentences are:

1. We waited in line for a *ticket*.
2. Sally thinks we should give the bird its *food*.
3. My mother said she would write a *letter*.

To ensure that children comprehended the sentences (i.e., processed their meaning) and did not merely treat the task as one of short-term memory, they were required to answer a question after each group of sentences was presented. For the three-sentence set, for example, they were asked "Where did we wait?" The results of this study suggest that LD readers' working memory is inferior to NLD readers. Thus, studies that suggest that LD students' memory deficiencies are localized to a short-term store system must be reevaluated within the context of a model that incorporates the operations of working memory.

Long-Term Memory

The amount of information, as well as the form of information, transferred to long-term memory is primarily a function of control processes (e.g., rehearsal). Long-term memory is a permanent storage of information of unlimited capacity. How information is stored is determined by the uses of links, associations, and general organizational plans. Information stored in long-term memory is primarily semantic. Forgetting occurs because of item decay (loss of information) or interference.

In comparison to the volume of research on short-term memory processes, research on LD students' long-term memory is sparse. The available research, however, provides considerable support for the assertion that storage and retrieval problems are primary sources of individual differences in long-term memory performance (e.g., Brainerd, Kingma, & Howe, 1987; Swanson, 1987). Numerous studies have also shown that LD students are less skilled than NLD peers in the use of rehearsal strategies used to store information in long-term memory (Bauer, 1979a, 1979b; Tarver, Hallahan, Kauffman, & Ball, 1976; Torgesen & Goldman, 1977). The main source of evidence for the inference of rehearsal deficits in LD students is the diminished primacy effect (i.e., better recall of items at the beginning of a list over the middle items of the list) of the serial position curve (Bauer, 1979b). Primacy performance is a measure of the accessibility of items placed in long-term storage. Thus, the primacy effect is thought to reflect greater rehearsal of those items at the beginning of the list.

In terms of retrieving information from long-term memory, LD students can use organized strategies for selecting retrieval cues (Wong, 1982) and word attributes (e.g., graphophonic, syntactic, semantic) to guide retrieval (Blumenthal, 1980); however, they appear to select less efficient strategies, to conduct a less exhaustive search for retrieval cues, and to lack self-checking skills in the selection of retrieval cues (Wong, 1982). Swanson (1984b, 1987) also provided evidence suggesting that long-term memory deficits may arise from failure to integrate visual and verbal memory traces of visually presented stimuli at the time of storage or retrieval. His findings suggested that semantic memory limitations contribute to LD children's failure to integrate verbal and visual codes. Ceci, Ringstrom and Lea (1980) presented data that suggested that there are separate pathways for auditory and visual inputs to the semantic memory system and that LD students may have an impairment in one or both of these pathways. They found that for students with visual and auditory impairments the recall deficit arises in both storage and retrieval. When only one modality is impaired, the long-term memory deficit is hypothesized to arise at the time of storage. Furthermore, semantic-orienting tasks were found to ameliorate the recall deficits of the students with single modality impairments, but not those with impairments in both visual and verbal modalities (Ceci et al., 1980; Experiment 2).

Other investigators (for a review, see Worden, 1986) have suggested that LD students' long-term memory is intact, but the strategies necessary to gain access to this information are impaired. This notion has been challenged (e.g., Baker, Ceci, & Herrmann, 1987), and some evidence suggests that LD students' long-term memory for tasks that require semantic processing is clearly deficient when compared with that of NLD peers (Swanson, 1986). Moreover, some experimental evidence suggests that LD students may have problems in the structural component of information processing (e.g., Baker et al., 1987; Cohen, 1981; Swanson, 1987; Torgesen & Houck, 1980). Specifically, Torgesen and Houck (1980), in a seminal study, administered a series of eight experiments in which subgroups of LD and NLD students were compared on a digit span task (see Torgesen et al., 1991 for replication studies). Treatment variations among the eight experimental conditions included manipulations of rehearsal, incentives, and related mnemonic activities. Not all LD subjects benefited from strategy intervention, suggesting that structural or capacity difficulties may exist in some students with LD (also see Swanson, 1986, 1989).

Taken as a whole, the selective results reviewed here suggest that the cognitive processes involved in entering a memory trace into the long-term store may account for weaknesses in LD students' long-term recall. Additional research to discover methods for remediating these deficits is warranted.

Executive Function

An executive function is a cognitive activity that determines the order in which processes will be performed. In other words, it is the organizational directive for various memory strategies. The executive function does not perform the searching task, nor organize, nor sort out material; instead, it directs the various mental activities to a goal.

Neisser (1967) sums up some important points related to executive processing:

1. Retrieval of information consists of many programmed searches simultaneously and independently (parallel search or multiple search).
2. Control of parallel and sequential processes is directed by the executive routine.
3. Executive function and search processes are learned and based on earlier processing, the implication being that:
    a. Individuals learn to organize and retrieve
    b. There are individual styles of organization
4. Failure to recall is failure to access, the implication being that there is a misguided search strategy.

Measures of executive processing usually included dual-processing tasks (e.g., see Swanson, Cochran, & Ewers, 1990) that vary the processing load (difficulty of material) and type of processing required (verbal, nonverbal). Although executive functioning has been researched with respect to its importance and application to mentally retarded students' memory (Belmont, Butterfield, & Ferretti, 1982; Campione, Brown, Ferrara, Jones, & Sternberg, 1985), its application to LD is just emerging (Borkowski, Estrada, Milstead, & Hale, 1989; Palincsar & Brown, 1984; Pressley et al., 1989; Swanson, 1990a; in press). A focus on executive processing is an important area of research because planning activities prior to solving a problem, monitoring behavior in action, reorganizing strategies, and evaluating the outcomes of any strategic action have characterized LD students' functioning in a number of academic domains (e.g., Bos & Anders, 1990; Palincsar & Brown, 1984). Strategy deficits in LD learners have been noted in terms of failing to monitor cognitive progress or to notice important task differences in learning tasks (for a review, see Pressley et al., 1989). The focus of research has been to determine whether or not LD students can review their own cognitive strategies, select and reject them appropriately, and persist in searching for the most suitable task strategies at various stages of performance (Palincsar & Brown, 1984; Pressley, Johnson, & Symons, 1987). Evidence for possible problems in LD students' executive functioning can be found in studies where such students have difficulty checking, planning, and monitoring control processes (e.g., Gelheizer, et al., 1983; Palincsar & Brown, 1984; Wong, 1982; Wong & Jones, 1982). This type of research focuses on how decisions or strategies are prioritized, the kinds of decisions LD students make at a specific point to carry out a strategy, and how they make decisions related to an unresolved processing stage (e.g., cannot understand the gist of the passage).

Summary

Overall, current research suggests that LD students experience problems with several information processing components. The majority of research has focused on problems in short-term memory, which may very likely influence processes related to working memory, long-term memory, and executive processes. As yet, research has not identified the independent effects and contributions of various components to LD students' overall memory functioning. Thus, it is best to view their cognitive difficulties as reflecting interactive problems between and among various cognitive-processing components.

Cognitive Correlates

Another approach to assessing LD students' abilities is to compile a list of cognitive components related to psychometric instruments. That is, cognitive processes are identified that underlie the factor structure of psychometric measures. Unfortunately, this approach has not been systematically investigated in the field of learning disabilities, but has much to offer in assessing cognitive processing. For example, Carroll (1976) has compiled a list of component processes that arbitrarily define academic and intellectual domains in terms of information processing (see Kyllonen & Christal, 1990, Exp. 3, for a recent application). To assess the cognitive components that may account for some of the variance on psychometric measures, French, Ekstrom, and Price's (1963) Kit of Reference Tests for Cognitive Factors may be appropriate. This set includes 24 factors of cognitive abilities, further categorized by information processing operations (i.e., strategies) that must be performed if the task is to be mastered successfully. These operations are of three kinds: attentional (visual searches, e.g., as measured by eye movements), memorial (storing, searching, and retrieving), and executive (judgments about stimulus attributes).

Within the cognitive-correlate framework, traditional psychometric measures (e.g., standardized intelligence and achievement tests) administered in isolation are viewed as providing little insight into the nature of cognitive mechanisms that account for LD students' poor performance (e.g., see Wagner & Sternberg, 1984, for a review). However, this does not preclude using psychometric measures for predictive purposes. Unfortunately, such measures fail to identify the internal processes that account for poor academic performance. Within this context it becomes necessary to suggest some measures to assess cognitive processing that can be used concurrently with psychometric measures. Some of the contemporary methodological procedures discussed here are interviews, protocol analysis, ethnographic assessment, and utilizing non-entrenched tasks and psychophysiological measures.

Interviews

Interviews are a common method of gathering information about the child's knowledge concerning the cognitive processes he/she is using on various psychometric tasks (e.g., Swanson, 1990b). Students' knowledge about their own cognitive processes and the compatibility between their perceptions of self as a learner and the learning situation is called *metacognition*. The metacognitive difficulties of LD students and its implication for assessment have been well documented (e.g., see Wong, 1991, for a review). Unfortunately, such interviews suffer from reliability and validity difficulties and variations of subjects' language skills. Some of these difficulties have been overcome by converting such interviews to questionnaires (see Paris, Cross, & Lipson, 1984). Additional criticism of metacognitive interviewing, however, has been directed toward the practice of asking students questions prior to or after task performance. Students tend to verbalize what they think they ought to do during task performance, rather than what they actually do. One means of control for this problem has been to use several types of probe questions during actual task performance. This procedure allows for the assessment of interim decision making. Further, students are not required to verbalize all thoughts during task performance, which may interfere with performance, but to verbalize only intermittently (See Ericsson & Simon, 1980, for a review of the advantages and disadvantages of verbal reports as data).

Protocol Analysis

Recently, there has been an emphasis on protocol methods (i.e., the talking aloud procedure and the clinical interview technique in which taped recordings or written transcripts provide information on students' overt thinking) as a basis for understanding academic and intellectual performance of students (e.g., see Ginsburg, Kossan, Schwartz, & Swanson, 1983; and Garner, 1988, for a review). The protocols are used to draw inferences about underlying cognitive processes involved in academic and/or intellectual activities. The usefulness of students' verbalizations as data for testing theoretical models is based upon the assumption that students' thinking can be assessed through a process of inquiry during academic performance or problem solving and that thinking aloud is one means of understanding and identifying information processing components. Procedures for utilizing a protocol analysis usually involve transforming transcripts of raw data (e.g., verbal report of an interview conducted while the child is performing the task). In addition, interviewing procedures are defined a priori, as are explicit sets of subject attributes for which scores are derived. That is, scores are derived from specified codes that may represent a category or subcategory of cognitive processing. Each subject is videotaped or interviewed by several individuals. Interview information is transcribed so that several raters read each transcript and determine the score of each subject. Traditional concepts of reliability and validity apply (e.g., interrater reliability) to such procedures (see Garner, 1988, for a review). Accuracy of inferences can be correlated with concurrent measures (e.g., arithmetic achievement, reading comprehension performance, observation of problem solving, eye-movement data). [See study by Swanson (1988) utilizing "think aloud" procedures to measure LD students' cognitive abilities].

Ethnographic Assessment

Ethnographic assessment in this context focuses on the interactions of teaching and learning (e.g., Goetz & LeCompte, 1984). Employing audio or audio-visual equipment, the researcher examines academically related behavior thoroughly and repeatedly. Because the social interactions associated with academic accomplishments are complex, merely gathering cognitive performance data for a few points in time is questionable. It is only when information is reviewed repeatedly that a complete and accurate description of academic behavior occurs. Ethnographic methodology includes such procedures as participant observation, interviews, case studies, and audio and videotape equipment. One variation of participant observation is when the experimenter assumes an indirect role in the natural setting (i.e., naturalistic observation).

The underlying rationale for the naturalistic observational approach is consistent with the processing analysis discussed earlier. By representative sampling (e.g., using LD students) of environment-subject interactions involving achievement-related behavior, it is possible to identify more accurately what variables and processes characterize the various degrees of academic success and failure. Such a representative sample of behavior would lead to an expansion of the existing domain of academic performance assessment to include aspects not conventionally associated with academic achievement (e.g., contextual or emotional factors that directly influence performance). An example of a naturalistic observational study during instructional activities (reading and math) is provided by Swanson (1984a; Swanson, Reffel, & Trahan, 1990; also see Moely, Hart, Santulli, Leal, Johnson, & Roa, 1986, for sample observational form).

Nonentrenched Tasks

Some authors (e.g., Sternberg, 1981) have suggested that intellectual and achievement-related behaviors can best be understood through the use of novel (nonentrenched) tasks. These tasks are designed to allow students to form strategies that differ in kind from those associated with traditional psychometric measures. For example, a projection task utilized in Sternberg's (1981) study allowed for the assessment of metacognitive components directly linked to intellectual functioning.

Other Procedures

During the last decade there have been a number of other major analytical and methodological approaches to the study of LD children's learning processes. These procedures have been essentially a rediscovery of paradigms and methods used in adult studies (e.g., Donders' subtraction method logic, the additive-factor method, mathematical modeling, computer simulation). Some example extensions of these methods in the study of children's learning include Sternberg's componential analysis (see Kolligian & Sternberg, 1987; Sternberg, 1987) and Calfee and Hedges' (1980) generalization of the additive-factor method, and Brainerd and Reyna's (1991) Markov adaptations. Our purpose in mentioning these is to indicate that substantial methodological work needs to be done in order to understand the link between LD students' cognitive processes and academic performance.

Domain-Specific Processes

Another approach to assessing LD students' cognitive processing is to identify specific processes that are thought to be critical to learning in a specific academic domain (e.g., reading, spelling, or mathematics). Since the learning disabilities tradition is based upon the assumption of a deficit in one or more specific processes (Foorman, 1989; Stanovich, 1988), findings derived from this approach have important theoretical and practical implications. As an illustration of this approach, we present a brief review of the literature on phonological awareness, since this is one of the most researched areas on the cognitive deficits of the learning disabled in the last decade.

There are four factors that make the relationship between phonological awareness and reading of critical importance in understanding the cognitive processing abilities of LD students. First, converging evidence suggests there is a causal relationship between skills in phonological awareness and reading achievement (see Adams, 1990; Barron, in press). Second, phonological awareness can be distinguished from other linguistic skills associated with reading because of its independence of IQ (Bradley & Bryant, 1983; Olson, Wise, Conners, Rack, & Fulker, 1989; Stanovich, Cunningham, & Cramer, 1984; Tunmer, Herriman, & Teasdale, 1988). Third, behavioral genetic studies have presented evidence that phonological awareness is genetically in heritable whereas orthographic awareness is environmentally determined (Olson et al., 1989; Olson, Wise, Conners, & Rack, 1990). Finally, phonological awareness is an important causal and core factor that distinguishes normally developing readers from dyslexic readers (Adams, 1990; Juel, 1988; Stanovich, 1986, 1988).

Over the last three decades several tests of phonological awareness have been developed, each with varying cognitive demands, reliability, and predictive validity. Although it is difficult to make comparisons across studies with so much variability, there appears to be some agreement regarding the relative difficulty of various categories of phonological awareness tests (Adams, 1990). The following is an attempt to synthesize some of these findings.

1. Rhyme/Rime

The easiest category of phonological awareness tasks is the rhyme category (Adams, 1990; Yopp, 1988). MacLean, Bryant, and Bradley (1987) found that many children as young as 3 years of age could successfully perform a nursery rhyme production, rhyme detection, and rhyme alliteration task. For the nursery rhyme task, students were asked to recite familiar nursery rhymes (e.g., Humpty-Dumpty). In the rhyme detection task they were asked to tell which words did not rhyme. In the rhyme alliteration task, students were asked to identify the word that did not start with the same initial sound (e.g., *pin, pig, tree*). Olson et al. (1989) asked their adult subjects to perform a rhyme fluency task. Subjects were asked to list as many words as possible that rhymed, for instance, with *eel* in one minute. Although this test had the advantage of avoiding ceiling effects, it did not distinguish the dyslexic from younger reading level controls.

2.   Synthesis and Analysis/Blending and Segmenting

Synthesis or blending tasks have been found to be easier than analysis or segmentation tasks (Perfetti, Beck, Bell, & Hughes, 1987) and analyzing words into syllables is thought to be easier than segmenting words into phonemes (Blachman, 1984; Morais, Bertelson, Cary, & Algeria, 1986; Yopp, 1988). One of the easiest forms of phoneme segmentation is the classic phoneme tapping or phoneme counting task (Yopp, 1988).

3.   Phoneme Manipulation

Among the most difficult phoneme tasks are those that require some manipulation such as adding, deleting, and moving phonemes within and around words (Adams, 1990). One of the most difficult phoneme manipulation tasks that has been used with adults (Olson et al., 1989; Pennington, Van Orden, Smith, Green, & Haith, 1990) requires subjects to play the traditional children's Pig Latin game. To create a Pig Latin word for *dog*, one removes the initial consonant *d* then puts it at the end of the word and follows it with the sound *ay* to create *ogday*.

Some investigators have concluded that despite a range of difficulty levels in the tasks noted above, the tasks tend to be measuring the same underlying construct (Pennington et al., 1990; Stanovich et al., 1984; Yopp, 1988). Morais et al. (1986), however, found that rhyme detection and speech segmentation tasks administered to adult illiterates were not significantly correlated. Similar findings with children have led Lundberg, Frost, and Peterson (1988) to conclude that rhyme and segmentation tasks involve different mechanisms.

When selecting phonological awareness tasks for experimental investigations of LD students' cognitive abilities, one needs to be aware of the ceiling effects of the various tasks. Fox and Routh (1975), for instance, found that performance on both word and syllable segmentation tasks reached ceiling at around 4 years of age, while phoneme segmentation tasks reached ceiling around 6 years of age. With a reading disabled sample the ceiling on the latter task was reached at age 9 (Fox & Routh, 1983). In order to circumvent ceiling effects, Stanovich (1988) informed his subjects that they were to execute a rhyme production and odd-sound-out task as fast as possible. Both accuracy and response latencies were recorded. Stanovich reasoned that speed might have some "diagnosticity" (p. 593) that accuracy could not detect and that the speed instructions would force subjects to make more errors than they would in an untimed condition.

It is difficult to determine which phonological awareness tasks are the most reliable in diagnosing LD students' abilities, because few investigators have included this information in their reports. Moreover, among those who have reported reliability coefficients, there are wide variations in the tasks that have been employed and in the age of the subjects (Blachman, 1984; Bryant, MacLean, Bradley, & Crossland, 1990; Cunningham & Stanovich, 1990; Juel, 1988; Pratt & Brady, 1988; Stanovich et al., 1984; Yopp, 1988). Bryant et al. (1990) attempted to determine the extent to which their phonological awareness tasks satisfied the specificity criteria. They concluded that the classic phoneme tapping task may not be a pure measure of phonological awareness since it was found to correlate with both reading and arithmetic tasks. In contrast, rhyming tasks and phoneme deletion tasks correlated only with reading and spelling. Since this group of investigators appears to be the only one that has tested for specificity across academic domains, it is difficult to know how far this result can be generalized.

Reading Disabilities and Phonological Awareness

Stanovich (1988) has recently advanced an individual-differences model of reading disabilities/dyslexia that features phonological deficits as the "core" feature in the pattern of performance in dyslexic readers. Drawing on the theoretical notions of modularity in language (Fodor, 1983), Stanovich posits that the "key deficit in dyslexia must be a vertical (domain specific) faculty rather than a horizontal faculty" (p. 592). Moreover, evidence for a specific deficit must be derived from demonstrations that students with reading disabilities are superior to "garden variety" readers in more global skills but inferior to reading level IQ matches on specific phonological skills.

Although there are many demonstrations of the strong relationship between phonological awareness and reading in samples of average and poor readers, there are few studies that have included severely disabled readers in their sample. Two notable exceptions are a study by Fox and Routh (1983) and a study by Lovett (1987). In both studies, the most impaired readers were found to be deficient on sound analysis tasks.

Two studies of dyslexics, which have used reading-level designs, are of particular interest because they lend support to the specificity hypothesis. Olson et al. (1989) compared a group of older dyslexics (mean age 15) with a younger group of reading-level controls (mean age 10) and found that the dyslexics were inferior to the reading level (word recognition scores) on a Pig Latin test of phoneme segmentation, but not on rhyming fluency. Pennington et al. (1990), using both reading level and age matched controls, reported similar findings. The dyslexics were inferior to the reading-level controls on a Pig Latin test, but not on articulatory speed, lexical retrieval (naming) by initial consonant, nor articulatory speed.

In sum, although an understanding of cognitive processing by LD students is relatively well developed in reading, and to some extent in spelling, it does not appear to be well developed in mathematics, likely because of the research that indicates that the majority of children with math disabilities also have difficulties in reading. There may be some value, however, in exploring specific processes in students whose learning disability is restricted to the mathematics domain despite their small numbers (see Morrison & Siegel, 1991; Siegel & Ryan, 1989 for a review of promising research).

Stage and Sequence of Processing

A final approach to assess cognitive processes in LD students is to select dependent measures in terms of a *series* of operations that reflect the flow of information. We briefly list some of these tasks in Table 13.1, in hopes of facilitating the inclusion of such measures in future assessment studies. The set of tasks was gleaned from the LD literature with several criteria in mind:

1. The task has to have a history within the information processing literature and have empirical support as a device for determining individual differences.
2. There has to be a theoretical rationale for the task (e.g., construct validity) and that task must assess some elementary processing mechanism.
3. The task must be adaptable to moderately language-handicapped students as well as lend itself to paper-and-pencil format, computer simulation, and/or group administration.
4. The tasks must be logically interrelated to performance on several academic tasks.

In general, all tasks included in Table 13.1 can be described in a series of operations outlined by several authors (e.g., Schneider & Pressley, 1989; Swanson, 1991). The operations that are assumed to be important to assessment include the following:

1. *Encoding* is a process by which input information is initially analyzed. The child merely matches the input against past learning. This process also involves the extraction of different types of information from a stimulus. For example, consider a child who is presented with a series of words to be remembered for a spelling test. The child may process the words by their orthographic features, or the phonological features represented by the printed word, or the semantic features represented by the meaning of the word.
2. *Elaboration* is a process by which connections are made—either with the material to be learned, or between the material to be learned and other information previously stored. For example, when students are presented spelling words to remember, they form associations to those words by use of extra ways of mediating the information (visualize the

word *boy*, i.e., the process of imagery), proposing or answering questions about the word (e.g., "Is a boy the same as a man?"), and categorizing information (e.g., the word *boy* represents one of two genders), or associating the word with a context (e.g., the teacher uses the word *boy* in several sentences).

3. *Transformation* is a process by which rules, algorithms, or heuristics are applied to the incoming information (the word *perceive* follows the *i* after *c* rule). In contrast to encoding and elaboration, this process requires the child to apply some previously stored rules about information processing.

4. *Storage* is a process by which input information is added to the existing information within the mental system. This process forms a memory trace. Forgetting this memory trace can be attributed to an interference from other learning (e.g., the child has difficulty remembering how to spell the word *perceived* for the present spelling test because the week before the spelling test included the word *received*, i.e., proactive interference). The effects of interference can be assessed by the degree to which the child has overlearned and reviewed the material.

5. *Retrieval* is a process by which information that was previously stored can be made available. The process generally requires the reproduction of information with minimal aids (i.e., free recall, serial recall). For example, the child is asked to write down a spelling word with all letters in their correct order.

6. *Searching* is a process by which information is accessed by determining the presence or absence of additional properties. For example, a child is asked if any of the word spellings that were forgotten rhyme with the word *receive* (i.e., cued recall). The child may internally develop an aid to help him/her remember the word or the aid may be external (e.g., teacher induced).

7. *Comparing* is a process in which information is judged or recognized to be either old or new, same or different, and so forth, relative to information that has been previously stored. For example, a child is asked to pick out 10 words for a review spelling test from a list of 20 words in which 10 words are new. Recognizing new and old words is generally easier than cued or free recall situations. That is, free recall places more demands on retrieval than cued recall and cued recall places more demands upon retrieval than recognition.

8. *Reconstruction* is a process in which information recall is based on concepts that tie together fragments or pieces of stored information. More specifically, the information recalled is not a duplicate of information that was encoded. For example, a child may incorrectly associate fragments of encoded information with information stored in long-term memory. Thus, recall would represent only partially or possibly incorrectly the original input information.

TABLE 13.1. Components of various tasks for assessing cognitive processes.

Task (sample)	Encode	Elaboration	Transformation	Storage	Retrieval	Search	Compare	Reconstruct
Central incidental recall task (e.g., Tarver, Hallahan, Kauffman, & Ball, 1976)	Encode pictures				Serial and incidental recall			
Letter classification Posner task (e.g., Sergeant & Scholten, 1983)	Encode letters						Recognize letter rate (reaction time) with increases in memory load	
Continuous performance task (e.g., Swanson, 1983a)	Encode letters						Judge accuracy of target items over time	
Orienting task (e.g., Swanson, 1989)	Encode words	Focus on semantic and nonsemantic aspects of words			Free recall of words			
Sorting tasks (e.g., Gelzheiser, Cort, & Shepard, 1987; Wong, 1982)	Encode items (pictures)	Sort by categories			Free recall of items	Organization of retrieval (clustering)		
Recognition paradigm (Morrison et al., 1977)	Presentation of letters, geometric patterns			Storage and retrieval of auditory and visual information				
Sternberg memory scanning task (e.g., Elbert, 1984)	Encoding of target letters or words (measured by intercept values)						Reaction time linear function of set size (slope values)	

Free recall of words (e.g., Bauer, 1977)	Encode words		Serial recall: primacy reflects rehearsal and recency reflects attention and stimulus recognition		
Prose paradigm (e.g., Worden & Nakamura, 1983)	Encode stories	Categorize stories	Recall main idea units		Main ideas units reflect elaboration, substitutions, or notstated propositions of fragmented information
Rule learning task (e.g., Swanson, 1982)	Encode dimension of stimulus	Apply conjuctive, disjunctive, and conditional rule			
Digit span (e.g., Torgesen & Houck, 1980)	Encode numbers		Recall numbers in order		
Lexical decision task (e.g., Manis, 1985)	Encode letter string	Construct phonemic representation		Search in LTM word and word rules	
Cued recall/Math model analysis (e.g., Brainerd & Reyna, 1991; Ceci et al., 1980)	Encode unrelated words	Memory trace analyses		Cued recall for several trails	

These processes may be tied to several dependent measures that assess students' information processing. The dependent measures and processes that are represented are provided in Table 13.1. The reader is referred to the citations for a detailed description of each task. It is hypothesized that some of these tasks involve certain processes while others do not. Inferences about the validity of such processing constructs are based upon empirical studies. To further validate a model, however, a general linear procedure is necessary. That is, a best fit model could be evaluated in terms of the obtained multiple R^2 (i.e., the proportion of variance accounted for in the entire set of tasks) or exploratory/confirmatory factor analysis.

Summary and Conclusion

The major implication of this chapter is that if any understanding is to occur related to LD students' cognitive abilities, a fine-grained analysis is necessary. We have outlined four approaches to assessing the cognitive processes of LD students. These approaches are not mutually exclusive, but stress the importance of cognitive operations or mechanisms that facilitate the acquisition of information. Within this framework, LD students, as well as their normally achieving counterparts, are perceived as learning through various intervening stages of cognition (e.g., encoding, organizing, storing), domain-relevant processes (e.g., phonological coding), and structures (e.g., short-term memory). At present, research on LD students' poor academic performance is best conceptualized as an interaction between their deficient cognitive processes and a multitude of external variables (instruction, context, etc.).

Acknowledgments. This chapter was partially supported by an SSHRC grant from the University of British Columbia to the first author. Address: H.L. Swanson, School of Education, University of California, Riverside, CA., 92521.

References

Adams, M.J. (1990). *Beginning to read: Thinking and learning about print.* Cambridge, MA: M.I.T. Press.

Anderson, J. (1990). *Cognitive psychology and its implications.* New York: Freeman.

Baddeley, A.D. (1986). *Working memory.* London: Oxford University Press.

Baker, J.G., Ceci, S.J., & Herrmann, N.D. (1987). Semantic structure and processing: Implications for the learning disabled child. In H.L. Swanson (Ed.), *Memory and learning disabilities* (pp. 83–110). Greenwich, CT: JAI Press.

Barron, R.W. (in press). Proto-literacy, literacy, and the acquisition of phonological awareness. *Learning and Individual Differences, 3,* 243–255.

Bauer, R.H. (1977). Memory processes in children with learning disabilities: Evidence for deficient rehearsal. *Journal of Experimental Child Psychology, 24*(3), 419–430.

Bauer, R.H. (1979a). Memory processes in children with learning disabilities: Evidence for deficient rehearsal. *Journal of Experimental Child Psychology*, *24*, 415–430.

Bauer, R.H. (1979b). Memory, acquisition, and category clustering in learning disabled children. *Journal of Experimental Child Psychology*, *27*, 365–383.

Bauer, R.H. & Embert, J. (1984). Information processing in reading-disabled and nondisabled children. *Journal of Experimental Child Psychology*, *37*, 271–281.

Belmont, J.M., Butterfield, E.C., & Ferretti, R.P. (1982). To secure transfer of training instruct self-management skills. In D.K. Detterman & R.J. Sternberg (Eds.), *How and how much can intelligence be increased?* Norwood, NJ: Ablex.

Blachman, B.A. (1984). Relationship of rapid naming ability and language analysis skills to kindergarten and first-grade reading achievement. *Journal of Educational Psychology*, *76*, 610–622.

Blumenthal, S.H. (1980). A study of the relationship between speed of retrieval of verbal information and patterns of oral reading errors. *Journal of Learning Disabilities*, *3*, 568–570.

Borkowski, J.G., Estrada, M., Milstead, M., & Hale, C.A. (1989). General problem-solving skills: Relations between metacognition and strategic processing. *Learning Disability Quarterly*, *12*, 57–70.

Bos, C.S. & Anders, P.L. (1990). Toward an interactive model: Teaching test-based concepts to learning disabled students. In H.L. Swanson & B.K. Keogh (Eds.), *Learning Disabilities: Theoretical and research issues* (pp. 247–261). Hillsdale, NJ: Erlbaum.

Bradley, L. & Bryant, P.E. (1983). Categorizing sounds and learning to read—A causal connection. *Nature*, *301*, 419–421.

Brainerd, C.J., Kingma, J., & Howe, M.L. (1987). Long-term memory development and learning disability: Storage and retrieval loci of disabled/nondisabled differences. In S. Ceci (Ed.), *Handbook on cognitive social, and neurological aspects of learning disabilities* (pp. 161–184). Hillsdale, NJ: Erlbaum.

Brainerd, C.J. & Reyna, V.F. (1991). Acquisition and forgetting processes in normal and learning-disabled children: A disintegration/reintegration theory. In J. Obrzut & G.W. Hynd (Eds.), *Neuropsychological foundations of learning disabilities* (pp. 147–175). New York: Academic Press.

Bryant, P.E., MacLean, M., Bradley, L.L., & Crossland, J. (1990). Rhyme and alliteration, phoneme detection, and learning to read. *Developmental Psychology*, *26*, 429–438.

Calfee, R.C. & Hedges, L.V. (1980). Independent process analysis of aptitude-treatment interactions. In R. Snow, P. Frederico, & W. Montague (Eds.), *Aptitude, learning and instruction* (Vol. 1, pp. 193–314). Hillsdale, NJ: Erlbaum.

Campione, J.C., Brown, A.L., Ferrara, F.A., Jones, R.S., & Steinberg, E. (1985). Breakdown in flexible use of information: Intelligence related differences in transfer following equivalent learning performances. *Intelligence*, *9*, 297–315.

Carroll, J.B. (1976). Psychometric tests as cognitive tasks: A new structure of intellect. In L.B. Resnick (Ed.), *The nature of intelligence* (pp. 27–57). Hillsdale, NJ: Erlbaum.

Ceci, S.J. (1986). Developmental study of learning disabilities and memory. *Journal of Experimental Child Psychology*, *38*, 352–371.

Ceci, S.J., Ringstrom, M.D., & Lea, S.E.G. (1980). Coding characteristics of normal and learning-disabled 10 year olds: Evidence for dual pathways to the cognitive system. *Journal of Experimental Psychology: Human Learning & Memory*, *6*, 785–797.

Cohen, R.L. (1981). Short-term memory deficits in reading disabled children in the absence of opportunity for rehearsal strategies. *Intelligence*, *5*, 69–76.

Cooney, J.B. & Swanson, H.L. (1987). Overview of research on learning disabled children's memory development. In H.L. Swanson (Ed.), *Memory and learning disabilities* (pp. 2–40). Greenwich, CT: JAI Press.

Cunningham, A.E. & Stanovich, K.E. (1990). Assessing print exposure and orthographic processing skill in children: A quick measure of reading experience. *Journal of Educational Psychology*, *82*, 733–740.

Dallego, M.P. & Moely, B.E. (1980). Free recall in boys of normal and poor reading levels as a function of task manipulation. *Journal of Experimental Child Psychology*, *30*, 62–78.

Daneman, M. & Carpenter, P.A. (1980). Individual differences in working memory and reading. *Journal of Verbal Learning and Behavior*, *19*, 450–466.

Daneman, M. & Carpenter, P.A. (1983). Individual differences in integrating information between and within sentences. *Journal of Experimental Psychology: Learning, Memory & Cognition*, *9*, 561–584.

Dawson, M.H., Hallahan, D.P., Reeve, R.E., & Ball, D.W. (1980). The effect of reinforcement and verbal rehearsal on selective attention in learning-disabled children. *Journal of Abnormal Child Psychology*, *8*, 133–144.

Dempster, F.N. & Cooney, J.B. (1982). Individual differences in digit span, susceptibility to proactive interference, and aptitude/achievement test scores. *Intelligence*, *6*, 399–416.

Elbert, J.C. (1984). Short-term memory encoding and memory search in the word recognition of learning-disabled children. *Journal of Learning Disabilities*, *17*, 342–345.

Ericsson, K.A. & Simon, H.A. (1980). Verbal reports as data. *Psychological Review*, *87*, 215–251.

Fodor, J. (1983). *Modularity of mind*. Cambridge, MA: M.I.T. Press.

Foorman, B.R. (1989). What's specific about reading disability: An introduction to the special series. *Journal of Learning Disabilities*, *22*, 332–333.

Fox, B. & Routh, D.K. (1975). Analyzing spoken language into words, syllables and phonemes: A developmental study. *Journal of Psycholinguistic Research*, *4*, 331–342.

Fox, B. & Routh, D.K. (1983). Reading disability, phonemic analysis and dysphonetic spelling: A follow-up study. *Journal of Clinical Child Psychology*, *12*, 28–32.

French, J.W., Ekstrom, R., & Price, L. (1963). *Kit of reference tests for cognitive factors*. Princeton, NJ: Educational Testing Service.

Garner, R. (1988). Verbal report data on cognitive and metacognitive strategies. In C. Weinsteinn, E. Goetz, & P. Alexander (Eds.), *Learning and study strategies: Issues in assessment, instruction, and evaluation* (pp. 63–76). San Diego: Academic Press.

Gelzheiser, L.M., Cort, R., & Shephard, M.J. (1987). Is minimal strategy instruction sufficient for learning disabled students? *Learning Disability Quarterly*, *10*, 267–275.

Gelzheiser, L.M., Solar, R.A., Shephard, M.J., & Wozniak, R.H. (1983). Teaching learning disabled children to memorize: Rationale for plans and practice. *Journal of Learning Disabilities, 16,* 421–425.

Ginsburg, H.P., Kossan, N.E., Schwartz, R., & Swanson, D. (1983). Protocol methods in research on mathematical thinking. In H.P. Ginsburg (Ed.), *The development of mathematical thinking* (pp. 8–46). Orlando, FL: Academic Press.

Glass, G. (1977). Integrating findings: The meta-analysis of research. *Review of research in education* (Vol. 5, pp. 351–379).

Goetz, J.P. & LeCompte, M.D. (1984). *Ethnographic and qualitative designs in educational research.* Orlando, FL: Academic Press.

Haines, D. & Torgesen, J.K. (1979). The effects of incentives on short-term memory and rehearsal in reading disabled children. *Learning Disability Quarterly, 2,* 18–55.

Hall, J., Wilson, K., Humphreys, M., Tinzmann, M., & Bowyer, P. (1983). Phonemic-similarity effects in good vs poor readers. *Memory & Cognition, 11,* 520–527.

Hallahan, D.P. & Reeve, R. (1980). Selective attention and distractibility. In B. Keogh (Ed.), *Advances in special education* (pp. 141–182). Greenwich, CT: JAI Press.

Johnson, R.S., Rugg, M., & Scott, T. (1987). Phonological similarity effects, memory span and developmental reading disorders. *British Journal of Psychology, 78,* 205–211.

Jorm, A.F. (1983). Specific reading retardation and work memory: A review. *British Journal of Psychology, 74,* 311–342.

Juel, C. (1988). Learning to read and write: A longtitudinal study of fifty-four children from first through fourth grade. *Journal of Educational Psychology, 80,* 437–447.

Kolligian, J. & Sternberg, R.J. (1987). Intelligence, information processing, and specific learning disabilities: A triarchic synthesis. *Journal of Learning Disabilities, 20,* 8–17.

Koorland, M.A. & Wolking, W.D. (1982). Effect of reinforcement on modality of stimulus control in learning. *Learning Disability Quarterly, 5,* 264–273.

Kyllonen, P.C. & Christal, R.E. (1990). Reasoning ability is (little more than) working-memory capacity?! *Intelligence, 14,* 389–433.

Lehman, E.B. & Brady, K.M. (1982). Presentation modality and taxonomic category as encoding dimensions from good and poor readers. *Journal of Learning Disabilities, 15,* 103–105.

Lovett, M.W. (1987). A developmental approach to reading disability: Accuracy and speed criteria of normal and deficient reading skill. *Child Development, 58,* 234–260.

Lundberg, I., Frost, J., & Peterson, O.P. (1988). Effects of an extensive program for stimulating phonological awareness in preschool children. *Reading Research Quarterly, 23,* 264–284.

MacLean, M., Bryant, P., & Bradley, L. (1987). Rhymes, nursery rhymes, and reading in early childhood. *Merrill-Palmer Quarterly, 33,* 255–281.

Manis, F.R. (1985). Acquisition of word identification skills in normal and disabled readers. *Journal of Educational Psychology, 27,* 28–90.

Mazer, S.R., McIntyre, C.W., Murray, M.E., Till, R.E., & Blackwell, S.L. (1983). Visual persistence and information pick-up in learning disabled children. *Journal of Learning Disabilities*, *16*, 221–225.

McIntyre, C.W., Murray, M.E., Coronin, C.M., & Blackwell, S.L. (1978). Span of apprehension in learning disabled boys. *Journal of Learning Disabilities*, *11*, 13–20.

Moely, B.E., Hart, S.S., Santulli, K., Leal, L., Johnson, T., & Rao, N. (1986). How do teachers teach memory skill? *Educational Psychologist*, *21*, 55–57.

Morais, J., Bertelson, P., Cary, L., & Algeria, J. (1986). Literacy training and speech segmentation. *Cognition*, *24*, 45–64.

Morrison, F.J., Giordani, B., & Nagy, J. (1977). Reading disability: An information processing analysis. *Science*, *196*, 77–79.

Morrison, S.R. & Siegel, L.S. (1991). Arithmetic disability: Theoretical considerations and empirical evidence for this subtype. In L.V. Feagans, E.J. Short, & L.J. Meltzer (Eds.), *Subtypes of learning disabilities: Theoretical perspectives and research* (pp. 189–209). Hillsdale, NJ: Erlbaum.

Neisser, U. (1967). *Cognitive psychology*. New York: Appleton-Century-Crofts.

Olson, R.K., Wise, B., Conners, F., Rack, J., & Fulker, D. (1989). Specific deficits in component reading and language skills: Genetic and environmental influences. *Journal of Learning Disabilities*, *22*, 339–348.

Olson, R.K., Wise, B., Conners, F., & Rack, J. (1990). Organization, heritability, and remediation of component word recognition and language skills in disabled readers. In J.A. Carr & B.A. Levy (Eds.), *Reading and its development: Component skills approaches*. New York: Academic Press.

Palinscar, A.S. & Brown, A.L. (1984). Reciprocal teaching of comprehension-fostering and comprehension-monitoring activities. *Cognition and Instruction*, *1*, 117–175.

Paris, S.G., Cross, D.R., & Lipson, M.Y. (1984). Informed strategies for learning: A program to improve children's reading awareness and comprehension. *Journal of Educational Psychology*, *76*, 1239–1252.

Pennington, B.F., Van Orden, G.C., Smith, S.D., Green, P.A., & Haith, M.M. (1990). Phonological processing skills and deficits in adult dyslexics. *Child Development*, *61*, 1753–1778.

Perfetti, C.A., Beck, I., Bell, L.C., & Hughes, C. (1987). Phonemic knowledge and learning to read are reciprocal: A longitudinal study of first grade children. *Merrill-Palmer Quarterly*, *33*, 283–319.

Pratt, A.C. & Brady, S. (1988). Relation of phonological awareness to reading disability in children and adults. *Journal of Educational Psychology*, *80*, 319–323.

Pressley, M., Johnson, C.J., & Symons, S. (1987). Elaborating to learn and learning to elaborate. *Journal of Learning Disabilities*, *20*, 76–91.

Pressley, M., Scruggs, T.E., & Mastropieri, M.A. (1989). Memory strategy research in learning disabilities: Present and future directions. *Learning Disabilities Research*, *4*, 68–77.

Richie, D. & Aten, J. (1976). Auditory retention of nonverbal and verbal sequential stimuli in children with reading disabilities. *Journal of Learning Disabilities*, *9*, 54–60.

Samuels, S.J. (1987a). Information processing and reading. *Journal of Learning Disabilities*, *20*, 18–22.

Samuels, S.J. (1987b). Why is it difficult to characterize the underlying cognitive deficits in special education populations? *Exceptional Children*, *54*, 60–62.

Schneider, W. & Pressley, M. (1989). *Memory development between 2 and 20.* New York: Springer-Verlag.

Scruggs, T.E. & Mastropieri, M.A. (1989). Mnemonic instruction of LD students: A field-based evaluation. *Learning Disability Quarterly, 12,* 119–125.

Scruggs, T.E., Mastropieri, M.A., Levin, J.R., & Gaffney, J.S. (1987). Facilitating the acquisition of science facts in learning disabled students. *American Educational Research Journal, 22,* 575–586.

Sergeant, J.A. & Scholten, C.A. (1983). A stages-of-information approach to hyperactivity. *Journal of Child Psychology and Psychiatry and Allied Disciplines, 24*(1), 49–60.

Shankweiler, D., Liberman, I.Y., Mark, S.L., Fowler, L.A., & Fischer, F.W. (1979). The speech code and learning to read. *Journal of Experimental Psychology: Human, Learning, & Memory, 5,* 531–545.

Shephard, M., Gelzheiser, L., & Solar, R. (1985). How good is the evidence for a production deficiency among learning disabled students? *Journal of Educational Psychology, 77,* 533–561.

Siegel, L.S. & Linder, B.A. (1984). Short-term memory processing in children with reading and arithmetic learning disabilities, *Developmental Psychology, 20,* 200–207.

Siegel, L.S. & Ryan, E.B. (1988). Development of grammatical-sensitivity, phonological, and short-term memory skills in normally achieving and learning disabled children. *Developmental Psychology, 24,* 28–37.

Siegel, L.S. & Ryan, E.B. (1989). The development of working memory in normally achieving and subtypes of learning disabled children. *Child Development, 60,* 973–980.

Stanovich, K.E. (1986). Matthew effects in reading: Some consequences of individual differences in the acquisition of literacy. *Reading Research Quarterly, 21,* 360–407.

Stanovich, K.E. (1988). Explaining the differences between the dyslexic and the garden-variety poor reader: The phonological-core variable-difference model. *Journal of Learning Disabilities, 21,* 590–605.

Stanovich, K.E., Cunningham, A.E., & Cramer, B.C. (1984). Assessing phonological awareness in kindergarten children: Issues of task comparability. *Journal of Experimental Child Psychology, 38,* 175–190.

Sternberg, R.J. (1981). Intelligence and nonentrenchment. *Journal of Educational Psychology, 73,* 1–16.

Sternberg, R.J. (1987). A unified theory of intellectual exceptionality. In J.D. Day & Borkowski, J. (Eds.), *Intelligence and exceptionality: New directions for theory, assessment, and instructional practices* (pp. 135–172). Norwood, NJ: Ablex.

Swanson, H.L. (1978). Verbal coding effects on the visual short-term memory of learning disabled and normal readers. *Journal of Educational Psychology, 70,* 539–544.

Swanson, H.L. (1981). Vigilance deficit in learning disabled children: A signal detection analysis. *Journal of Child Psychology and Psychiatry, 22,* 393–399.

Swanson, H.L. (1982). Conceptual process as a function of age and enforced attention in learning-disabled children. *Contemporary Educational Psychology, 7,* 152–160.

Swanson, H.L. (1983a). A developmental study of vigilance in learning disabled and non-disabled children. *Journal of Abnormal Child Psychology, 11,* 415–429.

Swanson, H.L. (1983b). A study of nonstrategic linguistic coding on visual recall of learning disabled and normal readers. *Journal of Learning Disabilities*, *16*, 209–216.

Swanson, H.L. (1983c). Relations among metamemory, rehearsal activity and word recall in learning disabled and nondisabled readers. *British Journal of Educational Psychology*, *53*, 186–194.

Swanson, H.L. (1984a). Does theory guide teaching practice? *Remedial and Special Education*, *5*, 7–16.

Swanson, H.L. (1984b). Effects of cognitive effort and word distinctiveness on learning disabled and nondisabled readers' recall. *Journal of Educational Psychology*, *76*, 894–908.

Swanson, H.L. (1986). Do semantic memory deficiencies underlie disabled readers' encoding processes? *Journal of Experimental Child Psychology*, *41*, 461–488.

Swanson, H.L. (1987). Verbal coding deficits in the recall of pictorial information in learning disabled readers: The influence of a lexical system. *American Educational Research Journal*, *24*, 143–170.

Swanson, H.L. (1988). Learning disabled children's problem solving: Identifying mental processes underlying intelligent performances. *Intelligence*, *12*, 261–278.

Swanson, H.L. (1989). Central processing strategy differences in gifted, average, learning disabled, and mentally retarded children. *Journal of Experimental Child Psychology*, *47*, 370–397.

Swanson, H.L. (1990a). Intelligence and learning disabilities. In H.L. Swanson & B.K. Keogh (Eds.), *Learning disabilities and research issues* (pp. 97–113). Hillsdale, NJ: Erlbaum.

Swanson, H.L. (1990b). Influence of metacognitive knowledge and aptitude on problem solving. *Journal of Educational Psychology*, *82*, 306–314.

Swanson, H.L. (1991). A subgroup analysis of learning-disabled and skilled readers' working memory: In search of a model of reading comprehension. In L.V. Feagans, E.J. Short, & L.J. Meltzer (Eds.), *Subtypes of learning disabilities: Theoretical perspectives and research* (pp. 209–228). Hillsdale, NJ: Erlbaum.

Swanson, H.L. (in preparation). Metaanalysis of memory research on children with learning disabilities. University of California-Riverside.

Swanson, H.L. (in press). Executive processing in learning disabled readers. *Intelligence*.

Swanson, H.L. (1992). The generability and modifiability of working memory in skilled and less-skilled readers. *Journal of Educational Psychology*, *84*, 473–488.

Swanson, H.L., Cochran, K.F., & Ewers, C.A. (1989). Working memory and reading disabilities. *Journal of Abnormal Child Psychology*, *17*, 745–756.

Swanson, H.L., Cochran, K.F., & Ewers, C.A. (1990). Can learning disabilities be determined from working memory performance? *Journal of Learning Disabilities*, *23*, 59–67.

Swanson, H.L. & Cooney, J.B. (1991). Learning disabilities and memory. In B.Y.L. Wong (Ed.), *Learning about learning disabilities* (pp. 104–122). San Diego, CA: Academic Press.

Swanson, H.L. & Rathgeber, A. (1986). The effects of organizational dimensions on learning disabled readers' recall. *Journal of Educational Research*, *79*, 155–162.

Swanson, H.L., Reffel, J., & Trahan, M. (1990). Naturalistic memory in learning disabled and skilled readers. *Journal of Abnormal Child Psychology, 19,* 117–148.

Swanson, H.L. & Trahan, M. (1992). Learning disabled readers' comprehension of computer mediated text: The influence of working memory, metacognition, and attribution, *Learning Disability Research & Practice, 7,* 74–86.

Tarver, S.G., Hallahan, D.P., Kauffman, J.M., & Ball, D.W. (1976). Verbal rehearsal and selective attention in children with learning disabilities: A developmental lag. *Journal of Experimental Child Psychology, 22,* 375–385.

Torgesen, J.K. (1978). Memorization process in reading-disabled children. *Journal of Educational Psychology, 69,* 571–578.

Torgesen, J.K. (1988). Studies of children with learning disabilities who perform poorly on memory span tasks. *Journal of Learning Disabilities, 21,* 605–612.

Torgesen, J.K. & Goldman, T. (1977). Rehearsal and short-term memory in second-grade reading disabled children. *Child Development, 48,* 56–61.

Torgesen, J.K. & Houck, D.G. (1980). Processing deficiencies of learning-disabled children who perform poorly on the digit span test. *Journal of Educational Psychology, 72*(2), 141–160.

Torgesen, J.K., Rashotte, J., Greenstein, J., & Portes, P. (1991). Further studies of learning disabled children with severe performance problems on the digit span test. *Learning Disabilities: Research & Practice, 6,* 134–145.

Tunmer, W.E., Herriman, M.L., & Teasdale, A.R. (1988). Metalinguistic abilities and beginning reading. *Reading Research Quarterly, 23,* 134–158.

Wagner, R. & Sternberg, R.J. (1984). Alternative conceptions of intelligence and their implications for education. *Review of Educational Research, 54,* 179–223.

Wong, B.Y.L. (1982). Strategic behaviors in selecting retrieval cues in gifted, normal achieving and learning disabled children. *Journal of Learning Disabilities, 15,* 33–37.

Wong, B.Y.L. (1991). Assessment of metacognitive research in learning disabilities: Theory, research and practice. In H.L. Swanson (Ed.), *Handbook on the assessment of learning disabilities: Theory, research and practice* (pp. 265–284). Austin TX: PRO-ED.

Wong, B.Y.L. & Jones, W. (1982). Increasing metacomprehension in learning-disabled and normally-achieving students through self-questioning training. *Learning Disability Quarterly, 5,* 228–240.

Wong, B.Y.L., Wong, R., & Foth, D. (1977). Recall and clustering of verbal materials among normal and poor readers. *Bulletin of the Psychonomic Society, 10,* 375–378.

Worden, P.E. (1986). Comprehension and memory for prose in the learning disabled. In S.J. Ceci (Ed.), *Handbook of cognitive social and neuropsychological aspects of learning disabilities* (Vol. 1, pp. 241–262). Hillsdale, NJ: Erlbaum.

Worden, P.E. & Nakamura, G.V. (1983). Story comprehension and recall in learning-disabled vs. normal college students. *Journal of Educational Psychology, 74,* 633–639.

Yopp, H.K. (1988). The validity and reliability of phonemic awareness tests. *Reading Research Quarterly, 23,* 159–177.

14
Social Assessments of Students with Learning Disabilities: Do They Measure Up?

Sharon Vaughn and Diane Haager

This chapter examines social assessments frequently used with students with learning disabilities. While there are a number of teacher and parent rating scales of social skills and behavior problems, this chapter will not address these measures (see for review, Gresham, 1986). Instead, this chapter will examine assessment procedures that relate to three increasingly important factors of childhood social competence: peer ratings and nominations, observations, and measures of self-perception.

Peer Reports: Ratings and Nominations of Social Competence

The resurgence of interest in the social functioning of children that has occurred in the last 10 years (Hartup, 1990) has resulted in an increased interest in the application and interpretation of sociometrics. Peer reports have been used as indices of aggression, social status, social skills, and overall social functioning (LaGreca, 1990). Peers provide a very important perspective on the social competence of youngsters, and their perspective is predictive of later outcomes such as adjustment, school success, and success in the workplace (see for review, Parker & Asher, 1987). In a classic study conducted by Cowen, Pederson, Babigian, Izzo, and Trost (1973), early peer rejection was the best predictor of later psychiatric problems; a better predictor than even teacher ratings, self-report data, achievement scores, and evaluations by mental health professionals. The results of this study have supplied significant credence to peers' evaluations. Also, adults are not always able to directly observe social interactions among peers, and thus peers are better able to reflect on social behaviors of which adults may be unaware (Lancelotta & Vaughn, 1989).

Peer reports, specifically sociometrics, have been identified as the criterion measure by which social skills training programs should be evaluated (Gresham, 1986; McIntosh, Vaughn, & Zaragoza, 1991). Since students who have poor skills in interacting with peers are often the targets for social skills training, the ultimate test of the effects of the social skills training might very well be increased positive perceptions by peers. Thus, procedures for assessing peers' perceptions of the social functioning of others in their social group are an important source for assessing social functioning and evaluating the effects of social intervention programs.

Definition of Sociometrics

There are many definitions of sociometry. Moreno (1934), considered the father of sociometry, restricted the criteria to requiring the students to make an emotional response, and the referent to include a real-life situation. According to Moreno, a sentence such as "Name the child in your class you would most like to have spend the night," would qualify because it contains an emotional response ("like"), and a real-life referent ("spending the night"). While these two criteria frequently occur in present-day application of sociometrics, there are examples of using sociometric ratings with only one criterion. For example, "Tell me the names of the three classmates you like best," includes an emotional response ("like"), but does not include a referent. Similar to the definitions proposed by others (e.g., McConnell & Odom, 1986), the definition of sociometry we suggest is *preferential responses to the social functioning of known peers*. Children's preferential responses to the social functioning of their peers are frequently obtained in one of two ways: peer ratings and peer nominations.

Peer Ratings of Social Acceptance

Ratings of peer likability are the most frequent application of peer sociometrics for assessing the social acceptance of youngsters. Peer ratings require youngsters to rate their feelings about selected peers on a Likert-type scale indicating how much they like the target peer. Each rating scale is assigned a weighted value that ranges from 3 points to 7 points. In our own work, we use a 3-point scale with younger children (through first grade) and then convert to a 4-point scale (after first grade, e.g., Vaughn, Haager, Hogan, & Kouzehanani, 1992). With young children (kindergarten and younger) we show them three pictures; a happy face, a neutral face, and an unhappy face. Using familiar examples such as food, cartoon characters, and activities (e.g., swimming), students are given trial examples to indicate the extent to which they like the example by pointing at the picture that best represents how they feel. For example: "Point to the face that indicates how much you like to eat ice cream. Now, point to the face that shows how much you like to clean your room." After the students understand the procedures, they are asked to indicate, by pointing at the faces, how they feel about selected classmates. Each of the faces is assigned a weighted value and the child's response to each of the selected peers is recorded. Each target student's level of acceptance is computed as the mean of all of the raters. Children who are in second grade or older are supplied a roster of names and asked to indicate how much they like each of the target students by circling the number that best indicates their preference on a Likert-type scale.

Peer sociometric rating scales have been found to be a valid and reliable index of peer relations for both preschool and elementary school children (Asher & Hymel, 1981; Asher, Markell, & Hymel, 1981; Drewry & Clark, 1983; Hayvren & Hymel, 1984). The Peer Acceptance Scale, used with students with learning disabilities as well as mentally retarded and nonhandicapped youngsters, revealed a stability coefficient above .75 (Sainato, Zigmond, & Strain, 1983). Overall, rating scale scores appear to be more reliable than nominations (Thompson & Powell, 1951) in assessing social functioning.

Despite the widespread use of ratings of peer acceptance, there are several considerations regarding their use, particularly with their application to students with learning disabilities (LD). One potential difficulty is the effect of the "stem" on children's ratings of students. To illustrate how the "stem" might influence children's ratings, consider whether the following stems would yield the same response: "How much do you like the following children? How much would you like to be friends with each of the following children? How much would you like to play with each child? How much would you like to work with each child?" The effects of the stem on students' ratings of others has not been empirically investigated, but is likely to be important when attaining sociometric information about students with learning disabilities. It is quite possible that students with learning disabilities would be highly liked by their peers, but receive low ratings for how much their peers would like to work with them because of their low academic functioning. It seems that "like" and "play with" questions would yield similar responses, but the results may be influenced by other factors such as sex and age and ability in selected areas. For example, one would expect that with middle elementary and older boys, responses to "play with" questions would be influenced by the peer's ability to succeed in sports. Again, it may be that a male student with learning disabilities is well liked but is extremely unsuccessful in sports. Thus, it would be expected that this student's scores on how much others would like to "play with" him might be deflated, and not give a true score of how well the student was accepted by peers. We suggest that if one is addressing the extent to which students are accepted by classmates, a stem such as "How much do you like——" would be the most useful. In summary, researchers need to consider carefully the possible multiple interpretations to their questions and thus how these interpretations could influence outcomes.

The most frequent use of peer rating scales is to determine how a target child (e.g., LD child) is perceived by classmates. Typically, the mean rating for the LD student is compared with mean ratings for others in the class. This information indicates how the LD student on the average is perceived by classmates and how the LD student's rating compares with others in the same group. Mean peer rating data, however, does not inform as to whether the student has peers who like him a lot or dislike him a lot. Using a 5-point Likert scale one student could receive ratings of 2s, 3s, and 4s, obtaining an average of 3.0. Another student could obtain several 5s and several 1s, also obtaining an average of 3.0, but demonstrating a completely different friendship pattern than the first student. Thus it is important to consider more than just the target student's mean rating; the frequency of extreme scores (like a lot; dislike a lot) also provide valuable information about the student's level of acceptance.

Other than determining how the target student is perceived on the average by others, additional information of importance can be addressed with peer rating scales. One issue is the notion of reciprocal friendships. A reciprocal friendship is when the same two students provide similarly high ratings of each other in terms of likability, or in the case of nominations (discussed in the next section), choose each other as best friends. A single reciprocal friendship may ease the negative consequences associated with low peer acceptance or rejection from other peers. Howes (1987) reports that rejected children with reciprocal friendships had easier entry into play groups than rejected students who did not have reciprocal friendships. Little is known about the reciprocal friendships of students with learning disabilities, and the impact of a single reciprocal friendship on their social support, self-perception, and overall adjustment. We feel that this is an important area for future research, as a single reciprocal friendship may "buffer" the negative effects associated with low peer acceptance from others.

Peer Nominations

Nominations differ from ratings in that all students in the social group are not rated and the rater must identify a specified number of peers who fit the criteria. The Guess Who? technique is a frequently used peer assessment in which a number of attributes of hypothetical students are provided and students are asked to write the name of the student they know who best fits the description (Lesser, 1959; Shapiro & Sobel, 1981). For example, in a study conducted by Lancelotta and Vaughn (1989), they applied the Guess Who procedures of Lesser (1959) to identify subtypes of aggressive children (see Table 14.1).

Nominations are most frequently used to determine the social status of students. Social status refers to the youngster's social type: popular, rejected, neglected, controversial. Children from the child's peer group (frequently his/her class) are asked to nominate their 3 best friends and

TABLE 14.1. Subtypes of aggression: Guess who? nominations.

Provoked physical aggression
This boy or girl will fight, but only if someone picks on him or her.
This classmate will always fight back if you hit him or her.

Outburst aggression
This classmate gets very, very mad at times all of a sudden.
This classmate gets so mad at times that he or she doesn't know what they are doing.

Unprovoked physical aggression
This classmate starts a fight for no reason.
This classmate gets mad while he or she is playing and ends up in a fight.
This classmate is always looking for a fight.

Verbal aggression
This boy or girl often threatens other kids.
This classmate always puts others down when playing a game with other kids.

Indirect aggression
This boy or girl tattles to the teacher about what other kids do.
This classmate breaks things on purpose that belong to others.

the 3 students they like least. Peery (1979) identified *social impact* as a measure of the influence the child has on the peer group and *calculated social impact* by adding the number of positive and negative nominations. *Social preference* was identified as the extent to which the child, overall, was liked by peers. Based on social impact and social preference, types of social status could be identified: popular (high impact, high preference) and rejected (low impact, low preference). Coie, Dodge, and Coppotelli (1982) extended the work of Peery (1979) and identified other social status types: neglected (low impact, low preference) and controversial (high impact, low preference).

In a recent study assessing the stability of peer nominations in kindergartners, Wasik (1987) reported a 5-month test-retest correlation of .76 for negative nominations and .57 for positive nominations. For elementary age and older students peer nominations have been reported as moderately stable for a 1- to 2-year period ($rs = .52$ and $.42$) (Roff, Sells, & Golden, 1972), and for a 4-year period ($r = .89$) (Northway, 1969). Gresham (1981), however, reports considerably lower test-retest correlations across a 6-week period ranging from .19 to .62.

Gresham (1981) and Asher and Taylor (1981) have empirically demonstrated that peer ratings and peer nominations do not measure the same thing. Thus, it has been recommended by several sources (Asher & Taylor, 1981; McConnell & Odom, 1986) that if you are interested in studying social acceptance you should use peer ratings, and if you are interested in studying social status types (e.g., popularity and rejection) you should use nominations.

Ratings of Social Skills

Considerable attention has focused on the development and interpretation of peer friendship ratings and nominations (see for reviews, Landau & Milich, 1990; McConnell & Odom, 1986). Surprisingly little work, however, has addressed peers' perceptions of the social behaviors of children in their social group. While teacher and parent measures of social and behavioral adjustment abound (Achenbach, 1990; Gresham & Elliott, 1990; Quay & Peterson, 1987; Walker & McConnell, 1988), few if any scales to assess peers' ratings of the social behaviors of their classmates have been developed or used.

In an attempt to provide a basis for peer assessment, Walker (1990) developed a peer rating of prosocial behavior (PRPB). The PRPB scale was based on an adapted version (Vaughn & Hogan, 1990) of the Social Skills Rating Scale for Teachers (Gresham & Elliott, 1986) and included items that represented two dimensions of social skills: outgoing/initiating and cooperating/responding. Three items from each of the two dimensions of the adapted version of the Social Skills Rating Scale for Teachers that had the highest factor loadings were selected and reworded for peer evaluation. Walker (1990) reports reliability for the PRPB scale of .85. Each student rates every other student on a 1 (*never*) to 4 (*all of the time*) scale on the extent to which they feel the target child demonstrates the identified prosocial behaviors. The six behaviors used in this scale are provided in Table 14.2. Since adults may have a different interpretation of the social behaviors of children, peers' perspectives on their social behavior provides further information on their social functioning. This information might be particularly valuable in determining the types of social behaviors target students need to learn.

Peer ratings and nominations are frequently used measures that demonstrate high reliability, validity, and predictive power with respect

TABLE 14.2. Peer ratings of prosocial behavior.

Directions: Children are to rate each target peer on the frequency with which they feel the target child demonstrates the prosocial behaviors that follow.

1 = Never; 2 = Not very often; 3 = Pretty much; 4 = All of the time

1. This child invites others to play with him/her.
2. This child makes friends easily.
3. This child plays/participates in games with other children.
4. This child can control his/her temper (doesn't get real angry) when he/she disagrees with others.
5. This child does something else instead of hitting when other children tease him/her.
6. This child can control himself/herself when other children tell lies about him/her.

Items 1–3 correspond with the Outgoing/Initiating Dimension
Items 4–6 correspond with the Cooperating/Responding Dimension

to such important outcomes as adjustment and later school and work success. Despite their importance there are several points that should be considered when using peer ratings and nominations.

Issues Related to the Use of Sociometrics with Students with Learning Disabilities

While considerable research support for the negative effects of low peer acceptance with children exists (for review, see Parker & Asher, 1987), the targets of this research have not been youngsters with learning disabilities and thus the extent to which these results generalize to LD students is unknown. While there is no compelling evidence that previous research with non–learning disabled groups does not apply, there simply has been no test of its application to this population. We have an insufficient data base to determine the impact of low peer acceptance on the later functioning of students with learning disabilities. Additionally, we know little about the variables that mediate the negative effects of poor peer acceptance with students with learning disabilities. It is possible, for example, that such variables as social support from the family or a single, long-lasting reciprocal friendship could mediate the impact of low peer acceptance.

When using nominations, one of the major disadvantages is that each child rates relatively few other children. For example, if you are interested in friendship, each student usually nominates his/her three best friends and the three persons they least like. Thus, we know how the student feels about six children in the group but we know little about how the student feels about the other children.

Another concern with nominations is the use of negative nominations. Many school personnel are concerned with the possible negative side effects from asking students to identify classmates they like least, or the possibility that by requesting dislike nominations they are condoning the behavior (Asher & Hymel, 1981). Though this concern is highly reasonable, there appears to be little evidence to suggest that there are negative outcomes from the process (Bell-Dorlan, Foster, & Sikora, 1989; Hayvren & Hymel, 1984). Students' negative interactions do not increase following the administration of peer sociometrics, and children report that they enjoy participating in studies involving sociometrics (Bell-Dorlan, Foster, & Sikora, 1989).

Sampling problems are particulary troublesome when gathering peer measures. Most peer ratings are conducted within the child's classroom. Thus, parent permission from all students in the class to participate in the study is an extremely important factor. In an elementary classroom with 25 students and a high permission return rate to participate in the study, say 75%, or about 19 students, would participate. If there are equal numbers of boys and girls, and if you are examining same-sex nominations, there are approximately 9 students for the child to select from as his/her best or least liked friend. Often, nominations are used with even fewer students, 6–8, thus most of the students in the candidate pool must be ranked as either best or least liked friend. If you are interested in reciprocal friendships, particularly with students who are rejected, the problem of not having permission for all students in the peer group to participate becomes a bigger problem. If one reciprocal friendship can potentially "buffer" the negative effects of rejection, knowing if a student has a single other person who likes him/her in the same way he/she is liked by the target student is essential information. Without full class participation, reciprocal friendships are limited to those students who participate; thus it is impossible to rule out the possibility that a reciprocal friendship exists.

An important issue when interpreting sociometrics with students with learning disabilities is to consider the extent to which the target student is known by the classmates who are completing the evaluation. This is more likely an issue with students with learning disabilities than with non–LD students, because LD students are frequently out of the room for as much as 50% of the school day and during instructional time (Gelzheiser & Meyers, 1991). Thus, when conducting sociometrics with students with learning disabilities it is important to determine how well they know the target student, as well as how they feel about the target student, because the implications for intervention would then be quite different.

For example, if a student was not very well known and received low ratings of peer acceptance, an intervention that focused on increasing classmates' knowledge of the target student, such as the mutual interest group (Fox, 1989), would be an appropriate intervention. Fox (1989) hypothesized that when students were more familiar with each other and knew more about each other's likes and dislikes, hobbies, and interests, they would be more likely to view the other person positively because they would be able to identify ways that they and the target student were alike. She paired low-accepted LD students with high-accepted classmates for approximately 40 minutes once each week. During these sessions student pairs interviewed each other on preassigned topics such as entertainment, hobbies, and sports. Following the interview each partner wrote three items he/she discovered he/she had in common with his/her partner about the topic. They also participated in art exercises and journal-keeping that focused on getting to know each partner better. Partners who participated in the mutual interest group demonstrated higher ratings of their partners over time than did partners in a control group. It is possible that the low acceptance of many students with learning disabilities can be attributed to their being less well known by their classmates, and thus intervention programs like the one described by Fox are effective with students who meet that criteria.

However, if the student is reasonably well known but is low accepted then it is likely that the student would benefit from learning social skills that would enhance his/her ability to make and maintain friends (Hazel Schumaker, Sherman, & Sheldon, 1982). Hazel, et al. (1982) have identified eight critical social skills (giving positive feedback, giving negative feedback, resisting peer pressure, problem solving, negotiation, following directions, and conversation) and nine basic steps for teaching each of the social skills (review, explain, provide rationale, give example, examine, model, verbal rehearsal, behavioral rehearsal, and homework). If a student appeared to need to get to know others in the social group better, as well as increase social skills, then an intervention that combines both would be more appropriate (see for example, Vaughn, McIntosh, & Spencer-Rowe, 1991).

An example of a peer rating form that includes ratings of both how well the student is known and how well the student is liked is contained in Table 14.3.

Determining the extent to which the rater knows the target student is an important aspect of using and interpreting sociometrics with LD students. A second important aspect of using and interpreting sociometrics with LD students is considering who should be doing the rating of the LD student (e.g., regular classroom classmates, special education classmates). The answer to this question depends a lot on the research question addressed. If the research question concerns how the LD student is perceived by classmates from the perspective of students in the regular classroom, then the raters are regular classroom peers. If, however, the research question involves identifying the extent to which the LD student has friends or is liked by others, then a broader rating pool that includes both students from the regular classroom and students from the resource room would be appropriate. If possible, the extent to which the target student with learning disabilities has friends outside of the school setting would also provide additional valuable data sources. Few studies have considered multiple sources and settings for obtaining peer acceptance ratings on students with learning disabilities (Coben & Zigmond, 1986).

By far the greatest number of sociometric studies have been conducted with LD elementary students, with considerably fewer conducted with middle and high school students (see for review, Dudley-Marling & Edmiaston, 1985). There are many difficulties to overcome when evaluating the social status of secondary students. The most formidable might be selecting the setting in which to conduct the social status evaluations. With secondary students there is no single cohort of students who spend an extensive amount of time together, so the researcher must decide if he/she is going to randomly select a content area class (with academic performance bias as the result), the homeroom class (with the possibility that others in the class have little or no contact with the target student), or conduct ratings in a physical education (PE) class, which might provide

TABLE 14.3. Peer rating: How well do you know, how well do you like.

School ————————————————— Teacher —————————————————

Your name ————————————————— Male ——————— Female ———————

Directions: Please circle the number that best represents each person listed below. Cross out
your own name.

> 1—not at all
> 2—not much
> 3—pretty much
> 4—very much

Child's name	How well do you know				How much do you LIKE			
1.	1	2	3	4	1	2	3	4
2.	1	2	3	4	1	2	3	4
3.	1	2	3	4	1	2	3	4
4.	1	2	3	4	1	2	3	4
5.	1	2	3	4	1	2	3	4
6.	1	2	3	4	1	2	3	4
7.	1	2	3	4	1	2	3	4
8.	1	2	3	4	1	2	3	4
9.	1	2	3	4	1	2	3	4
10.	1	2	3	4	1	2	3	4
11.	1	2	3	4	1	2	3	4
12.	1	2	3	4	1	2	3	4
13.	1	2	3	4	1	2	3	4
14.	1	2	3	4	1	2	3	4
15.	1	2	3	4	1	2	3	4
16.	1	2	3	4	1	2	3	4
17.	1	2	3	4	1	2	3	4
18.	1	2	3	4	1	2	3	4
19.	1	2	3	4	1	2	3	4
20.	1	2	3	4	1	2	3	4

bias against students who do not perform well in motor activities. Sabornie
and colleagues (Sabornie & Kauffman, 1986; Sabornie, Marshall, & Ellis,
1990) have selected PE classes for data collection with secondary students.

While few studies have been conducted investigating the social status of
secondary students (Perlmutter, Crocker, Cordray, & Garstecki, 1983;

TABLE 14.4. Summary of issues related to the application of sociometrics with students with learning disabilities.

1. Long-term effects of low peer acceptance are documented for non–learning disabled populations only (See Parker & Asher, 1987). The long-term effects of low peer acceptance for students with learning disabilities have not been empirically supported.
2. A major disadvantage to the use of peer nominations is that each student rates relatively few other children.
3. School personnel and parents are frequently concerned about the use of negative nominations for fear it will appear as though they condone students' low regard for other students. Little empirical support for negative consequences associated with the use of negative nominations.
4. Peer ratings and nominations are highly influenced by the participation rate among the cohorts of students providing the evaluation.
5. The extent to which the target student is "known" by the classmates providing the sociometric rating is an important factor when interpreting the target student's overall peer acceptance.
6. The "stem" that is used to assess peer acceptance is likely to influence the peer ratings received by students with learning disabilities. Such stems as, "How much would you like to play with _____," and "How much would you like to work with _____," are likely to yield different results from "How much would you like to be friends with _____."
7. Few studies have been conducted evaluating the peer sociometrics of secondary students with learning disabilities. Procedures for conducting sociometrics with secondary students with learning disabilities are complicated because it is difficult to identify which peer group should evaluate the target student.

Sabornie & Kauffman, 1986), even less is known about the social functioning of adults with learning disabilities, and LD preschoolers and early elementary students (Vaughn, Hogan, Kouzekanani, & Shapiro, 1990). Furthermore, since the social functioning of students with learning disabilities has largely been evaluated in school settings, we are unsure of the extent to which their social difficulties generalize to other settings. A summary of the issues related to the application of sociometrics with students with learning disabilities are provided in Table 14.4.

While peer reports are often considered the sine qua non of social functioning, another important assessment procedure is observation. Though naturalistic observations are difficult to obtain, they can be a valuable source of information on the social functioning of youngsters.

Observation of Social Behavior

Observation as a method of data collection usually involves the direct observation and recording of specific behaviors. Methods of observing social behavior include observation in naturalistic settings, using either time sampling or checklists, and analogue or simulated situations designed to elicit specific responses or behaviors. Though direct observation has been widely used in developmental research with non-LD subjects, it is less common in research with students with learning disabilities. Observation research methods have typically been used to obtain information about the frequency or quality of children's interactions with peers or adults, to investigate the correlates of related variables such as social status or social acceptance, and to evaluate the effectiveness of social or behavioral interventions.

Since observations are both time-consuming and costly to obtain and analyze, consideration should be given to the advantages and disadvantages of their use. An obvious advantage is that behavioral observations are usually less biased than teacher or parent ratings. Secondly, control of the data report is in the hands of the experimenter, unlike the subject's or a third party's (such as teacher or parent) report, and thus reliability can be enhanced by rigorous training and code refinement. Thirdly, with an increasing trend in learning disabilities research to obtain contextual or qualitative information in addition to quantitative data, observation methods provide the ability to focus on classmates, teachers, and environmental factors as well as subjects' behavior. Observational methods are not without limitations, however. A substantial investment of time and effort are required to obtain reliable data. Forness and Guthrie (1977) found that at least four successive observations were necessary to obtain a reliable sample of behavior with 30 kindergartners. This is generally thought to be standard for other populations as well, though it has not been specifically determined with samples of older school-age students and/or students with learning disabilities.

Naturalistic Observation

In naturalistic observation, the focus is on the target behavior(s) in a naturally occurring environment (e.g., classroom, playground, or home settings). Behavioral observation in a naturalistic setting offers the best face validity of all the social measures (Asher & Hymel, 1981; Gresham, 1986; LaGreca & Stark, 1986). Additionally, it is naturalistic observation that best allows for a contextual examination of social behavior (Asher & Hymel, 1981; Bryan, 1974; Gresham, 1981, 1986; Hops, 1983), whereby the time and setting of specific social behaviors behaviors as well as antecedent and subsequent behaviors on the parts of subjects, peers and/or teachers may be observed as they occur naturally.

In early investigations, the frequency or rate of children's social interactions was recorded. This procedure, though it provides ease of data collection, establishment of interrater reliability, and data analysis, is quite limited in scope, providing little information as to the nature or quality of the interactions or the context in which they occurred. Specifically, using this procedure, positive and negative interactions are recorded equally in a frequency count of occurrences of interactions with no regard to the nature of the interaction. Thus, a negative behavior such as gently hitting another child would be coded equivalent with beating up on another child. Therefore, in many subsequent investigations using naturalistic observation, behavioral categories were developed to obtain qualitative as well as quantitative information about children's social behaviors and interactions.

Several of the investigations employing naturalistic observation techniques to compare handicapped with nonhandicapped children have focused on preschool children's positive and negative social interactions. Guralnick (1980) developed a coding procedure in which both the frequency and nature of communicative interactions during free-play times were examined. The frequency of interactions in four communicative categories (positive verbal and nonverbal, and negative verbal and nonverbal), for target children both giving and receiving communication, were recorded using a systematic time-sampling method, revealing that nonhandicapped and mildly handicapped preschoolers interacted with each other more often than with moderately or severely handicapped children. In another study investigating the social interactions of handicapped and nonhandicapped preschoolers, six behavioral categories were used (DeKlyen & Odom, 1989) to record children's social behavior during structured and unstructured play: interaction with peer, negative interaction with peer, proximal play, unoccupied/isolate, and teacher interaction. Using a cyclical scanning procedure, the observer watched a target child for 2 seconds, recorded the behavior, located the next target child during the next 4 seconds, and then repeated the steps, thereby obtaining 10 samples of behavior of 12 children during 12 minutes. Results indicated that the amount of peer interaction for both the handicapped and nonhandicapped groups increased during structured play activities.

The lack of opportunity to observe free play or open interaction in a highly structured and task-oriented environment presents a major difficulty in using naturalistic observation with school-age children. Problems with collecting naturalistic observation data help explain the few studies conducted in which naturalistic observational methods were used with samples of students with learning disabilities (see Table 14.5a for a summary).

Most of the observational research involving students with learning disabilities has been in the area of behavior problems. However, some information about social behaviors can be discerned from this literature. For example, in an investigation of teacher-student interactions in regular classrooms (Dorval, McKinney, & Feagans, 1982), the student-initiated interactions of students with learning disabilities tended to be situationally inappropriate. Teacher-initiated interactions with LD students tended to be related to behavior management due to the students' inattentiveness and rule infractions. In contrast, Slate and Saudargas (1986) observed the classroom behavior of fourth and fifth grade male students with learning

TABLE 14.5a. Summary of research using observation of social behavior of students with learning disabilities in naturalistic settings.

Authors	Sample	Observation method	Other measures	Findings
Bryan (1974)	5 LD boys, 5 NLD boys from same 3rd grade classroom	Observation of LD and NLD pair was rotated every 5 minutes, for a total of five school days. LD students were observed in both regular and special education classes. Behaviors coded: 1. Task-oriented behavior 2. Non–task-oriented behavior 3. Social interactions 4. Waiting	No other measures	There were no group differences in proportion of time spent in either student-teacher interactions or student-peer interactions. There were differences in the patterns of interactions: Teachers were 3 times more likely to respond to verbal initiation of NLD than LD student; peers were more likely to ignore LD than NLD.
Bryan & Bryan (1978)	25 LD students, 25 NLD students matched on sex and ethnicity from same 4th and 5th grade classrooms	Focus was verbal communication: One observer recorded subjects' statements and another recorded peers' statements for periods of 5 minutes. Behaviors coded: 1. Rejection statements 2. Requests for information and materials 3. Self-image 4. Helping/Cooperation/giving Material 5. Positive reinforcement/Social/Consideration 6. Egocentric/Self–comments 7. Reactivity Observations were conducted in physical education and art classes where communication was more free to occur. A total of 30 minutes were recorded for each subject.	Sociometric ratings yielding Social Attraction and Social Rejection scores were used.	LD students more frequently emitted "nasty" statements than NLD; LD students were more often the recipient of rejection statements than NLD; LD received less votes of Social Attraction on the sociometric measure.

Table continued

TABLE 14.5a. *Continued*

Authors	Sample	Observation method	Other measures	Findings
Bryan, Wheeler, Felcan, & Henek (1976)	17 LD and 17 NLD matched on sex and grade from grades 3, 4, and 5	Focus was verbal communication: one observer recorded subjects' statements and another recorded peers' statements for periods of 5 minutes. Behaviors coded: 1. Rejection statements 2. Information source (e.g., asking for advice, directions, permission; or asking for factual information). 3. Self-image 4. Cooperation 5. Competition 6. Helping 7. Consideration 8. Intrusiveness (bossy, shouting, taking over)	Measures of attitudes toward altruism and willingness to donate money were also obtained.	LD students emitted more competitive statements; LD students received less consideration statements from peers; other categories were nonsignificant.
Schumaker, Wildgen, & Sherman (1982)	47 same-sex pairs of LD and NLD, NLD were teacher-identified as "model students," in grades 7–9	Focus on social behaviors: target students' interactions with teachers and peers in the classroom, with the exception of study behaviors such as class discussions. Target student behaviors coded: 1. Attending to teacher 2. Statement to peer/teacher		LD students interacted with peers with the same frequency and duration as NLD. They spoke as often and to as many different peers as NLD. Teacher-student interaction was also very similar for the two groups, with the only difference being that the LD were less attentive.

3. Conversation with peer/teacher
4. Touching peer/teacher
5. Laughing
6. Asking a question to teacher
7. Requesting feedback from teacher
8. Requesting help from teacher
9. Requesting permission from teacher
10. Hand gestures to peer/teacher
11. Posture
12. Grooming appearance
13. General attractiveness
14. Clothing appearance
15. Facial expression
16. Physical abnormalities

Peer/teacher behaviors coded:

1. Statement to target student or the class as a whole
2. Touching target student
3. Positive feedback from teacher
4. Negative feedback from teacher

A larger percentage of the LD students demonstrated physical appearance problems related to grooming, dress, etc.

TABLE 14.5b. Summary of research using observation of social behavior of students with learning disabilities in simulated or role-play situations.

Authors	Sample	Observation method	Other measures	Findings
Bryan, Donahue, & Pearl (1981)	54 LD and 46 NLD matched on sex and grade, in grades 5–8	Observations were conducted in a laboratory setting with a one-way mirror and video recording equipment. Given a group problem-solving task, videotaped transactions were coded for: 1. Persuasion (match between the subject's independent choice and group choice) 2. Discourse strategies (communicative function of conversational turn) 3. Conversational housekeeping (keeping the conversation on task) 4. Affect (positive and negative statements about themselves and others)	No other measures	LD students were less persuasive; i.e., LD students' choices were less likely to be group's choices. LD students were more likely to agree with the group and less likely to argue or disagree. LD students engaged in less "conversational housekeeping."
Bryan, Donahue, Pearl, & Sturm (1981)	20 LD, 20 NLD matched on sex and grade, grades 2 and 4	Role-play situation: "TV talk show." Subject was given socially dominant role of talk show host. Talk show guests were randomly selected peers. Turn-taking, discourse strategies (i.e., questions, responses, confirmations, and conversational devices), and discomfort (i.e., nonverbal behaviors associated with tension or anxiety) were coded in the observations of videotapes.	No other measures	LD "hosts" contributed the same amount of conversation as NLD "hosts"; however, the manner of conversation differed. LD students demonstrated less skill in initiating and maintaining the conversation. LD students asked less process questions which elicit more elaborate responses from the listener.

Hazel, Schumaker, Sherman, & Sheldon (1982)	7 LD adolescents (6 males, 1 female) with behavior problems (truancy, noncompliance); 7 NLD adolescents (all female) with similar behavior problems; 7 adolescents (5 males, 2 females) on probation with a juvenile court	Role-play test consisted of problem situations requiring the use of specific social skills: 1. Giving positive feedback 2. Giving negative feedback 3. Accepting negative feedback 4. Resisting peer pressure 5. Negotiation 6. Personal problem solving Behavioral checklists of the components of each skill were used during the role-play test. A tester acted out the situations with the subject. Intervention consisted of group social skills training. Subjects were tested with novel situations during each training session.	No other measures	A multiple baseline across skills design allowed for continuous evaluation of effectiveness of training. Prior to training, LD and NLD were similarly deficient in social skills. LD and NLD youths acquired social skills at the same rate except for problem-solving skill.
Schumaker, Hazel, Sherman, & Sheldon (1982)	119 LD students in grades 10–12; 60 NLD in high school band, grades 10–12; 57 court-adjudicated youth (JD) ages 13–17	Eight social skills were tested with checklists consisting of the steps required to perform the skills. Role-play situations designed to elicit the skills were administered by observer-testers who acted out the role-play with the subjects. Social skills tested: 1. Accepting negative feedback 2. Conversation 3. Following instructions 4. Giving positive feedback 5. Giving negative feedback 6. Negotiation 7. Problem solving 8. Resisting peer pressure	No other measures	Group differences were found for total skill performance and for all separate skills except following directions. Differences were between the NLD and both the LD and JD youths with NLD performing skills significantly better. LD performed resisting peer pressure tasks better than JD. A discriminant function analysis indicated that NLD and JD youths were classified correctly more often with these variables, suggesting heterogeneity in the LD group with respect to social skills.

disabilities and average students, finding that *student* classroom behaviors did not discriminate among the groups. Teacher behaviors and the combination of teacher and student behaviors produced significant group differences.

Bryan and colleagues conducted several investigations of the nature of elementary-age LD children's social communications and interactions using naturalistic observation techniques (Bryan, 1974; Bryan & Bryan, 1978; Bryan & Wheeler, 1972; Bryan, Wheeler, Felcan, & Henek, 1976). LD children did not differ from matched nonhandicapped subjects in the amount of interaction with teachers and peers, but the nature of interactions was substantially different. For example, the teacher was three times as likely to respond to the nonhandicapped children as to the LD children and peers were more likely to ignore initiations made by LD students (Bryan, 1974). Also, LD students emitted more competitive and less considerate statements than nonhandicapped students (Bryan et al., 1976). Students with learning disabilities were rated by peers as less popular and also emitted and received more hostility and rejection statements in their communications with peers.

We have recently completed an investigation examining teacher and student factors that occur in regular classrooms that differentially affect students with learning disabilities and nonhandicapped students (McIntosh, Vaughn, Schumm, Haager, & Lee, 1991). Using the Classroom Climate Scale (CCS) observations were conducted in classrooms of 60 teachers identified by principals or department chairpersons as "planful" in teaching and making adaptations for mainstreamed special education students. There were 20 teachers in each of three grade groupings: elementary, middle school, and high school. At least one student with learning disabilities was enrolled in each class. Findings indicated that, overall, the teachers' use of praise, monitoring student performance, and the use of modifications were rated the same for students with learning disabilities and nonhandicapped students. Teachers tended to use whole-group activities and individualize or group students for instruction very little. The target students, however, did respond differentially. The students with LD who were mainstreamed volunteered to answer questions, asked for help, and interfered with the activity of others significantly less than their nonhandicapped peers. Additionally, their engagement in activities and the frequency of their interactions with the teacher and peers was substantially less than that of nonhandicapped students.

Observational studies conducted to examine the frequency of positive interactions with peers reveal that high levels of positive initiations are highly related to peer acceptance with nonhandicapped populations (Dodge, 1983; Gresham, 1981, 1982; Hartup, Glazer, & Charlesworth, 1967). Little has been done to replicate these findings with children with learning disabilities. Bryan and Bryan (1978) found that sociometric scores were related in the following manner. Attraction was negatively correlated with the failure of students with learning disabilities to respond to peers and rejection statements made by peers to students with learning disabilities. However, attraction was also negatively correlated with peers' positive social reinforcement/social statements, a confusing result for which no conceptual or empirical explanation emerges other than that the observation coding scheme may not have provided enough contextual information. Rejection scores were positively correlated with peers' making nasty statements to subjects, and negatively correlated with subjects' helping/cooperation behavior and to peers' positive reinforcement/ social statements to subjects. Since the Bryan studies of the late 1970's, few, if any, observational studies of social competence factors have been conducted with students with learning disabilities. If for no other reason than to confirm the behavioral correlates of social status found in developmental research, further research is needed.

Analogue or Behavioral Role-Play Methods of Observation

Role-play in simulated situations exhibit some advantages over naturalistic observation. A major strength of analogue methods of observation is that the researcher is able to structure or contrive settings that facilitate social behaviors or events that are difficult to study because they occur infrequently in the classroom setting or may typically occur in the home or other environment. Analogue settings also offer the researcher control over the context in which a behavior occurs, to other potentially confounding variables, thus permitting standardization across subjects and settings. Videotopes of simulated behavior are easily made, facilitating the use of elaborate coding schemes and careful study of actual behavior, and thus enhancing the likelihood of reliable scoring. Additionally, role-play methods are less expensive and time-consuming than naturalistic observations.

With nonhandicapped populations, behaviors observed in analogue settings have shown low relations with social outcomes such as social status or social acceptance, or with the same behaviors observed in naturalistic settings (Asher & Hymel, 1981; Gresham, 1986). This is likely due to the fact that classroom structures do not typically allow for a wide range of social behaviors to be represented, whereas role-play activities are structured so that all target social behaviors performed (Asher & Hymel, 1981; Vosk, Forehand, Parker, & Rickard, 1982). It is not always possible to generalize behaviors observed in simulated settings to the natural environment and to postulate that skills demonstrated in the simulated situation are used in a natural environment, unless the specific procedures used have demonstrated adequate concurrent validity with naturalistic observation. Gresham (1986) suggests that analogue research may be useful in determining social skills deficits (i.e., subjects' inability to perform social tasks) rather than in determining performance deficits (i.e., subjects' lack of use of social skills in natural environments). For a summary of research using simulated or role-play situations, see Table 14.5b.

Two studies demonstrated the use of behavioral role-play social assessment with individuals with learning disabilities. Schumaker, Hazel Sherman, and Sheldon (1982) compared adolescents with learning disabilities with a nonhandicapped group and a court-adjudicated group using a behavioral role-play test which consisted of eight role-play situations designed to demonstrate eight social skills. The nonhandicapped group performed significantly better than the other two groups on seven of the eight skills; the students with learning disabilities performed better than the court-adjudicated group on only one skill, resisting peer pressure. The group with learning disabilities was found to be heterogeneous with respect to social skills performance. Another study applied the same behavioral roly-play test as an outcome measure for an intervention program designed to teach the targeted social skills (Hazel et al., 1982). Subjects included a group of adolescents with learning disabilities who had been referred to an alternative school due to behavior problems such as truancy and noncompliance, a nonhandicapped group of adolescents with similar behavior problems, and a nonhandicapped group on probation with juvenile court. All groups showed an increase in all targeted social skills, except for the cognitive problem-solving skill on which the students with learning disabilities showed only a slight gain as compared to the other groups. A major limitation of analogue assessment is illustrated by this study in that the relation between the observation of role-play and other measures of social skills was not established, thus it is difficult to determine if skill gains generalize to actual use in other settings.

Validity and Reliability of Observational Data

Criterion-related validity of observation methods has not been well established. For example, Forness, Guthrie, and Hall (1976) reported only moderate predictive validity of an observation code disigned to examine classroom behaviors and interactions in kindergarten class. The observation rating scale consisted of four categories: Verbal Positive, Attend, Not Attend, and Disrupt. Correlations between the observation categories and first-grade achievement were similar to those between the observation categories and first-grade teacher ratings of academic and social abilities, ranging from $-.45$ to $.42$. We can only conclude from this, however, that these observation categories do not adequately predict achievement or teacher ratings. It may be a comparison of apples and oranges in that the observation code and the outcome measures are inherently dissimilar. Future research might address predictive validity with more highly related vaiables.

Moderate concurrent validity was reported by Gresham (1981, 1982) using peer ratings, peer nominations, and behavioral observations with a commonly used coding of positive and negative interactions given and received, peer ratings, and peer nominations. A factor analysis revealed that the social observations comprised a separate factor from the sociometric measures (Gresham, 1981), suggesting that the observations measured a different aspect of social competence, labeled social interaction, from the sociometric measures, thus limiting the validity coefficient. Reliability of observational data is essential. Asher and Hymel (1981) note that, typically, the duration of observations ranges from 30 minutes to 2 hours, but that to capture low frequency behaviors or events, this may not be adequate. When examining low frequency behaviors, it is often suggested that simulated situations or analogue measures in which children role-play may be more useful. On the average, four consecutive observations are needed to obtain reliable samples of social behavior with very young children (Forness & Guthrie, 1977). There is some evidence that with older students reliability of the data may be achieved more quickly (McIntosh et al., in press).

Observer accuracy and interobserver agreement are two important reliability issues. Observer drift occurs when the observer gradually shifts from the original behavioral code definition (i.e., the same behavior is coded differently at different times), resulting in inaccuracy of observer reports and preventing comparison of observations across time. Interobserver agreement refers to the degree to which two or more observers agree on how specific occurrences are coded. To ensure reliability across raters, reliability checks must be planned. Chance also plays a role in interobserver reliability. High frequency bahaviors can inflate percentage agreements (Repp, Nieminen, Olinger, & Brusca, 1988). In the McIntosh et al. study, observer accuracy and interobserver reliability were enhanced by rigorous training and the development of performance indicators in which the items of the observation code were clearly defined and examples of the target behaviors were provided. Raters were trained using videotapes. During training sessions, coding procedures were clarified and interobserver disagreement was resolved through discussion and review of the videotapes.

Another consideration in observational research in classrooms is the degree of reactivity caused by the observer's presence (see Haynes & Horn, 1982, for a review). Subjects who are aware of the observer's presence or of videotaping procedures may engage in more socially desirable behavior than they would normally (Repp et al., 1988), thus affecting both internal and external validity. In our own research, teachers have reported after videotaping that they were "a bit nervous," and that students either "hammed it up" or "were on their best behavior," even after practice videotaping sessions (Schumm, Vaughn, Haager, & Rothlein, in review). When it is impossible to have an observer unobtrusively secluded behind a one-way mirror, attempts to minimize reactivity include the use of adaptation periods in which observers visit the environment or conduct practice videotape sessions. Another possible method is to use participant observers, who become or already are a naturally occurring part of the environment. There are two ways of thinking about participant observers: They may enhance the quality of the data by knowing the subjects and providing information about possible motivations for subjects' and other people's behavior, as well as about environmental or contextual factors; or, participant observers may provide less than objective observations of behavior, thereby "reading into" behaviors based on their own assumptions and experiences in the environment.

Issues Related to the Use of Observations with Students with Learning Disabilities

It is important to recognize how few observation studies have been conducted with students with learning disabilities. Of particular importance is to note how little replication has been done with the observation categories developed within studies. Table 14.4 reveals that the categories differed for every study. Also summarized in Table 14.4 is the relatively small sample sizes used in the studies. This is surely related to the immense investment required to conduct observational research. However, with an increased interest in the social behavior of individuals with learning disabilities, further studies that observe the social behavior of students with LD in a naturalistic setting are needed. It is also important to note that the studies summarized in Table 14.4 involve observation of students in academically structured regular classroom environments. No studies observed the students in the resource room where the students are on equal academic footing with each other. Additionally, no studies observed students in a setting outside of the school environment.

Observation methodology exhibits both promise and limitations for social assessment with learning disabled populations. With the research community increasingly attracted to context-based research, naturalistic observation methodology will be a key research tool. However, with the substantial investment of time and effort required to conduct observations, the researcher may want some assurance that the information yielded from the selected methodology is both appropriate and important.

The setting in which the observation is conducted is of primary importance. Consideration should be given to conducting observations outside of the structured classroom settings or during the most socially interactive times of the school day. It is also important to observe students who attend resource classes in both the regular classroom and resource settings. Ideally, information regarding the target students' social functioning should also be obtained outside of the school setting. We assume that students who are not particularly popular in school suffer from social rejection or neglect. This may not be accurate when the student has a strong social support system outside of the school setting.

Important considerations in assessing social competence in students with learning disabilities include such factors as language abilities and achievement differences (La Greca & Stark, 1986). These factors are highly related to the ability to communicate and interact. Students' ability to communicate would surely influence their performance in role-play situations. We need to consider students' language competence, and to the extent possible, assess its affects on students' social behavior.

Methodologies developed with nonhandicapped populations need to be reestablished as sound techniques for use with special populations. In the same vein, conclusions drawn from the use of observation with nonhandicapped populations must be verified with students with learning disabilities.

We have recently endeavored to develop an observational approach to assessing social skills (Haager & Vaughn, 1991), and have encountered several issues. First and foremost is the decision to invest the time and effort necessary to obtain a reliable observation. The refinement of observation categories involves the development of succinct definitions and arduous training of observers. We were most interested in assuring that the observations provide information that is unavailable by other means which are less burdensome to the researcher (e.g., interviews and rating scales). We were also concerned that the observation be conducted in a setting that would provide for maximum student control over the social interactions. These settings occur infrequently, if at all during the school day. In summary, observation data provides an opportunity to record the social functioning of individuals with learning disabilities in a natural setting. However, as the few observation studies with LD students demonstrate, they are time-consuming and difficult to conduct. Up to this point in the chapter peer ratings and observations have been discussed. A third perspective, the child's, is important for obtaining a full understanding of a youngster's social functioning. The most frequently used measure of self-respect is self-concept.

Social Self-Report as a Measure of Social Functioning

The majority of research examining the social functioning of students with learning disabilities demonstrates that the social difficulties of LD students are more extensive than their non-LD peers. Thus, it is reasonable to question the extent to which their peer acceptance difficulties have influenced their self-perception. Self-perceptions and self-concept are attractive constructs in that they theoretically provide a window in which to examine children's own perceptions about their social relationships.

The research on self-concepts of students with learning disabilities is fraught with contradiction. Many studies report lower self-esteem for students with learning disabilities than for nonhandicapped students (e.g., Battle & Blowers, 1982; Rogers & Saklofske, 1985; Silverman & Zigmond, 1983), while others report no difference in the self-perceptions of children with learning disabilities and their normally achieving peers (e.g., Winne, Woodlands, & Wong, 1982). The apparent contradiction is somewhat resolved by examining the ages of the samples and the measures used (see Table 14.6).

There is evidence that self-evaluations are domain-specific (Harter & Pike, 1984; Winne et al., 1982), and that results differ depending on whether the self-appraisal is tapping feelings of general self-worth or feelings about specific domains of development, usually academic or social development. When assessments of global self-worth or self-perceptions of academic ability are used to compare individuals with learning disabilities with nonhandicapped students, the results tend to show marked differences, especially with older students. It is often thought that academic-oriented items influence ratings of global self-worth in students with learning disabilities. This was confirmed, in fact, when differences in global self-worth between students with learning disabilities and a normally achieving comparison group diminished after removing the academic component of the measure (Cooley & Ayres, 1988). Self-concept tends to become more differentiated with age, with a general decline in self-ratings through the childhood years (Marsh, 1989; Marsh, Byrne, & Shavelson, 1988). A review by Chapman (1988) provides the interested reader with a compilation of the research on general and academic self-concepts of students with learning disabilities. When non-academic, domain-specific self-evaluations are measured, results have varied. This section will address only research methods for investigating the social self-perceptions of students with learning disabilities.

Self-reports of social skills, social behavior, or social acceptance have been included in several studies for the purpose of comparison to other measures such as teacher reports or peer ratings of popularity or accep-tance. Garrett and Crump (1980), for example, compared actual peer acceptance with perceived peer acceptance of elementary students in grades 4–6 with learning disabilities and nonhandicapped students. Peer acceptance was a nomination task in which children were asked to name 3 classmates that they would select for free-play time and 3 classmates that they would not select. The self-appraisal of social status was a 3-point self-rating of how they anticipated other children would rate them. For each classmate on the list, the target student was asked whether he/she thought that classmate had nominated him/her on the peer nomination

TABLE 14.6. Summary of research using measures of self-perceptions of social acceptance with students with learning disabilities.

Authors	Sample	Self-report measure	Other measures	Findings
Bruininks (1978)	16 LD, 16 NLD; grades 1–5	Peer Acceptance Scale, used for measuring peer acceptance, was utilized to ask students to self-report. Subjects were asked to indicate how they felt each of their classmates regarded them. Mean ratings were computed.	Peer Acceptance Scale: to assess peer acceptance	LD subjects scored significantly lower on peer acceptance than comparison group and total class. Perceived peer status (self-report) for LD students was similar to that of comparison group. However, perceived acceptance was significantly higher than actual peer acceptance.
Bursuck (1989)	8 LD, 8 low-achieving matched on classroom and reading achievement, and 8 higher achieving matched on classroom; all were from grades 2–5.	MESSY (Matson Evaluation of Social Skills with Youngsters), four factors: Inappropriate Social Skills, Inappropriate Assertiveness, Impulsive/Recalcitrant, and Overconfident. Contains 92 items, 5-point rating scale. Matson, J.L., Rotatori, A.F., & Helsel, W.J. (1983). Development of a rating scale to measure social skills in children: The Matson Evaluation of Social Skills with Youngsters (MESSY). *Behavior Research Therapy*, *21*(4), 335–340.	Sociometric measures: "play with" rating scale, limited-choice friendship nomination inventory, peer behavior nomination inventory. MESSY teacher rating scale (parallel to self-report measure), teacher rating of behavior problems (BPC).	LD students were significantly less accepted than low-achieving and high-achieving students. LD students were less positively nominated for friendship than high-achieving but not less than low-achieving students. Similarly, peers rated LD as having more behavior problems than others. Teachers rated LD as having more behavioral and social problems than high-achieving students but not low-achieving students.
Cooley & Ayres (1988)	46 LD, 47 NLD, ages 10–14 from same classroom	Piers-Harris Children's Self-concept Scale (Piers, 1984). Subscales: Behavior (problematic) Intellectual and school status Physical appearance Anxiety Popularity	Questionnaire: depicting success and failure attributions	Self-report showed no significant differences between groups. Lower overall self-concepts for LD with differences primarily due to Intellectual and school status and Behavior subscales. Attributions did not differentiate the groups.

Table continued

TABLE 14.6. Continued

Authors	Sample	Self-report measure	Other measures	Findings
Durrant, Cunningham, & Voelker (1990)	60 LD subjects, ages 8–13, from a private clinic, were classified into the following subgroups: LD-normals (non-behavior disordered), LD-Externalizing Disorders, LD-Internalizing and Externalizing (mixed symptomatology), 15 control non-LD)	Perceived Competence Scale for Children (Harter, 1979), with the following subscales: Cognitive competence Social competence General self-esteem Harter, S. (1982). Perceived competence scale for children (Manual, Form O). Denver, CO: University of Denver.	Child Behavior Checklist used for classification of groups	Overall self-concept scores: LD-Ext. and LD-Int. obtained lower ratings than LD-nomral or non-LD groups. When groups were collapsed into BD (behavior disorder) and non-BD, the BD group obtained lower scores on the Social Competence than the non-BD group.
Garrett & Crump (1980)	100 LD, 100 NLD, grades 4, 5, and 6	Self-appraisal of social status, modified from Peer Acceptance Scale. A self-report of how each subject felt classmates had rated him/her on the Peer Acceptance Scale.	Peer Acceptance Scale: Subjects were asked to nominate 3 classmates they would choose to play with and 3 classmates they would not choose. Yielded social status score. Teacher Preference Score: Q-sort technique.	LD significantly lower on social status and teacher preference. In comparing actual and perceived social status, LD more accurate in self-appraisal, NLD underrated social status.

| Priel & Leshem (1990) | 44 LD, 36 NLD, grades 1 and 2 | Translate Hebrew version of Pictorial Scale of Perceived Competence and Social Acceptance (Harter & Pike, 1984).

Subscales:

Physical competence
Cognitive competence
Peer acceptance
Mother acceptance | Teachers' rating of Children's Competence and Acceptance (parallels self-rating on 3 of 4 factors). Standardized reading and math tests. Peer rating. | LD lower on teacher rating of all but physical competence.
  LD lower on cognitive competence ratings only with self-ratings. LD self-ratings were significantly higher than teacher ratings and peer ratings. |
| Renick & Harter (1989) | 86 LD, grades 3–8 | Perceived Competence Scale for Children (Harter, 1982).

Subscales:

Scholastic competence
Athletic competence
Social acceptance
Global self-worth | | Mean scholastic competence ratings for LD students in regular education setting were significantly lower than in special education settings. Developmental trends were explored with scholastic competence ratings. When comparing themselves with regular education peers, LD students' self-ratings showed a developmental decline across grade levels. When comparing themselves with special education peers, no decline in academic competence ratings was evident. Across domains of competence, scholastic competence ratings were significantly lower than social competence, athletic competence, and global self-worth, all of which were similar to each other. |

Table continued

TABLE 14.6. *Continued*

Authors	Sample	Self-report measure	Other measures	Findings
Vaughn, Haager, Hogan, & Kouzekanani (1992)	10 LD, 10 low achievers (matched with LD on reading and math achievement), 10 average/high achievers, all matched with LD on ethnicity, sex, and age; followed longitudinally from kindergarten through 4th grade	The Pictorial Scale of Perceived Competence and Social Acceptance for Young Children (Harter & Pike, 1984); an adapted version for 2nd, 3rd, and 4th grade. Subscales for kindergarten and 1st grade: Social acceptance, Academic competence. Subscales for 2–4 grade's: Social acceptance Academic competence Global self-worth	Peer ratings of acceptance	This was a longitudinal, prospective study in which the measures were administered every year for 5 years. Since LD students were identified and placed into services during 2nd grade, but measures had been collected since entering kindergarten, data represents both prior to and following the identification and placement of LD students. Results indicated no differences between groups on any self-concept subscale. There was a significant decline in overall academic competence scores from kindergarten to grade 1. The average/high-achieving group was significantly higher in peer acceptance than the low-achieving group only. A significant overall decline in peer acceptance scores occurred from 2nd to 3rd grade.
Vaughn, Hogan, Kouzekanani, & Shapiro (1990)	10 LD students prior to identification, 10 low achievers, 10 average achievers, 10 high achievers, kindergarten grade	The Pictorial Scale of Perceived Competence and Social Acceptance for Young Children (Harter & Pick, 1984). Subscales: social acceptance.	Revised Behavior Problem Checklist, Social Skills Rating Scale for Teachers, Peer ratings and nominations	As early as 8 weeks into kindergarten, students with learning disabilities prior to their identification (LDPI) received significantly fewer positive peer nominations than average or high achievers; had significantly higher behavior problem scores than low, average, or high achievers; yet had higher self-perception scores than average and high achievers.

task, had listed them on the "would not select" list, or had not listed them at all. The peer acceptance ratings of the two groups were consistent with other findings of lower peer status for students with learning disabilities. The self-appraisal, however, yielded no significant differences between groups. Perceived status for the students with learning disabilities was almost identical to actual status. The nonhandicapped students had underestimated their perceived status. The authors interpreted this, not as an indication that students with learning disabilities were more accurate in their self-perceptions of social status, but that the normally achieving comparison group demonstrated socially appropriate modesty in their self-ratings.

Others have confirmed the tendency for the self-perceptions of students with learning disabilities to reflect their lowered peer status or peer acceptance. LaGreca and Stone (1990) reported lowered self-perceptions of social acceptance and self-worth, as well as lowered peer acceptance and status, for both low achievers and students with learning disabilities. In contrast, using a self-report measure that paralleled a teacher measure of prosocial and problem behaviors, Bursuck (1989) found the self-ratings and teacher ratings not to reflect lowered peer ratings for the students with learning disabilities and not to be different for any group. The apparent conflict in the findings of these two studies may be explained as an effect of age differences. The subjects in the Bursuck (1989) study were in grades 2, 3, and 4, whereas in the LaGreca and Stone (1990) study, the subjects were in grades 4, 5, and 6. This is consistent with child development literature in that self-concept generally declines and that children's sense of self becomes more refined with age (Harter & Pike, 1984; Marsh, 1989; Marsh et al., 1988; Nicholls, 1978, 1979).

Two studies have examined the self-perceptions of students with learning disabilities prior to their identification and placement for services as part of a longitudinal, prospective research project investigating risk factors associated with academic and social difficulties. Vaughn et al. (1990) compared the peer, teacher, and self-assessments in the fall and spring of the kindergarten year for low achievers, average achievers, high achievers, and LD students prior to identification. As early as the second month of kindergarten, teachers and peers rated the students with learning disabilities as lower than the other comparison groups; however, the self-perceptions, using a domain-specific measure designed for very young children (Harter & Pike, 1984), did not indicate any acknowledgement on the part of the students with learning disabilities of lowered regard by others. Following the original cohort through third grade on the peer ratings and fourth grade on the self-concept measures (Vaughn et al., 1992), the differences in peer acceptance became evident only for the average/high achievers and low achievers, with the combined average/ high group demonstrating significantly higher scores than the low-achieving group only. A significant time effect indicated a general decline in peer acceptance scores for all groups from kindergarten through third grade. At no time from kindergarten through fourth grade did the self-perception scores yield any significant differences between groups for either academic, social, or global self-concepts. Though real group differences may not have been discerned due to such factors as a small sample size (from the original cohort of 239 entering kindergartners, there were 10 students with learning disabilities), the longitudinal, prospective design of this project has laid the groundwork for considering this population from a developmental perspective.

Issues in Using Self-Perceptions with Students with Learning Disabilities

One very important issue that is raised by the longitudinal studies reported above is a developmental one. We assume that developmental trends in normally achieving and developing populations apply to the special population of individuals with learning disabilities, when in fact, this population is quite heterogeneous with respect to academic, behavioral, and social factors. Little has been done to track this population developmentally or to explore the extent to which social difficulties are related to developmental, cognitive, or other differences. A few studies have examined the self-perceptions of very young children in the early school grades. Generally, consonant with the developmental literature, self-perceptions before the ages of 7 or 8 are not well-defined or differentiated (Priel & Leshem, 1990; Vaughn et al., 1990, Vaughn et al., 1992).

The tendency for self ratings to be biased by social desirability is inherent in any self-report measure. This probably explains why other measures, such as peer or teacher reports, are often used in tandem with self-ratings. It is difficult to discern if self-reports accurately reflect true self-perceptions.

Some self-report measures are highly dependent on language or cognitive abilities. It may be desirable to build in a control for achievement, cognitive ability, or language ability. Using an achievement control group is one possible method for understanding the role played by academic differences between groups (Bursuck, 1989; La Greca & Stone, 1990; Vaughn et al., 1990; Vaughn et al., 1992).

References

Achenbach, T.M. (1990). *Child behavior checklist*. Burlington, Vermont. University of Vermont.

Asher, S.R. & Hymel, S. (1981). Children's social competence in peer relations: Sociometric and behavioral assessment. In J.D. Wine & M.D. Smye (Eds.), *Social competence* (pp. 125–157). New York: Guilford.

Asher, S.R., Markell, R.A., & Hymel, S. (1981). Identifying children at risk in peer relations: A critique of the rate-of-interaction approach to assessment. *Child Development*, *52*, 1239–1245.

Asher, S.R. & Taylor, A.R. (1981). Social outcomes of mainstreaming: Sociometric assessment and beyond. *Exceptional Education Quarterly*, *1*, 13–30.

Battle, J. & Blowers, J. (1982). A longitudinal comparative study of the self-esteem of students in regular and special education classes. *Journal of Learning Disabilities*, *15*, 100–102.

Bell-Dorlan, D.J., Foster, S.L., & Sikora, D.M. (1989). Effects of sociometric testing on children's behavior and loneliness in school. *Developmental Psychology*, *25*, 306–311.

Bruininks, V.L. (1978a). Actual and perceived peer status of learning disabled students in mainstream programs. *Journal of Special Education*, *12*, 51–58.

Bryan, T.H. (1974). An observational analysis of classroom behaviors of children with learning disabilities. *Journal of Learning Disabilities*, *7*, 35–43.

Bryan, T.H. & Bryan, J.H. (1978). Social interactions of learning disabled children. *Learning Disability Quarterly*, *1*, 33–37.

Bryan, T., Donahue, M., & Pearl, R. (1981). Learning disabled children's peer interactions during a small-group problem-solving task. *Learning Disability Quarterly*, *4*(1), 13–22.

Bryan, T., Donahue, M., Pearl, R., & Sturm, C. (1981). Learning disabled children's conversational skills—the "TV talk show." *Learning Disabilities Quarterly*, *4*(3), 250–259.

Bryan, T. & Wheeler, R. (1972). Perception of children with learning disabilities: The eye of the observer. *Journal of Learning Disabilities*, *5*, 199–206.

Bryan, T., Wheeler, R., Felcan, J., & Henek, T. (1976). "Come on, Dummy": An observational study of children's communications. *Journal of Learning Disabilities*, *9*, 53–61.

Bursuck, W. (1989). A comparison of students with learning disabilities to low achieving and higher achieving students on three dimensions of social competence. *Journal of Learning Disabilities*, *22*, 188–194.

Chapman, J.W. (1988). Learning disabled children's self-concepts. *Review of Educational Research*, *58*, 347–371.

Coben, S.C. & Zigmond, N. (1986). The social integration of learning disabled students from self-contained to mainstream elementary school settings. *Journal of Learning Disabilities*, *19*, 614–618.

Coie, J.D., Dodge, K.A., & Coppotelli, H. (1982). Dimensions and types of social status: A cross-age perspective. *Developmental Psychology*, *18*, 557–570.

Cooley, E.J. & Ayres, R.R. (1988). Self-concept and success-failure attributions of nonhandicapped students and students with learning disabilities. *Journal of Learning Disabilities*, *21*, 174–178.

Cowen, E., Pederson, A., Babigian, H., Izzo, L., & Trost, M. (1973). Long-term follow-up of early detected vulnerable children. *Journal of Consulting and Clinical Psychology*, *41*, 438–446.

DeKlyen, M. & Odom, S.L. (1989). Activity structure and social interactions with peers in developmentally integrated play groups. *Journal of Early Intervention*, *13*, 342–352.

Dodge, K.A. (1983). Behavioral antecedents of peer social status. *Child Development*, *54*, 1386–1399.

Dorval, B., McKinney, J.D., & Feagans, L. (1982). Teachers' interaction with learning disabled children and average achievers. *Journal of Pediatric Psychology, 17*, 317–330.

Drewry, D.L. & Clark, M.L. (1983). Factors important in the formation of preschoolers' friendships. *Journal of Genetic Psychology, 146*, 37–44.

Dudley-Marling, C.C. & Edmiaston, R. (1985). Social status of learning disabled children and adolescents: A review. *Learning Disabilities Quarterly, 8*, 189–204.

Durrant, J.E., Cunningham, C.E., & Voelker, S. (1990). Academic, social, and general self-concepts of behavioral subgroups of learning disabled children. *Journal of Educational psychology, 82*(4), 657–663.

Forness, S.R. & Guthrie, D. (1977). Stability of pupil behavior in short-term classroom observations. *Psychology in the Schools, 14*, 116–120.

Forness, S.R., Guthrie, D., & Hall, R.J. (1976). Follow-up of high-risk children identified in kindergarten through direct classroom observation. *Psychology in the Schools, 13*, 45–49.

Fox, C. (1989). Peer acceptance of learning disabled children in the regular classroom. *Exceptional Children, 56*(1), 50–57.

Garrett, M.K. & Crump, D. (1980). Peer acceptance, teacher preference, and self-appraisal of social status among learning disabled students. *Learning Disability Quarterly, 3*, 42–48.

Gelzheiser, L.M. & Meyers, J. (1991, April). What do students miss during pullout? Paper presented at American Educational Research Association (AERA), Chicago.

Gresham, F.M. (1981). Validity of social skills measures for assessing social competence in low-status children: A multivariate investigation. *Developmental Psychology, 17*, 390–398.

Gresham, F.M. (1982). Social interactions as predictors of children's likability and friendship patterns: A multiple regression analysis. *Journal of Behavioral Assessment, 4*, 39–54.

Gresham, F.M. (1986). Conceptual issues in the assessment of social competence in children. In P.S. Strain, M.J. Guralnick, & H.M. Walker (Eds.), *Children's Social Behavior* (pp. 143–179). Orlando, FL: Academic Press.

Gresham, F.M. & Elliott, S.N. (1986). Social skills rating scale for teachers. Baton Rouge: Louisiana State University.

Gresham, F.M. & Elliott, S.N. (1990). *Social skills rating system manual.* Circle Pines, MN: American Guidance Service.

Guralnick, M.J. (1980). Social interactions among preschool children. *Exceptional Children, 46*, 248–253.

Haager, D. & Vaughn, S. (1991). *Assessment of social skills: An observational approach.* Manuscript in preparation.

Harter, S. & Pike, R. (1984). The pictorial scale of perceived competence and social acceptance for young children. *Child Development, 55*, 1969–1982.

Hartup, W.W. (1990). A final note (Editorial). *Child Development, 61*(6), 1659–1660.

Hartup, W.W., Glazer, J.A., & Charlesworth, R. (1967). Peer reinforcement and sociometric status. *Child Development, 38*, 1017–1024.

Haynes, S.N. & Horn, W.F. (1982). Reactivity in behavioral observation: A review. *Behavioral Assessment, 4*, 369–385.

Hayvren, M. & Hymel, S. (1984). Ethical issues in sociometric testing: The impact of sociometric measures on interaction behavior. *Developmental Psychology, 20*, 844–849.

Hazel, J.S., Schumaker, J.B., Sherman, J.A., & Sheldon, J. (1982). Application of a group training program in social skills and problem solving to learning disabled and non-learning disabled youth. *Learning Disability Quarterly, 5*, 398–408.

Hops, H. (1983). Children's social competence and skill: Current research practices and future directions. *Behavior Therapy, 14*, 3–18.

Howes, C. (1987). Peer interaction of young children. *Monographs of the Society for Research in Child Development, 53*, (1, Serial No. 217).

LaGreca, A.M. (Ed.). (1990). *Through the eyes of the child*. Needham Heights, MA: Allyn & Bacon.

LaGreca, A.M. & Stark, P. (1986). Naturalistic observations of children's social behavior. In P.S. Strain, M.J. Guralnick, & H.M. Walker (Eds.), *Children's social behavior: Development, assessment, and modification* (pp. 181–213). Orlando, FL: Academic Press.

LaGreca, A.M. & Stone, W.L. (1990). LD status and achievement: Confounding variables in the study of children's social status, self-esteem, and behavioral functioning. *Journal of Learning Disabilities, 23*, 483–490.

Lancelotta, G.X. & Vaughn, S. (1989). Relation between types of aggression and sociometric status: Peer and teacher perceptions. *Journal of Educational Psychology, 81*(1), 86–90.

Landau, S. & Milich, R. (1990). Assessment of children's social status and peer relations . In A.M. LaGreca (Ed.), *Through the eyes of the child* (pp. 259–291). Needham Heights, MA: Allyn & Bacon.

Lesser, G.S. (1959). The relationship between various forms of aggression and popularity among lower class children. *Journal of Educational Psychology, 50*, 20–25.

Marsh, H.W. (1989). Age and sex effects in multiple dimensions of self-concept: Preadolescence to early adulthood. *Journal of Educational Psychology, 81*, 417–430.

Marsh, H.W., Byrne, B.M., & Shavelson, R.J. (1988). A multifaceted academic self-concept: Its hierarchical structure and its relation to academic achievement. *Journal of Educational Psychology, 80*, 366–380.

McConnell, S.R. & Odom, S.L. (1986). Sociometrics: Peer-referenced measures and the assessment of social competence. In P.S. Strain, M.J. Guralnick, & H.M. Walker (Eds.), *Children's social behavior* (pp. 215–284). Orlando, FL: Academic Press.

McIntosh, R., Vaughn, S., Schumm, J.S., Haager, D. & Lee. O. (in press). Observations of students with learning disabilities in general education classrooms: You don't bother me and I won't bother you. *Exceptional Children*.

McIntosh, R., Vaughn, S., & Zaragoza, N. (1991). A review of social skills interventions for students with learning disabilities. *Journal of Learning Disabilities, 24*(8), 451–458.

Moreno, J.L. (1934). *Who shall survive? A new approach to the problem of human interrelations*. Washington, DC: Nervous and Mental Disease Publishing Co.

Nicholls, J.G. (1978). The development of the concepts of effort and ability: Perceptions of academic attainment and the understanding that difficult tasks require more ability. *Child Development, 49*, 800–814.

Nicholls, J.G. (1979). The development of perceptions of one's own attainment and causal attributions for success and failure in reading. *Journal of Educational Psychology, 71*, 94–99.

Northway, M.L. (1969). The stability of young children's social relationships. *Educational Research, 11*, 54–57.

Parker, J.G. & Asher, S.R. (1987). Peer relations and later personal adjustment: Are low-accepted children at risk? *Psychological Bulletin, 102*, 357–389.

Peery, J.C. (1979). Popular, amiable, isolated, rejected: A reconceptualization of sociometric status in preschool children. *Child Development, 50*, 1231–1234.

Perlmutter, B.F., Crocker, J., Cordray, D., & Garstecki, D. (1983). Sociometric status and related personality characteristics of mainstreamed learning disabled adolescents. *Learning Disability Quarterly, 6*, 344–346.

Priel, B. & Leshem, T. (1990). Self-perceptions of first- and second-grade children with learning disabilities. *Journal of Learning Disabilities, 23*, 637–642.

Quay, H.C. & Peterson, D.R. (1987). *Manual for the revised behavior problem checklist*. Coral Gables FL: University of Miami Press.

Renick, M.J. & Harter, S. (1989). Impact of social comparisons on the developing self-perceptions of learning disabled students. *Journal of Educational Psychology, 81*(4), 631–638.

Repp, A.C., Nieminen, G.S., Olinger, E., & Brusca, R. (1988). Direct observation: Factors affecting the accuracy of observers. *Exceptional Children, 55*, 29–36.

Roff, M., Sells, B., & Golden, M.M. (1972). *Social adjustment and personality development in children*. Minneapolis: University of Minnesota Press.

Rogers, H. & Saklofske, D.H. (1985). Self-concept, locus of control, and performance expectations of learning disabled children. *Journal of Learning Disabilities, 18*, 273–278.

Sabornie, E.J. & Kauffman, J.M. (1986). Social acceptance of learning disabled adolescents. *Learning Disability Quarterly, 9*, 55–60.

Sabornie, E.J., Marshall, K.J., & Ellis, E.S. (1990). Restructuring of mainstream sociometry with learning disabled and nonhandicapped students. *Exceptional Children, 56*(4), 314–323.

Sainato, D.M., Zigmond, N., & Strain, P.S. (1983). Social status and initiations of interactions by learning disabled students in regular education settings. *Analysis and Intervention in Developmental Disabilities, 3*, 71–88.

Schumaker, J.B., Hazel, J.S., Sherman, J.A., & Sheldon, J. (1982). Social skill performances of learning disabled, non-learning disabled, and delinquent adolescents. *Learning Disability Quarterly, 5*, 388–397.

Schumaker, J.B., Wildgen, J.S., & Sherman, J.A. (1982). Social interaction of learning disabled junior high students in their regular classrooms: An observational analysis. *Journal of Learning Disabilities, 15*(6), 355–358.

Schumm, J.S., Vaughn, S., Haager, D., & Rothlein, L. (in review). *Teacher planning and adaptations for mainstreamed students: A case study report*. Manuscript submitted for publication.

Shapiro, S.B. & Sobel, M. (1981). Two multinominal random sociometric voting models. *Journal of Educational Statistics, 6*, 287–310.

Silverman, R. & Zigmond, N. (1983). Self-concept in learning disabled adolescents. *Journal of Learning Disabilities, 16*, 478–482.

Slate, J.R. & Saudargas, R.A. (1986). Differences in learning disabled and average students' classroom behaviors. *Learning Disability Quarterly, 9*, 61–67.

Thompson, G.G. & Powell, M. (1951). An investigation of the rating scale approach to the measurement of social status. *Educational and Psychological Measurement, 11*, 440–445.

Vaughn, S., Haager, D., Hogan, A., & Kouzekanani, K. (1992). Self-concept and peer acceptance in students with learning disabilities: A four to five year prospective study. *Journal of Educational Psychology, 84*, 43–50.

Vaughn, S. & Hogan, A. (1990). Social competence and learning disabilities: A prospective study. In H.L. Swanson & B. Keogh (Eds.), *Learning disabilities: Theoretical and research issues* (pp. 175–191). Hillsdale, NJ: Erlbaum.

Vaughn, S., Hogan, A., Kouzekanani, K., & Shapiro, S. (1990). Peer acceptance, self-perceptions, and social skills of learning disabled students prior to identification. *Journal of Educational Psychology, 82*(1), 101–106.

Vaughn, S., McIntosh, R., & Spencer-Rowe, J. (1991). Peer rejection is a stubborn thing. *Learning Disabilities Research & Practice, 6*(2), 83–88.

Walker, J.J. (1990). *Social desirability response tendencies in young children: Relation to teacher, peer, and self-ratings of social competence.* Unpublished doctoral dissertation, University of Miami.

Wasik, B.H. (1987). Sociometric measures and peer descriptors of kindergarten children: A study of reliability and validity. *Journal of Clinical Child Psychology, 16*, 218–224.

Winne, P.H., Woodlands, M.J., & Wong, B.Y.L. (1982). Comparability of self-concept among learning disabled, normal, and gifted students. *Journal of Learning Disabilities, 15*, 470–475.

Part VI
Ethical Issues

15
Ethical Considerations When Conducting Research with Students with Learning Disabilities

SHARON VAUGHN AND G. REID LYON

It's not what we don't know that hurts, it's what we know that ain't so.
  —Will Rogers.

The overriding question guiding this chapter is, at what point does the researcher go astray to such a marked degree that the ethics of his/her research procedures and findings are in question? While key topics raised to address this question will be clearly within the boundaries of ethical principles, other issues are more broadly related to the conduct and interpretation of investigations. These issues are particularly interesting because ethical practices in research affect the foundation of the scientific process.

Learning disabilities is not the only discipline that needs to be concerned about ethical issues in conducting and interpreting research. Certainly, concerns about ethical practice have occurred historically and currently within all disciplines. Recently, Frank Sulloway, a professor of science history at the Massachusetts Institute of Technology, reported that the "kind of evidence we have now is extremely critical of Freud" ("Freudian Slip," 1991). Apparently one of Freud's major works is being questioned because when the patients were interviewed years later, the findings reported by Freud were not upheld and in fact his findings were found to misrepresent the facts ("Freudian Slip," 1991). Furthermore, many of the psychoanalytic practices that have been advocated because of the successes reported by Freud about his clients have been seriously questioned.

Concerns about scientific findings are certainly not limited to psychology, education, and medicine. Derek Freeman's (1983) challenge of Margaret Mead's classic work *Coming of Age in Samoa*, a best-selling book in anthropology, provides us with some understanding of how easy it is to accept the conclusions of researchers and how difficult it can be to obtain verification. After conducting extensive fieldwork and living with a Samoan family for several years, Freeman challenges Mead's conclusions that adolescence in Samoan society was easy and casual and without all of the stresses and conflicts characteristic of our society. He also provides

315

an account of why Mead may have felt pressured to interpret Samoan adolescence the way she did. While critical of Mead's findings, Freeman provides a sympathetic view on how easy it is for a researcher to go "astray" and be influenced by the perceptions of others; in this case by Boas, an influential anthropologist. It is interesting to observe what is necessary to reverse a commonly accepted "truth" in science. Despite years of research and very compelling evidence, few people outside of the field of anthropology are aware of Freeman's work, and general acceptance of the early findings of Mead regarding adolescence in Samoa continue.

As Parker (1990) states it, "Probably because altering or fabricating data is taboo among scientists, words like 'fudging' and 'trimming,' and 'cooking' are used to describe a researcher's unethical tampering with data" (p. 613). Apparently even Newton felt the political pressures to have numbers be more precise than the data supported and succumbed to the "fudge" factor (Westfall, 1973).

While issues that relate to the ethical collection and interpretation of data will be presented in this chapter, the chapter will address other ethical issues related to the treatment and identification of subjects; the beliefs and attitudes of the investigator; use and interpretation of assessments, data analysis, and interpretation; and ethical issues related to other research procedures.

Ethical Issues Related to the Treatment and Identification of Subjects

Ethical Issues Related to the Treatment of Subjects

Case studies with teachers are raising new issues about the role of anonymity in research. Many teachers, working collaboratively with researchers, want credit for the role they play in the study (Shulman, 1990). Qualitative research has traditionally had to deal with questions about protecting the rights and confidentiality of participants (Yin, 1985). Now, many participants are demanding that their role and identity be recognized. Central to this issue are the potential consequences associated with teachers' identification being known to their colleagues and administrators. When teachers relinquish anonymity they become very vulnerable to the disapproval of their colleagues and administrators. Shulman (1990) provides a case study of a cooperative research project in which teachers wrote essays about their experiences teaching in an inner-city school. The school district had agreed to publish their papers as part of preservice and in-service activities for teachers. Problems arose when teachers wanted to be associated with their writing and yet the potential for alienating fellow teachers, administrators, and perhaps even parents was quite high. Shulman's case study forecasts many potential difficulties as teachers rightfully assert recognition for their involvement in research studies.

In addition to ethical considerations when involving adults in research projects, issues arise on how to best protect children who participate in research. Ethical standards developed by the Council for Exceptional Children and Society for Research in Child Development provide little information about protecting the rights of subjects (particularly children) beyond good common sense. These ethical codes include statements that inform researchers not to use procedures that "may harm the child either physically or psychologically." From the code of ethics of the Council for Exceptional Children (Code of Ethics, 1991), we are informed that "special education professionals engage in professional activities which benefit exceptional individuals, their families, other colleagues, students, or research subjects." We would hope there would be no researcher who would have to check these guidelines to obtain this information.

The American Psychological Association has published 10 ethical principles of psychologists (Report of the Association, 1990). APA's ethical principles on research with human participants provide more specific information on several ethical issues in the conduct of research, including suggestions to plan a study to consider its ethical acceptability, considering the risk to a subject, respecting the individual's freedom to decline to participate or to withdraw with no penalties, protecting the participant from mental or physical discomfort, and providing participants with information about the study after the data are gathered.

Extensive room for interpretation is provided within these guidelines. Cook (1981) cautions us that the researcher is not able to remain objective about the prospective gain versus the "cost" because ostensibly the researcher would not be doing the research if they did not feel that it was valuable. Particularly when the study involves questionable risk, he suggests using an outside consultant to assist in evaluating cost and benefit. Also, the consultant can provide valuable guidelines for limiting risk.

According to Thompson (1990), "research ethics often begin from a common principle of respect for persons (a chief aspect of which is autonomy): treating persons as ends in themselves, never solely as means to an end" (p. 3). This principle includes researchers' respect for the wishes of the individual, his/her beliefs, attitudes, right to privacy, and right to withdraw from participation. It also includes treating the participant with dignity and respect, not coercing them or deceiving them without later explaining the purpose of the deception. Ramsay (1970) argues that based on this principle young children should not be involved in research that has no therapeutic value for them, because they are unable to provide consent and are therefore always a means to an end. A competing argument is that contributing to research and the common good is a moral responsibility of our society and we can assume that children would want to fulfill this responsibility. As you can imagine, this topic has aroused considerable interest and debate.

No matter where you stand on this issue, it is likely you will concede that children, particularly children with special needs, are uniquely vulnerable as research participants because they have very limited social power. If their parents provide consent, their teachers are supportive of the research project, and a usually unknown researcher with vested interests in their participation in the project requests their consent, to what extent is the child/student free to dissent? This brings up the whole issue of the rights of children. We know that permission from students over 7 is required even though parent permission has been obtained; however, how free is the student to withdraw from the research? Particularly when intervention research is conducted, is it possible for the teacher/researcher/parent to justify that the benefits exceed the harm and that the child's participation should continue even when the child requests to withdraw from the study? In general, persons who participate in research should gain something from it. General consensus exists that the means (procedures for collecting the data and handling the participants) cannot justify the end (acquisition of knowledge) and that appropriate and sensitive treatment of all subjects who participate in research projects is needed.

A second guiding principle on the ethics of child participation in research is that it is wrong to inflict harm on another. This second principle is easier to interpret and apply in nonclinical research than in biomedical or clinical research where the benefits accrued may outweigh the initial "harm" or pain. However, it is often very difficult to determine harm in nonclinical trials. For example, when students with learning disabilities are involved in a research study, to what extent is the researcher sensitive to calling undue attention to the student? When only students with learning disabilities or poor performing students are removed from the classroom to participate in a research study, to what extent does this further "mark" these individuals as different and therefore constitute harm? These are the types of questions investigators should consider when developing and implementing research studies.

We need to be concerned with minimizing stressors in research settings as part of our ethical obligations to the participants. Many researchers argue that the stress involved in research is minimal compared with the stress involved in everyday life and that while it should be considered, it is not grounds for eliminating a study.

A third principle for making ethical decisions about the participation of children in applied research is to "treat equally those who are equally situated and to treat differently those who differ in relevant ways" (Thompson, 1990, p. 4). This includes concern for the characteristics and backgrounds of participants and the need to provide nondifferential treatment based on these characteristics and backgrounds.

Ethical Issues Related to the Identification of Subjects for Research in Learning Disabilities

An ultimate goal of research conducted with students with learning disabilities (LD) is to obtain findings that are replicable and generalizable. However, attainment of this goal has been significantly impeded by the tendency of many researchers to identify samples of LD individuals from population sources that, while convenient, are clearly not appropriate due to biases inherent in referral and/or selection procedures: in particular, the selection of individuals for study who have been identified as LD on the basis of meeting diagnostic criteria mandated by public school policy. In the research literature, LD individuals identified in this manner are typically referred to as "school-identified" subjects.

From a methodological perspective, the selection of "school-identified" samples is problematic for several reasons, most of which are related to the ambiguities inherent in current exclusionary definitions of LD (Lyon, 1987). What is relevant for this chapter is that the methodological dangers of conducting research with school-identified LD individuals are so great and so well known that continuation of the practice reflects, in our view, a departure from ethical research standards. Before discussing sampling alternatives, a brief discussion of why school-identified samples are problematic is in order.

First, individuals who compose school-identified LD samples typically vary widely among themselves in terms of relevant classification criteria (e.g., IQ, age, SES). This substantial within-sample variability is referable to the highly ambiguous and "elastic" eligibility criteria inherent within policy-driven definitions of LD. If these within-subject differences are not accounted for and explained, any generalizations based upon the data would be spurious (Kavale & Forness, 1985; Lyon, 1987). Unfortunately, the majority of studies conducted to date with school-identified LD samples have provided only gross mean-level data; thus, important individual differences inherent within the sample have been masked, making generalization and replication of the data difficult.

In addition, and perhaps most importantly, school-identified samples frequently differ significantly from one another across identification and programmatic variables, depending upon the setting, school, or state from which the sample is selected (Keogh, Major-Kingsley, Omori-Gordon, & Reid, 1982). Similar to the issue raised with within-sample variability, these large between-sample differences are related clearly to the lack of specificity in current policy-driven definitions of LD. Unfortunately, such definitional ambiguity allows educational professionals in different states and school districts (and even within these catchment areas) to identify youngsters as LD according to an extraordinary range of eligibility criteria. Obviously, such variability in sample characteristics prohibit replicability and generalizability, the cornerstones of scientific inquiry.

Given the arbitrary nature of "school-identified" samples, it is unlikely that even an exhaustive study of these groups will culminate in coherent and useful information about LD. As Torgesen (1990) has pointed out, this situation will most likely not change since school-identified samples are usually defined by shifting political realities, local expediencies, and questionable psychometrics. Since school-identified samples do not provide a proper reference group for the scientific study of LD, it is the ethical responsibility of the investigator to apply sampling strategies and conditions that are known to enhance a researcher's ability to replicate and generalize findings. Some of these strategies are briefly discussed here.

It is our opinion that the way to study learning disabilities is through application of developmental, longitudinal designs. A major advantage in conducting research on LD from a longitudinal perspective is that there need not be any a priori assumptions about what LD is, thereby avoiding the pitfalls associated with school-identified samples. Within that context, individuals selected randomly from the general population (regardless of IQ and achievement levels, SES, race, and so on) could be studied over time across multiple assessment and teaching situations. In this manner, unbiased descriptions of the attributes of persons who are underachieving academically and socially could be obtained, thus identifying critical characteristics that may be manifested *in different ways at different age periods*. These characteristics could then serve as the relevant elements of a precise and reliable definition of LD that promotes replicability and generalizability of findings.

Given that longitudinal research studies will require financial, logistic, and professional commitments far beyond those available for typical studies of LD, it is unlikely that such strategies will be routinely implemented in the near future. As such, investigators must strive to account for sample heterogeneity and to increase awareness of sample distinctiveness. One way to do this is to provide descriptive benchmarks that allow determination of similarities and differences of subjects across research samples. Keogh and her coworkers (Keogh et al., 1982) have contributed significantly to the LD field in this regard by developing a system of *marker variables* that can be employed to identify descriptive, substantive, topical, and background characteristics of samples under study. While routine reporting of characteristics of LD samples using a common format of agreed-upon markers could reduce problems in interpreting findings, it should be understood that marker variables do not address issues related to sample selection bias. Only longitudinal investigations of randomly identified subjects or a priori specification of selection criteria can help in this regard.

Of all of the factors that have hindered our understanding of LD, failure to select samples according to known scientific principles and the use of convenience (school-identified) samples can be considered two of the major culprits. Since we now know a great deal about the dangers of such practices, failure to improve our practices in this area constitutes not only a departure from methodological common sense, but strains the ethics of conducting sound research.

School-identified samples are not verboten; it is imperative, however, that the investigator select from school-identified samples those students who meet the specific a priori established criteria for the investigation. It is not feasible to think that large cohorts of students could be tested to identify those who meet the investigator's criteria for population perimeters.

Ethical Issues Related to the Beliefs and Attitudes of the Investigator

Subjectivity

Subjectivity is the quality of an investigator that influences the results of an investigation. All researchers introduce subjectivity into their work; the task is to be aware of one's subjectivity and to establish formal procedures for monitoring it. Peshkin (1988) argues that it is impossible to obtain objectivity and therefore you should systematically seek to identify your own subjectivity that will bias all aspects of the research that you do. While subjectivity is most frequently associated with observational investigations, there is little question that researcher subjectivity influences all research. Peshkin (1988) states that "one's subjectivity is like a garment that cannot be removed. It is insistently present in both the research and nonresearch aspects of our life" (p. 17).

To illustrate the influence of subjectivity, Peshkin (1988) identified areas of subjectivity that influenced a recent field-based research study he conducted at a multiethnic high school. He warns us that these subjective influences occurred in this setting and may be repeated, or different influences might occur in other settings related to other topics. One of the six influences he presented was the Ethnic-Maintenance I. He felt that being Jewish shaped his "approval" of the retention of ethnicity in his observation of the persons in his study. For example, his approval of the positive aspects of identification with an ethnic group increased his interest and approval of a Mexican-American woman who identified with "her people," and a black American who identified with his development of an organization, Black Cultural League. He felt this same subjectivity could also set him up to ignore those who do not identify with their ethnic identity.

Subjectivity about the characteristics of the students we are testing or teaching (learning disabled versus non–learning disabled) is also likely to influence our behavior and eventually the data we obtain. We have beliefs and assumptions about learning disabilities that influence the measures we select and our interpretation of the results. We need to consider the extent to which these beliefs bias the way we collect data, the measures used, and our interpretation of the results. We think Peshkin is on the right track when he warns us that we are unable to remove all subjectivity, but we can attempt to identify our own and monitor its effect.

Related to subjectivity is the issue of why we conduct research. There is seldom one answer to this question. Interest in learning more about the topic, advancing science, and contributing to a knowledge base are likely factors. Also influencing our research are issues related to promoting our own career, such as job security (tenure), promotions and salary raises, and the perceptions of others. These issues are relevant to the extent that they influence ethical procedures in collecting, analyzing, and interpreting our research findings.

Researcher's and Clinician's Beliefs

The beliefs, attitudes, and expectations of outcome by the researcher influence how data will be interpreted and reported, particularly when the researcher has a great deal invested in the outcome.

The relationship between investigator/clinician preconceptions and their conclusions is well documented (Chapman & Chapman, 1967, 1969, 1971). In the main, it is known that our beliefs about a concept or topic modify our perceptions of cause and effect and correlation. Given this, it is our ethical responsibility to recognize that beliefs can interfere with objective analysis and reporting, and to explicitly remind ourselves of how such bias is typically manifested. Within this context a review of confirmatory bias is in order.

Confirmatory Bias

Confirmatory bias refers to the practice of maintaining beliefs despite counterevidence. In general, confirmatory bias can be seen in both research and clinical practice as the tendency to pay particular attention to evidence that supports a belief or hypothesis, to misinterpret ambiguous or even nonsupportive evidence as supportive of beliefs, and to disregard or dismiss counterevidence (Mahoney, 1977). Unless one is constantly aware that such bias is always possible, if not probable, even the most objective researcher can get "stuck" on an idea or belief and remain intractable despite overwhelming evidence that refutes their initial impression.

There are at least four aspects of confirmatory bias that researchers and clinicians should be familiar with in order to adequately defend against drawing false conclusions. Each are briefly discussed here.

Favoring Initial Hypotheses and Premature Closure

Wyatt and Campbell (1951) and Bruner and Potter (1964) discuss how preliminary hypotheses that are generated from inadequate data hinder the interpretation of subsequent and more informative data. This practice reflects a tendency to favor our initial hypotheses. For example, Bruner and Potter (1964) carried out an investigation in which one group was presented *slightly* blurred slides. Subjects within this group were still able to identify the objects pictured with a high degree of accuracy. A second group was shown the same slides but under different conditions. Specifically, for members of this second group the initial depictions were *very* blurry, but then focused so that the pictures were equal in clarity to those shown the first group. Despite this, members of the second group continued to make significantly more recognition errors than members in Group 1 primarily because they remained convinced that their initial observations were correct.

Related to this decision-making phenomenon is a tendency of researchers and clinicians to "jump to conclusions" early in the hypothesis-testing or diagnostic process and then close their minds to alternative interpretations despite evidence that other conclusions may be warranted. This resistance to correction is termed *premature closure*. The literature relevant to premature closure suggests that it may be the rare case that clinicians and researchers evaluate *all* of the existing information in an objective fashion before drawing final conclusions (Yager, 1977). For example, Robins and Helzer (1986) report that diagnosticians frequently select a diagnosis within the first few minutes and then spend the remainder of the time trying to confirm it, omitting that evidence which tends to disconfirm.

Why we tend to favor initial hypotheses or demonstrate premature closure is not clear. The important points, however, are that judgements based on new data frequently tend to be overly consistent with preliminary hypotheses and that many times we do not even consider the new data. We need to recognize these predictable biases if we are to draw valid conclusions from our research and clinical observation. Unfortunately, it is clear from discussions with clinicians as well as from even cursory review of the LD literature that the tendency to favor initial hypotheses and to demonstrate premature closure as forms of confirmatory bias are alive, well, and kicking within the LD enterprise.

Double Standards of Evidence

It is not uncommon among researchers and clinicians to hear or read about someone explaining away evidence that runs counter to a particular theoretical position or clinical conclusion. However, when one readily accepts information that supports their beliefs or conclusions but is much more strict and less accepting of information that disconfirms their theory or observation, the boundaries of intellectual honesty and ethical responsibility are stretched to their limits. Paul Meehl (1973) waxed eloquently about this aspect of confirmatory bias when he wrote: I have no objection if professionals choose to be extremely rigorous about their standards of evidence, but they should recognize that if they adopt that policy, many of the assertions made in a case conference ought not to be uttered because they cannot meet such a tough standard. Neither do I have any objection to freewheeling speculation . . . you can play it tight or you can play it loose. What I find objectionable . . . is a tendency to shift the criterion of tightness so that the evidence offered is upgraded or downgraded in the service of polemical interests" (p. 265).

In our experience, the use of different or double standards of evidence in the LD field is reflected sometimes in researchers or clinicians stating that the particular theories and/or measures that they employ are not well-suited to test via the scientific method because they are studying or working with "real-life" issues—not laboratory experiments. Another typical assertion frequently noted in clinical practice is that the lack of reliability and validity for test instruments used in a diagnostic evaluation is not important since the clinical task is to observe *how* the individual performs a task, not to obtain a score on the test per se. However, when the test scores support or confirm an initial clinical hypothesis, you can bet that the score is reported as if it had outstanding psychometric properties. The point is, you cannot have it both ways unless you want to push against the outer edge of ethical boundaries.

The Effects of Confirmatory Bias on Data Collection

Given the fact that confirmatory bias can lead one to eschew counterevidence, consider how this problem can become exacerbated if nonsupportive data is unlikely to be obtained in the first place. In clinical practice, this type of confirmatory bias is achieved by limiting the types of questions that are asked, by administering a set battery of tests known to yield particular patterns of performance, or through "channeling effects" (Robins & Helzer, 1986; Snyder, 1977). Unfortunately, in the behavioral sciences, behavior is so predictably variable and inconsistent that one can find an observation to support a particular impression if they wait long enough, give the right test, or ask the right question. Further, it is well known that clinicians and researchers can "channel" the behaviors of the individuals they are examining or studying so that they appear, albeit falsely, to conform with preconceived notions.

The only way to address these threats to objective clinical science and to professional ethics is to recognize that indeed systematic confirmatory bias exists in several forms and that we are all susceptible to its influence. In a sense, it may be wise to consider that we have met the enemy and they are our own naturally biased selves.

Ethical Issues Related to Measurement

Understanding the "true" meaning of a test score is essential to adequate interpretation. Using test scores that "work" in practice without some understanding of what they mean is like using a drug that works without knowing its properties and reactions. You may get some immediate relief, to be sure, but you had better ascertain and monitor the side effects. And although evaluation of side effects—or more generally, of the social consequences of the testing—contributes to score meaning, it is a weak substitute for score meaning in the rational justification of test use (Messick, 1989, p. 8).

This issue is particularly bothersome with respect to the role of measured intelligence as a criteria for learning disabilities. Stanovich (1991) identifies the bind we get into when we use a discrepancy between aptitude (intelligence) and achievement as a model for identifying reading and learning disabilities. There is a weak distinction between ability measures and achievement measures because "the acquisition of literacy skills fosters the very cognitive skills that are assessed on aptitude measures" (Stanovich, 1991, p. 7). The influence of literacy skills on cognitive functioning makes the use of a discrepancy between cognitive functioning as measured by intelligence tests and academic functioning, for example, reading, as measured by achievement tests, an unusable criteria for the identification of students with learning disabilities. Yet, government agencies (Kavanagh & Truss, 1988), professional organizations (Hammill, Leigh, McNutt, & Larsen, 1981), and researchers continue to use the discrepancy model as a criteria for identifying individuals with learning disabilities.

Ethical Issues Related to Intervention

In intervention research, ethical issues center around withholding the intervention from the control group, particularly if we have reason to believe the intervention is better than what is presently occurring. Some of these concerns have been addressed by providing the control group with the intervention following the experiment, but this is often not possible because the study includes a follow-up or a booster, or the students in the control group are no longer accessible to the investigator.

Many researchers justify the practice of a control group when conducting intervention research by indicating that even the experimental group would not be receiving the benefits of the intervention if the research study were not being conducted. These researchers reason that all students receive the school-based educational program available to them in their school and that the intervention program provided through the research study is a supplement.

In summary, the potential for withholding benefits from control group participants as an ethical question occurs in relatively few studies and these are studies in which the control group is somehow deprived of benefits that they would ordinarily receive. More frequently, the control group participants are receiving services no different from those students outside of the experiment, thus they are not perceived as being deprived of an intervention.

Summary and Conclusions

Research investigating issues related to learning disabilities seems to be particularly vulnerable to infractions related to ethical issues. Identification procedures, school-identified samples, the heterogeneity of the population, and measurement issues are but a few of the difficulties that make the conduct of research prone to biases, beliefs, and ethically

TABLE 15.1. Summary of ethical considerations.

Ethical issues related to the treatment and identification of subjects
+ Action research teams that involve teachers as participants in the research raise new questions about the "rights" of participants in research.
+ Protecting the rights of children who participate in research includes: respect for the child as an individual, consideration for what the child gains from participation, minimizing stress or undue attention to the child, and respecting the child's right to refuse participation.

Ethical issues related to the identification of subjects for research in learning disabilities
+ Consider criteria carefully for selecting subjects from school-identified samples of students with learning disabilities.
+ The use of developmental, longitudinal designs hold promise for investigating issues related to learning disabilities.
+ Use descriptive benchmarks or marker variables to determine similarities and differences of subjects across research samples.
+ Use a prior specification of selection criteria for subject selection.

Ethical issues related to the beliefs and attitudes of the investigator
+ Be aware of and document your subjectivity as it relates to the investigation.
+ Be aware of how your beliefs and attitudes guide all aspects of the investigation including identification of measures and interpretation of findings.
+ Be aware of confirmatory bias and the practice of maintaining beliefs despite counter-evidence.

Ethical issues related to measurement
+ Understand the measurement properties of tests used and interpret appropriately.
+ Consider whether the IQ-Achievement discrepancy model makes sense in your investigation of students with learning disabilities.

Ethical issues related to intervention
+ Consider ethical issues about withholding intervention from the control group.

questionable practices. See Table 15.1 for a summary of these points. As a research and clinical community we have our work set out for us and it requires an honest appraisal of what we know, and a critical eye about our ongoing findings, or what we think we are finding.

References

Bruner, J.S. & Potter, M.C. (1964). Interference in visual recognition. *Science, 144*, 424–425.

Chapman, I.J. & Chapman, J.P. (1967). Genesis of popular but erroneous psychodiagnostic observations. *Journal of Abnormal Psychology, 72*, 193–204.

Chapman, I.J. & Chapman, J.P. (1969). Illusory correlation as an obstacle to the use of valid psychodiagnostic signs. *Journal of Abnormal Psychology, 74*, 271–280.

Chapman, I.J. & Chapman, J.P. (1971, November). Test results are what you think they are. *Psychology Today*, p. 5.

Cook, S. (1981). Ethical Implications. In L.H. Kidder (Ed.), *Research methods in social relations* (pp. 365–417). New York: Holt, Rinehart & Winston.

Council for Exceptional Children. (1991, Winter). *Code of Ethics of the Council for Exceptional Children*. (Available from the Council for Exceptional Children, 1920 Association Drive, Reston, VA 22091-1589)

Freeman, D. (1983). *Margaret Mead and Samoa*. Cambridge, MA: Harvard University Press.

Freudian Slip? Father of psychoanalysis exaggerated claims, experts believe. (1991, February 19). *Miami Herald*, p. 1A.

Hammill, D.D., Leigh, J.E., McNutt, G., & Larsen, S.C. (1981). A new definition of learning disabilities. *Learning Disability Quarterly, 4*, 336–342.

Kavale, K.A. & Forness, S.R. (1985). *The science of learning disabilities*. San Diego: College-Hill Press.

Kavanagh, J.F. & Truss, T.J., Jr. (Eds.). (1988). *Learning disabilities: Proceedings of the national conference*. Parkston, MD: York Press.

Keogh, B.K., Major-Kingsley, S., Omori-Gordon, H., & Reid, H.P. (1982). *A system of marker variables for the field of learning disabilities*. Syracuse, NY: Syracuse University Press.

Lyon, G.R. (1987). Learning disabilities research: False starts and broken promises. In S. Vaughn & C.S. Bos (Eds.), *Research in learning disabilities* (pp. 69–85). San Diego: College-Hill Press.

Mahoney, M.J. (1977). Publication prejudices: An experimental study of confirmatory bias in the peer review system. *Cognitive Therapy and Research, 1*, 161–175.

Meehl, P.E. (1973). *Psychodiagnosis: Selected papers*. Minneapolis: University of Minnesota Press.

Messick, S. (1989). Meaning and values in test validation: The science and ethics of assessment. *Educational Researcher, 18*(2), 5–11.

Parker, R.M. (1990). Power, control, and validity in research. *Journal of Learning Disabilities, 23*(10), 613–620.

Peshkin, A. (1988). In search of subjectivity—one's own. *Educational Researcher, 17*(7), 17–22.

Ramsay, P. (1970). *The patient as a person*. New Haven, CT: Yale University Press.

Report of the American Psychological Association. (1990, June 2). Ethical principles of psychologists. *American Psychologist, 45*(3), 390–395.

Robins, L.N. & Helzer, J.E. (1986). Diagnosis and clinical assessment: The current state of psychiatric diagnosis. *Annual Review of Psychology, 37*, 409–432.

Shulman, J.H. (1990). Now you see them, now you don't: Anonymity versus visibility in case studies of teachers. *Educational Researcher, 19*(6), 11–15.

Snyder, C.R. (1977). A patient by any other name revisited: Maladjustment or attributional locus of problems? *Journal of Consulting and clinical Psychology, 45*, 101–103.

Stanovich, K.E. (1991). Discrepancy definitions of reading disability: Has intelligence led us astray? *Reading Research Quarterly, 26*(1), 7–29.

Thompson, R.A. (1990). Vulnerability in research: A developmental perspective on research risk. *Child Development, 61*, 1–16.

Torgesen, J.K. (1990, October). *Variations on theory in learning disabilities*. Paper presented at the National Institute of Child Health and Human Development (NICHD) Symposium on Learning Disabilities, Racine, Wisconsin.

Westfall, R.S. (1973). Newton and the fudge factor. *Science, 179*, 4075, 751–758.

Wyatt, D.F. & Campbell, D.T. (1951). On the liability of stereotype or hypothesis. *Journal of Abnormal and Social Psychology, 46*, 496–500.

Yager, J. (1977). Psychiatric Eclecticism: A cognitive view. *American Journal of Psychiatry, 134*, 736–741.

Yin, R.K. (1985). *Case study research: Design and methods*. Beverly Hills, CA: Sage.

16
Ethical Issues Related to Translating Research in Learning Disabilities into Practice

B. KEITH LENZ AND DONALD D. DESHLER

Introduction

As the field of learning disabilities (LD) emerged as a formal entity through the assistance of legislative initiatives in the late 1960s and early 1970s, expectations, especially by parents, were that the majority of any available resources be used to provide direct services to individuals with LD. Evidence of this was first seen following the passage in 1969 of Public Law 91-230, Title VI, Education of the Handicapped Act which included Part G, Special Programs for Children with Specific Learning Disabilities. This legislation made possible the expenditure of federal monies for, among other things, the following activities: funding of demonstration service centers for children and adolescents with LD; funding of teacher-training activities to prepare professionals to work with youth with LD; and funding to support research activities on issues related to populations with LD. Because parents and practitioners believed that students with LD had been denied services for such a long period of time, these groups strongly argued that service delivery programs be established at the federal level to assist this population. Consequently, a series of federally funded entitlement programs were established in response to these demands.

From its inception in 1969 through the mid-1970s, the majority of Title VI-G funding was channeled to providing direct services to students with LD. Secondarily, a significant portion of these funds were directed to teacher-training programs that focused on the preparation of teachers and university faculty members in the area of learning disabilities. Very little of the funds were devoted to research activities. The prevailing mind-set in the field's formative years was the following: "Let's do 'something' for these children who have been denied public school services for years, even if the 'something' has not been validated through research." Indeed, in those early years, very few of the assessment or instructional protocols used with populations with LD had been validated through research activities. Nonetheless, the prevailing paradigm was to provide services as quickly and as extensively as possible. Quantity, not quality, of services was the most highly valued attribute for measuring progress on behalf of individuals with LD. In short, validation of treatment methodologies was not a valued activity. It is interesting to compare this approach to service delivery with the model typically followed in other disciplines. For example, in medicine, regardless of the pressing need for a cure for a given disease (e.g., in the case of AIDS), research is required to precede the provision of services (in this example, the administration of a "promising, yet unvalidated" medication). Likewise in business and industry, the research and development model specifies that research activities on products take place *prior to* their entry into the market place.

As a means of providing services to students with LD, the majority of Title VI-G dollars were used to support Child Service Demonstration Centers (CSDCs). The CSDCs were to represent a variety of innovative service delivery models for students with learning disabilities. It was hoped that out of these centers would emerge several validated intervention routines. This hope was never quite realized (Deshler, 1978). As a result, many of the Title VI-G dollars were redirected and used to fund the five Institutes for Research in Learning Disabilities (Columbia University, University of Illinois, University of Kansas, University of Minnesota, and University of Virginia) that were in operation from 1977 through 1983. The University of Kansas Research Institute is still in existence. So, after several years of providing services to students with LD, a decision was made at the federal level to channel monies to support efforts to validate practice. The reallocation of these resources was significant in a symbolic sense in that it signaled an important role for researchers to play in the design and validation of assessment, instructional, and administrative practices used with individuals with LD. Regrettably, many of the materials that continue to dominate practice in the field of LD today have not been subjected to validation. Methods textbooks frequently list method after method without any mention of their validity. Commercial publishers of instructional materials and tests (and the authors they represent) often totally disregard the ethical responsibilities incumbent upon anyone engaged in the publication and dissemination process.

In order to ensure that services provided to individuals with LD are dominated by those practices that have been validated for the target population, it is important that all "stakeholders" who have an impact on individuals will share in the responsibility of advocating for the use of such practices. Included among this group would be: individuals with LD (as consumers/clients), parents of individuals with LD, teachers, policymakers, publishers, authors, teacher trainers, and researchers. The purpose of this chapter is to focus on the ethical responsibilities of the researcher who is involved in any of the processes of designing, validating, translating research into test protocols or instructional materials, or disseminating these products throughout the field.

This chapter will address the following topics: whether researchers have a role to play in product development, the importance of researchers adopting an ethical perspective, and factors that promote the translation of research to practice in an ethically responsible manner.

Do Researchers Have a Role to Play in Product Development?

There are those who have strongly questioned the contributions of researchers to efforts to improve schooling. Finn (1988), the former Assistant Secretary of Education, for example, has stated that "To put it simply, our labors haven't produced enough findings that Americans can use or even see the use of. . . . Education research has not fulfilled its role in the effort to improve our schools" (p. 5). Shavelson (1988) indicates that Finn's remarks echo the sentiments of many policymakers and practitioners, and much of the public as well. Questions about the value and ultimate contributions of social science research have been raised from many quarters (e.g., Goodwin, 1975; Weiss & Bucuvalas, 1980; Wilson, 1978). In Shavelson's 1988 Presidential Address to the American Educational Research Association (AERA) he argued against Finn's contention through the following points. (a) Social science does not directly and immediately influence policy or practice in the same way that physics might affect a space flight trajectory. The fields operate from markedly different models of inquiry, and hence expectations of each responding to problems in like manner is unrealistic. (b) Educational research *does* contribute to educational practice and policy by helping construct, challenge, and change the way policymakers and practitioners view particular problems. Shavelson cautioned, however, that the impact of educational research has not been as significant or frequent as it might be because researchers do not understand the cognition of policymakers and practitioners. He argues that researchers need to understand the *mindframes* of these stakeholders; a better understanding would enable researchers to more effectively communicate and translate research findings, and alter the way in which research questions are formulated and the way in which the actual research is conducted.

Shavelson (1988) contends that a first, and very significant, way to effectively translate research into practice is for researchers to understand how the mindframes of key educational stakeholders are quite dissimilar. The mismatch between the mindframes of researchers, policymakers, and practitioners accounts, in part, for the difficulty of translating research into practice. On the one hand, the researcher's mindframe is one that is dominated by the canons of disciplinary inquiry that reinforce a conservative posture in reporting and interpreting findings. A cautious and deliberate approach to problem solving, it can be argued, is fundamental to fulfilling the oft-cited adage of "do no harm." Typically, the researcher's primary referent group is fellow researchers. They strive to conduct research that warrants the attention of other researchers and contributes to theory. With reluctance, researchers make suggestions for applications of their findings to policy or practice. On the other hand, the mindframe of the policymaker and practitioner is dominated by a significantly different set of values. The pressures on these groups give rise to a mindframe that is more action oriented and goal directed. They seek information that contributes to pressing problems before them and they often view research findings as only one source of data in a complex decision-making process. Shavelson summarizes the different mindframes as follows: "Researchers use information to confirm or disconfirm theory, and policy makers and practitioners use information to guide actions with direct and indirect consequences for students and the public" (p. 11). The challenge to researchers is to seek a greater understanding of the mindframes of policymakers and practitioners: "by tackling policy-makers' and practitioners' mindframes, we might better formulate research questions, design studies, and translate our findings into the stuff that constructs, challenges, and changes policy-makers' and practitioners' cognition. In doing so we may just correct the common misperceptions held by many of those outside our research community" (Shavelson, 1988, p. 11).

Solutions to many of the pressing problems confronting the educational community today lie in the diversity of perspectives represented by different stakeholders. While Shavelson's counsel to researchers to seek a greater understanding of the mindframes of policymakers and practitioners is sound, he is not suggesting that researchers adopt their mindframes or canons of problem solving. To the contrary, the values and practices of researchers represent a useful tension in the educational arena. Policymakers and practitioners who do not frequently question the status quo for the purpose of upgrading practice through the infusion of validated methodology are acting as irresponsibly as the researcher who gives no thought to the potential applicability of his/her findings to practice. Researchers, however, can do much to improve existing practice by not only seeking to understand the educational problems facing policymakers and practitioners, but also by aggressively working to design and validate (using strict standards) improved assessment and instructional protocols that can be used by practitioners. By clearly translating field-test versions of procedures or protocols into forms that practitioners can readily use, researchers can play a vital role in the instructional development process (including product development) and, in turn, favorably impact practice. Prevailing practice in the field of learning disabilities is still dominated by the use of instructional procedures and materials that have not been validated. The availability of validated procedures and materials that sufficiently meet a criterion of "palatability" or usability by practitioners

(Deshler & Schumaker, 1988) would have a good probability of positively influencing existing practice.

The Importance of Researchers Adopting an Ethical Perspective

Rittel and Weber (1973) have argued that conducting scientific research on many of the problems in the social arena (including the design and validation of instructional materials) is exceedingly difficult because of the nature of these problems. They characterized these problems as being "wicked" problems, whereas the hard sciences largely deal with "tame" problems. Tame problems are ones that are usually definable and separable and may have solutions that are findable, whereas wicked problems have no definitive formulation, have no "stopping rules" (i.e., it is not clear when a problem has been solved), have no immediate or ultimate test of solution, and are usually unique in each case. These authors underscore the potential consequences of attempting to find solutions to wicked problems: *Every* implemented solution is consequential. It leaves "traces" that cannot be undone. One cannot build a freeway to see how it works, and then easily correct it after unsatisfactory performance. . . . the consequences they generate have long half-lives. . . . The effects of an experimental curriculum will follow pupils into their adult lives. Whenever actions are effectively irreversible and whenever the half-lives of the consequences are long, *every trial counts*. (p. 163) This analysis of wicked problems indicates that the potential costs associated with professionals' indiscriminately recommending products or procedures for use with populations with LD need to be more closely evaluated. Indeed, the risks of failing to carefully consider the cost-benefit factors can be great if the proposed solution fails to live up to its billing. Given the nature of the problems that researchers in the LD field encounter, it is exceedingly important that these problems be formulated and investigated within the context of ethical responsibility.

Frequently, marketing decisions are governed primarily by economic factors and legal and/or technical constraints (J. Reitz, personal communication, June, 1991). Much less often, however, does ethical responsibility enter the picture. Oftentimes, as an afterthought, the question is asked: "Is this the *right* thing to do?" (regardless of the economic or legal ramifications). In order to ensure that this question is answered, it is important for researchers' actions to be governed by a set of guiding principles that help them engage in and work through matters that require ethical deliberation. According to Benjamin and Curtis (1981), ethical deliberation seeks to answer the following question: What ought to be done under this set of circumstances, *when all things are considered?* Howe and Miramontes (1991) indicate that ethical deliberation must take into account an almost boundless array of considerations, including the facts and the law, as well as personal beliefs, attachments, feelings, and conceptions of "the good life." This renders ethical deliberation exceedingly complex, uncertain, and tentative. Furthermore, unlike the problem-solving in mathematics and physics, *everyone*, not just the experts, is afforded voice and possesses *expertise* when it comes to ethical deliberation. (p. 8) Thus for the researcher working toward models or protocols that result in better assessment, treatment, or service delivery systems for individuals with LD, it is imperative that they ensure that any solutions they propose do, in fact, result in a favorable outcome *when all things are considered.*

When researchers view their role in the larger context of being actively committed to ethical deliberation and responsibility, it is clear that they will be able to play a larger role in the school reform movement. By adopting a posture that says that only those products that meet prespecified standards of quality will be published and disseminated, researchers can do much to contribute to the overall improvement of the schooling process. Indeed, the success of educational reform may, in part, be related to the ability and willingness of researchers to adopt ethically responsible postures toward translating research into practice. Such a posture will necessitate that researchers reevaluate the time-honored practice of conducting research (either basic or applied) with the primary goal of *contributing* to the knolwedge base on teaching and learning, in the absence of *translating* research into practice. This traditional posture has been (and still is) consistent with the value system endorsed by colleges, universities, and other institutions involved in conducting research on learning and teaching. Embracing this new posture must be a carefully thought-out decision because it will have a significant impact on the researcher's time and the amount of resources required for successful engagement in the process. By committing to the process of translating research into practice, many of the barriers that have historically existed between researchers and practitioners will crumble. In order to make successful translations of research outcomes to practice, it is necessary for researchers and practitioners to team together for the purpose of refining the product in such a way as to maximize its usability in the classroom, and at the same time, to protect those features that the research has shown to be essential to its success. Collaborative efforts not only optimize the strengths of both the researcher and practitioner, but they reduce the attitudes of distrust and skepticism that have often characterized their relationships. In essence, the "we" and "them" dichotomy has been replaced and the resultant teaming has the potential of producing a synergistic relationship that has significantly more potential of addressing the school reform issue than would happen if each party was acting unilaterally (Covey, 1989).

One of the most obvious benefits of the teaming of researcher and practitioner in the translation of research to practice is that each party represents different perspectives and potentially independent judgments on the actions and decisions of the other. Multiple perspectives and opinions that are openly invited and listened to not only result in improved final outcomes but also increase the probability that ethically correct decisions will be made at critical junctures along the way. In essence, teaming relationships between researchers and practitioners represent an informal system of checks and balances. The significance of researchers adopting the posture described above is underscored by Ysseldyke and Algozzine (1982) in their analysis of the search by practitioners for solutions to the myriad of service delivery problems that they confront: "The critical issue . . . seems to be the demand for instant, simple solutions to incredibly complex problems . . . the demand for simple solutions has been so strong that it has created a receptive natural environment for those people who believe that they do have those answers" (p. 256). They cite several ads published in journals such as *Exceptional Children* and the *Journal of Learning Disabilities* to demonstrate the magnitude of unsubstantiated and ethically irresponsible claims made by publishers and authors (e.g., "Can your students become confident spellers in only 15 minutes per day? *Yes*, when you fill the time with lessons from————," or "All the instruments you'll ever need for evaluation and testing."). Obviously, researchers who design and validate procedures have a critical role to play in participating in a process that will provide practitioners with an alternative to those materials and practices that have not been subjected to a sound validation process.

Factors that Promote the Translation of Research to Practice in an Ethically Responsible Manner

What is ethically correct behavior for the researcher with regard to translating research into practice? While intentional deception, fraud, harm, and lies for the purpose of personal gain may be more easily judged as wrong, the more difficult ethical problems and questions revolve around the use of judgement in the absence of knowledge and in actions grounded in good intentions and integrity. The National Commission for the Protection of Human Subjects of Biomedical and Behavioral Research (1978), for example, concluded that the resolution of ethical dilemmas in research should be resolved by considering the values of beneficence (the avoidance of unnecessary suffering, injury or other harm, and the maximization of good outcomes), respect (a concern for the autonomy and dignity of persons), and justice (equitable distribution of social benefits and costs). It is our contention that there are a broad array of factors involved in the intricate process of translating research into practice. Researchers who intend to contribute to practice in an ethically appropriate way must give serious consideration to the factors discussed below.

Adopt a Set of Ethical Standards in Advance of Engaging in Research

It is important that a researcher's ethical position be clearly articulated *prior to* initiating any research so as to ensure that the translation of any research into practice meets appropriate standards of quality at every step along the way. Often, questions concerning whether something is "right" or not are only considered as an afterthought. If such questions are left to deliberations late during the research process, there is a higher probability that other factors (such as a pressure to publish a procedure or material to meet a pressing need in the field) will take precedence over issues of quality, appropriateness, and validity. Because in dealing with ethical concerns there are no simple answers, only broad principles can be applied to the process of translating research into practice. Among other things, a broad set of principles delineates the kinds of behavior that are indicative of researchers who act in an ethically responsible way. These researchers are ones who adopt an ethical position, explain that position to others (that is, they make their position public so there can be a source of external auditing), strive to act consistently within their ethical position, and change their position when new knowledge indicates that their current position is unethical.

An ethical position, for example, includes the standards that an individual adopts related to particular ethical questions in an area of ethical concern. In the areas of translating research into practice, sample questions that might be raised could include: "*How much* research is needed before research should be translated into practice?" or "*What type* of research should be conducted before research is translated into practice?" The answers that an individual gives to these questions represent ethical positions. For example: "At least five studies should be conducted on a practice before it is advocated for use by a practitioner," or "At least one study should be conducted in settings for which the practice is targeted by the type of practitioner who will be expected to use the practice." Similar questions and positions can be framed for each of the other areas (i.e., explaining one's position to others, acting consistently within a position, etc.). Figure 16.1 lists each of these dimensions and provides a definition and examples of ethical and unethical behaviors.

Use a "Participatory Research" Model

In order for research to have an impact on pressing educational problems, it must be conceptualized and framed to focus on those factors that are salient to the assessment of students or on the delivery of services in

Dimensions	Definition	The Ethical Response	The Unethical Response
1. Adoption	Takes a position on how research should be used beyond the study itself.	Adopts an ethical position on the application of research. *"I have found that special training is required to get the same results I got."*	Does not adopt an ethical position on the application of research. *"Sure, try it and see what happens."*
2. Justification	Explains why such a position is ethically necessary.	Empirically justifies the ethical position. *"When teachers were trained, 90% of the kids learned, but when we handed them the material, less than 10% learned."*	Does not empirically justify an ethical position. *"I feel that it is important for you to be trained."*
3. Enforcement	Persists in adhering to a stated ethical position.	Enforces a personal position on application of research. *"I will come and talk about my research, but there is not enough time for me to present the materials, and teachers will not be able to walk away being able to do this. Do you still want me to come?"*	Does not enforce a personal ethical position on the application of research. *"Sure, I will come. 60 minutes isn't much, but the teachers can take and use whatever they think will help."*
4. Respect	Recognizes the rights of others to adopt and enforce a personal ethical position.	Shows respect for the ethical positions and actions assumed by others. *"I would like to present the results of your work in my book...what can I write about at an awareness level and what procedures could be presented for direct application."*	Shows disrespect for the ethical positions and actions assumed by others. *"I think you are over-protective of your approaches...I have already described your procedures to teachers so that they can use them."*
5. Change	Modifies positions as new knowledge begins to undermine previously held ethical positions.	Positions, enforcements, and actions change as beliefs about ethical behavior change. *"It seems that the teachers can learn it this way...and we get good results, but they quit using it as soon as we leave...we better change our approach."*	Positions, enforcements, and actions do not change as beliefs about ethical behavior change *"It's too bad that they don't keep using it, but the data are publishable ...we have too much at stake to change our approach now."*

FIGURE 16.1. Dimensions of ethically responsible actions related to translating research into practice.

actual field settings. While much of the educational research that is formulated and conducted in laboratory settings is effective in controlling experimental variables, it often falls significantly short in the generalizability of its findings to actual problems in school settings. Oftentimes, the research results, as reported in a journal article on a new teaching procedure, appear to be quite encouraging. However, if the results have been achieved under conditions that are markedly different than those that exist in field settings, it may be difficult, if not impossible, for practitioners to replicate the findings. One way of narrowing the gap between research and practice is for researchers to team with practitioners during key phases of the research process. A "participatory research model" is based on the following assumptions: (a) The quality of instructional practices will be greatly enhanced when teachers and administrators are allowed and encouraged to be collaborators in the research and development process, and (b) The knowledge that teachers have about their content areas and about the students in their classrooms provides critical insights that can only be revealed over time (Lenz, Bulgren, Deshler, & Schumaker, 1989). By teaming together in conceptualizing the content of an intervention, as well as how it should be implemented in practice, practitioners can provide valuable knowledge to researchers regarding the nuances and realities of the teaching environment that must be built into any research and validation effort. Similarly, the researcher's unique perspective and knowledge base, when shared with practitioners during the participatory process, often sparks new thoughts and insights within the practitioner. In short, if carefully nurtured and developed over a sustained time, a synergistic relationship between researcher and practitioner will result which has the potential of being highly productive and relevant. The resultant research protocols will have a higher probability of yielding outcomes that can actually impact practice.

Another dimension of the participatory research model is to involve the clients themselves in the research process. A failure to do so implies that the researcher knows the mindframes and values of the client and can and will make decisions that are in the best interest of the client. Ayers' (1986) analysis of the language and posture of those in the helping professions captures the essence of a nonparticipatory model between professionals and clients: It is interesting to consider how much of the language of professionalism is a top-down and inaccessible language of mystification and distance. . . . From the traditional standpoint, professionals are the powerful ones, the ones with the special knowledge and training that allow them to control and solve other people's problems. Teachers teach; lawyers litigate; doctors heal. The professionals are the active ones. They bring culture to the masses, remove tumors, and prescribe cures. Their clients receive ministrations and services passively, are educated, acquitted, or cured" (p. 39). Along a similar vein, Adelman and Taylor (1983) delineate a set of issues related to the dynamics of the "helping relationship" that exists between professionals and clients with learning problems. They argue that the following implications be considered by anyone who sets out to help another (in the matters we are considering in this chapter, for example, designing educational materials "to help" students with learning disabilities): (a) Help is not always helpful; (b) Help is not always wanted, even though apparently needed; (c) Interventions designed to help usually have negative consequences and sometimes these outweigh the benefits; (d) Some ways of providing help are inappropriate even if effective in achieving desired ends; (e) What is defined as help by one person may not be seen as help by another; and (f) Sometimes interventions are used to serve the interests of one person or group at the expense of another (p. 273). They further contend that the "concept of *helping* represents a contrast to power both in terms of means and ends. In helping, all key decisions are 'ends' and should be controlled by the clients. To ensure that this is the case, the processes (means) used to arrive at decisions must be under the control of clients" (p. 279).

According to Sieber (1982), the research model used to conduct studies can have ethical ramifications on clients and practitioners. Sieber indicates that the most prevalent research model used in our culture is the "Analytic Scientist" model. She describes the analytic scientist as

a convergent thinker who focuses on impersonal external facts that are observed with certainty, and tests theory using classical logic. This scientist regards facts as separable both from values and from theories or ideas, and regards science as disinterested, impersonal, value free, precise, reliable, accurate, valid, reductionistic, causal, apolitical, cumulative, and progressive. According to this point of view, science contains clear standards for judgement, is realistic, antimystical, unambiguous, and exact. Inquiry proceeds by means of the controlled experiment. Knowledge is of value for its own sake, and the application of knowledge is not the scientist's concern. . . . Ethically, the overriding values are scientific freedom and validity of research (in the sense of whether their research design follows classical logical principles). Informed consent may be regarded as a legal formality that offers no possibility for increasing the validity of the research, but that seems to decrease validity by letting the subject in on the point of the study . . . experimental competence would refer to more factual, technical, and logical mastery than to interpersonal sensitivity. (pp. 20–21)

The need to involve clients in the research process is also clearly underscored by Sieber (1982) when she argues "that to be ethical, social scientists need to be aware of the goals of the persons whom they seek to study and assist" (p. 24), that persons involved with the problem should be involved in defining the problem, that choices should be provided to persons involved in resolving a problem, and that the benefits of a solution should be evaluated in terms of both long- and short-term outcomes and in terms of individual and social effects. A full range of research methodologies, including those associated with the Analytic Scientist model are required to accomplish this.

Use an Interactive System of Model Development

The production of high quality assessment or instructional materials for students with learning disabilities is facilitated if the research process follows a model that ensures the systematic building of a data base and multiple levels of validation and checks on fidelity of the treatment intervention. In the absence of such a model, most research efforts will tend to be fragmented. Any translations of findings from these (fragmented) research efforts to practice would be questionable from both an efficacy and ethical perspective. As an example, the model adopted by the University of Kansas Institute for Research in Learning Disabilities (KU-IRLD) to develop the Strategies Intervention Model will be presented (Schumaker, Deshler, & Ellis, 1986). This model is an interactive system of intervention model development that involves six stages (see Figure 16.2), some of which begin before others, but all of which run parallel and interact in a dynamic way to allow the gradual evolution of a data-based model that is responsive to the needs of adolescents with learning disabilities and other consumers of the model (e.g., teachers, parents, and administrators) (Talley, 1978).

The research conducted during Stage 1 (epidemiological research) provides a descriptive base on which subsequent research can be founded. Through epidemiological research, general and specific characteristics of students with LD and their environments are determined. From this

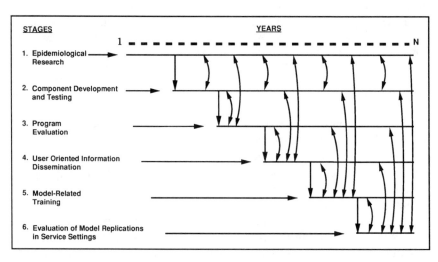

FIGURE 16.2. An interactive system of intervention model development, showing the six stages through which the Strategies Intervention Model has been developed.

information a theoretical working model is developed to frame future research problems, identify appropriate experimental designs, and set the direction for the development of specific interventions aimed at alleviating the deficits of students with LD, and which are appropriate for the settings in which the student will participate. Epidemiological research is used throughout the intervention development and testing process to understand the characteristics of those students for whom potential interventions may be most and least effective.

Within Stage 2 research (component development and testing), different interventions are developed, studied, and tested, using appropriate experimental designs. The results of these studies are then organized and integrated into specific *components* in a manner that has potential meaning to practitioners. As either epidemiological data or data from subsequent stages of the system (Stages 2–6) indicate a need for new intervention components or subcomponents, these new components are developed. Initially, each component is tested on a limited number of students and settings to establish its internal validity. Once the relative effectiveness of a component has been establised, attention is turned to questions concerning the component's broader generalizability.

Stage 3 research addresses the issue central to the validation of any intervention model: program evaluation. Once the successful components of the model have been combined within a single setting, program evaluation begins. This entails the monitoring of a number of measures to determine the overall impact of the model. Consumers of the model are regularly surveyed to determine their perceptions of the model. In addition, a host of outcomes measures, such as student adjustment and success in mainstream classes, are monitored.

Stage 4 of the interactive system deals with the dissemination of user-oriented information. During this stage, persons who are interested in using the model *and* who have influence in policy-making processes of their agencies or institutions are targeted for dissemination of the model. Precautions are taken during this stage to focus dissemination efforts primarily on those individuals willing to invest in the process of model adoption: in other words, those individuals and systems that are willing to make the necessary trade-offs and commitments to enable the new innovation to take root. In the absence of solid commitments, the probability of an effective translation from research to practice will be minimal. Hence, regardless of the quality of the validated innovation, implementation rates will be relatively low without the support and involvement of key stakeholders within the system.

The intent of Stage 5 (model-related training) is to prepare individuals and settings to adopt and implement the intervention model. The educational literature is replete with examples of interventions that have not been successfully adopted by the populace-at-large because of insufficient training in the target intervention. To prevent this from happening, the KU-IRLD has validated several staff development procedures that markedly enhance the probability of high adoption rates with fidelity being maintained in the instructional procedures (Schumaker & Clark, 1990).

Stage 6 (evaluation of model replications) is designed to address a variety of critical questions related to model replications such as: "Can the model be implemented under different administrative conditions?"; "Can the model be implemented in different types of service delivery settings?"; "In what ways must the model be flexible in order that it be usable in a wide variety of settings?" As results of evaluations in each stage are obtained, other stages of model development are, in turn, impacted. Thus, if a component of the model is found not to be suitable for certain settings, modifications may be required. Similarly, if certain students do not respond to a given intervention, subsequent epidemiological research may be needed to determine the characteristics and needs of those students. Subsequently, new model components would be developed to meet their needs.

This research system has been very helpful in facilitating the design and empirical validation of the Strategies Intervention Model. This system has forced KU-IRLD researchers to relate all research studies to a programmatic focus, to consider the broad array of issues related to intervention robustness and adoptability, and to make data-based decisions related to changing the model or determining at what point to translate a research finding into a material for use by a teacher or student. In addition, the interactive nature of the system has caused each component of the intervention model to be built on key population and setting attributes.

Finally, use of a research model such as the one described above necessitates a significant commitment on the part of the researcher to engage in the process of research translation over the long haul. It has been our experience that taking a research idea from the initial set of studies through the various stages described above requires several years of major investment (a minimum of 5). In order to ensure *appropriate* translation of research findings to practice, researchers must be strongly committed to the stages involving model testing, material development (in formats that are user-friendly), and sustained training efforts that ensure system adoption and routinization of the intervention. The allocation of time to these pursuits in order to assure appropriate translations come at the cost of making trade-offs with other professional undertakings. This fact was underscored to one of us about 4 years ago when he was attending a conference in Washington, DC for project directors of United States Office of Education (USOE) funded research projects. During a break between sessions he was approached by a colleague and asked: "Where have you been lately—I haven't seen many of your research articles in the journals lately!" When it was explained that a major emphasis by our Institute during the previous couple of years was being placed on the translation of some of our intervention procedures into teacher-use materials and training, the response was one that clearly implied that such activities were "nice but not as significant as actual research efforts"! The reward structure among fellow researchers is often not geared to reinforce those who are committed to the translation process.

Recognize Ethical Responsibilities across Various Research Roles

Researchers can perform a variety of roles; each is associated with a unique set of ethical issues and responsibilities. The salient factors related to three major roles that researchers can assume—producer, interpreter, and facilitator—will be discussed below.

Researcher as Producer

Researchers produce information and exert control over the availability of this information. This puts them in the position of determining when and under what circumstances information about a practice is made available to practitioners. Beyond the ethical questions of the integrity and quality of the research, the primary ethical question that researchers must face is when they must take an ethical position on the implications of findings related to direct use in practice.

Many researchers avoid this issue by publishing journal articles that describe the research process, findings, and limitations of their study. Some researchers do discuss the implications of the research for practice in their articles, and some journal editors require authors to include a section on implications for practice in the discussion section of the article. However, even when such information is provided, many articles conclude with the caveat that "more research is needed." As a result, even the few practitioners who are able to access and find the time to read the information presented in the article may not be able to determine whether the signal for practice is a "go," "stop," or "proceed with caution." To complicate matters, the information in the article related to the implementation of the practice may have been abbreviated for publication and may lead to poor implementation.

Avoiding the ethical responsibilities related to "producing" knowledge may, in itself, be unethical. Few programmatic lines of research currently exist in the field of learning disabilities (or in general education, for that matter). Lines of research are dictated by research interests and specific funding priorities. As a result, more research is not likely to follow, or is followed by research of another investigator who desires to give the research topic a unique twist or context to establish his or her work from the work of others.

The "producer" role of the researcher requires that researchers evaluate their ethical responsibilities to the practitioner. The responsibilities associated with this role go beyond making information available. These responsibilities include taking a position on (a) how much research is needed to recommend practice, (b) the nature and type of research that should be conducted as part of the required quantity of research, and (c) how information generated by research might be used by practitioners. It would seem that since many educational practices are based on no research, any research on a practice would be an improvement. However, the educational diversity of our country dictates that practices based on a single study with few subjects be viewed in the context of their validation. The producer is responsible for stating this limitation and making it clear that practitioners operating under different circumstances should only consider this practice for use after trial uses of the practice has demonstrated its benefits.

Researcher as Interpreter

No matter how comprehensive a methods textbook is or how detailed a journal article is written, the important practices that comprise the educational process are not easily translated for practice. Part of this dilemma may involve the expert decisions made by researchers in the development process. These expert decisions are not easily described or conveyed in text. Even when workshops on specific practices are provided, the rate of implementation for many educational practices and innovations does not increase. Since it is not clear what type of research to practice translation is successful, it is difficult to define the ethical responsibilities of the researcher in this area.

However, there seem to be a number of areas related to the translation of research that are important to evaluate. First, when implications for practice are known, this information should be made available in as detailed a form as possible. Articles that do not include these detailed procedures should announce the existence and availability of this information. Second, when research is described, the authors should make it clear whether or not the information provided on the practice in the article or textbook is sufficient for immediate use and replication. Third, when the research of others is described in articles or textbooks, the authors should indicate whether the information is for awareness of a practice and how the practitioner can obtain more information. This is an important challenge, since most methods textbooks are general and focus primarily on making the practitioner aware of educational practices.

The ethical roles associated with the "interpreter" become more complex as the researcher moves into the classroom and begins to describe research and interventions for teachers and prospective teachers in a manner that can be ethically responsible (Lenz & Deshler, 1990). Since classroom time usually focuses on selecting a few practices while relegating the rest of the practices to reading assignments, the basis for selecting the content of class discussion may also involve ethical questions. On what basis are practices selected? Are practices selected based on quantity of research or quality of research? Are practices discussed because they are novel or intriguing, or because they are in common use in the schools? Are practices taught thoroughly for expected use or casually for aware-ness? Are the teachers and prospective teachers aware of the basis for the selection of the content of classroom presentations and discussions?

Researcher as Facilitator

Whether the research is theirs or someone else's, most educational re-searchers involved in the process of translating research into practice work at some level toward promoting the implementation of research-based practices in schools. While there is a host of ethical issues related to conducting research in schools, a wide variety of ethical issues emerge as researchers move out of the environment of research and into the environment of everyday practice. The most significant issues emerge with regard to the researchers' respect for the individuals who work together in the school environment and the complex social interactions and performance demands that they must face each day and all year.

The legitimacy of the researcher involved in facilitating practice rests in their knowledge of a specific practice or set of practices. The degree to which researchers are able to help promote a practice is often contingent on their ability and willingness to understand how a new practice can become part of an existing environment. The prevailing problem is that neither the practitioner nor the researcher is willing to invest the time and energy to making this occur. Many practitioners are enamored with the idea of "new and improved," and many researchers are often unwilling to commit the time to ensuring that the practice is implemented in the manner that will bring about desired results.

Researchers interested in facilitating the implementation of research-based practices must ask themselves a number of questions: (a) How much time am I willing to invest in helping promote this practice? (b) Will my short-term involvement in promoting this practice do more harm than good? (c) What standards of implementation represent my position of what I believe is adequate implementation of this practice? (d) What standards will I place on myself to ensure the respect for the individuals in the school environment? (e) Am I qualified to facilitate the use of this practice in this school under these conditions?

Conclusion

The issues presented in this chapter are, by no means, meant to be exhaustive; rather, they are representative of the broad array of issues that must be seriously considered by researchers who desire to have an impact on educational practice by having the outcomes of their research translated in a meaningful way. Researchers in an applied field such as learning disabilities, despite the host of pressures and conflicting priorities, must take the responsibility for their actions and their impact. Adelman and Taylor (1983) contend that because of the relatively weak nature of the knowledge base in psychology and education, interveners should, at best, be viewed as having expertise, but not as being experts. This perspective underscores, even more emphatically, the importance of researchers raising their sensitivities to the broad range of ethical issues that surround the processes of conducting and translating research to practice for students with learning disabilities and their teachers. "In helping, the intention always is to behave ethically—to respect individual rights, liberties, dignity, and worth. Unfortunately, these rather straight-forward aims have proven easier to espouse in codes of professional ethics and standards for practice than they have been to accomplish in daily actions." (Adelman & Taylor, 1983, p. 285). Researchers who strive to construct research agendas that encompass ample provisions for ethical deliberation and review at all critical junctures will optimize the probability of meeting the maxim incorporated within the Hippocratic oath of "above all, do no harm." However, such agendas may, over time, end up doing considerable good because of the commitment to taking a measured and deliberate approach in translating research into practice.

References

Adelman, H.S. & Taylor, L. (1983). *Learning disabilities in perspective*. Glenview, IL: Scott, Foresman, & Company.

Ayers, W. (1986). On teachers and teaching. *Harvard Educational Review*, *27*(2), 35–38.

Benjamin, M. & Curtis, J. (1981). *Ethics in nursing*. New York: Oxford University Press.

Covey, S.R. (1989). *The seven habits of highly effective people*. New York: Simon & Schuster.

Deshler, D.D. (1978). New research institutes for the study of learning disabilities. *Learning Disability Quarterly*, *1*(1), 68–78.

Deshler, D.D. & Schumaker, J.B. (1988). An instructional model for teaching students how to learn. In J.L. Graden, J.E. Zins, & M.J. Curtis (Eds.), *Alternative educational delivery systems: Enhancing instructional options for all students* (pp. 391–411). Washington, DC: National Association of School Psychologists.

Finn, C.E., Jr. (1988). What ails education research? *Educational Researcher*, *17*(1), 5–8.

Goodwin, L. (1975). The relation of social research to practical affairs. *Journal of Applied Behavioral Science*, *11*, 7–13.

Howe, K.R. & Miramontes, O.B. (1991). A framework for ethical deliberation in special education. *The Journal of Special Education*, *25*(1), 7–25.

Lenz, B.K., Bulgren, J.A., Deshler, D.D., & Schumaker, J.B. (1989). *A proposal for collaborative research*. Lawrence, KS: University of Kansas Institute for Research in Learning Disabilities.

Lenz, B.K. & Deshler, D.D. (1990). Principles of strategies instruction as the basis of effective preservice teacher education. *Teacher Education and Special Education*, *13*(2), 82–95.

National Commission for the Protection of Human Subjects of Biomedical and Behavioral Research. (1978). *The Belmont report: Ethical principles and guidelines for the protection of human subjects of research* (DHEW Publication No. OS 78-0012). Washington, DC: U.S. Government Printing Office.

Rittel, H.W.J. & Webber, M.M. (1973). Dilemmas in a general threory of planning. *Policy Sciences*, *4*, 155–169.

Schumaker, J.B. & Clark, F.L. (1990). Achieving implementation of strategy instruction through effective inservice education. *Teacher Education and Special Education*, *13*(2), 105–116

Schumaker, J.B., Deshler, D.D., & Ellis, E.S. (1986). Intervention issues related to the education of LD adolescents. In J.K. Torgesen & B.Y.L. Wong (Eds.), *Learning disabilities: Some new perspectives* (pp. 329–365). New York: Academic Press.

Shavelson, R.J. (1988). Contributions of educational research to policy and practice: Constructing, challenging, changing cognition. *Educational Researcher*, *17*(3), 4–11.

Sieber, J.E. (1982). *The ethics of social research: Surveys and experiments*. New York: Springer-Verlag.

Talley, T.L. (1978, November). *Teaching family problems in a national perspective*. Keynote address presented at the National Teaching Family Association, Boys Town, NE.

Weiss, C.H. & Bucuvalas, M.J. (1980). *Social science research and decision-making*. New York: Columbia University Press.

Wilson, J.Q. (1978). Social sciences and public policy: A personal note. In L.E. Lynn (Ed.), *Knowledge and policy: The uncertain connection*. Washington, DC: National Academy of Sciences.

Ysseldyke, J.E. & Algozzine, B. (1982). *Critical issues in special and remedial education*. Boston: Houghton Mifflin.

Index